DEVELOPMENTAL NEUROPSYCHIATRY

Volume I

DEVELOPMENTAL NEUROPSYCHIATRY

The Fundamentals

VOLUME I

James C. Harris, M.D.

Director of Developmental Neuropsychiatry
Associate Professor of Psychiatry and Behavioral Sciences,
Pediatrics, and Mental Hygiene
Johns Hopkins University School of Medicine

New York   Oxford
OXFORD UNIVERSITY PRESS
1995

Oxford University Press

Oxford   New York
Athens   Auckland   Bangkok   Bombay
Calcutta   Cape Town   Dar es Salaam   Delhi
Florence   Hong Kong   Istanbul   Karachi
Kuala Lumpur   Madras   Madrid   Melbourne
Mexico City   Nairobi   Paris   Singapore
Taipei   Tokyo   Toronto

and associated companies in
Berlin   Ibadan

Library of Congress Cataloging-in-Publication Data
Harris, James C.
Developmental neuropsychiatry / James C. Harris.
p. cm.   Includes bibliographical references and index.
Contents: v. 1. Fundamentals — v. 2. Assessment, diagnosis, and
treatment of development disorders.
ISBN   0-19-506824-6 (v. 1)
1. Developmentally disabled children — Psychology. 2. Pediatric
neuropsychiatry. 3. Developmental neurology. I. Title.
[DNLM: 1. Child Psychiatry. 2. Child Development. 3. Child Development
Disorders. 4. Child Behavior Disorders. WS 350 H314d 1995]
RJ506.D47H37   1995
618.92'8 — dc20
DNLM/DLC   for Library of Congress   94-42699

Credits for copyrighted materials appear on page 263.

9 8 7 6 5 4 3 2 1

Printed in the United States of America
on acid-free paper

To Mary, Cathy, and Joan
Who made it all possible
and
To the memory of Leo Kanner
Scholar, Teacher, and Advocate
For all children with disabilities

FOREWORD

Although developmental concepts have held a prominent place in American psychiatry for over 50 years because of the dominance of psychodynamic theory, it is only in recent years that advances in neuroscience have begun to have an impact on developmental psychiatry. Two major factors have served as impediments to the incorporation of fruits of brain research in the understanding of the developmental aspects of psychopathology. First, the roots of child psychiatry in the United States can be traced back early in this century to the child guidance movement, which established free-standing community clinics that focused primarily on the psychosocial needs of youth. Thus, with a few exceptions, the primary sites for treatment and training in child psychiatry were isolated from medical school–affiliated departments of psychiatry where biobehavioral research began to flourish. Second, with the ascendance of psychoanalytic theory, the child guidance clinics were predisposed to embrace it as a coherent explanation of child psychopathology. This geographic segregation and the emphasis on psychosocial concepts of etiology rendered child psychiatry poorly prepared to incorporate neuroscientific advances that began to transform psychiatry in the 1970s.

Other barriers have impeded the comprehensive involvement of psychiatry in developmental disorders and mental retardation. The cognitive and communicational limitations of these patients rendered them poorly suited for psychodynamic psychotherapy, the main treatment modality of psychiatry in the past. Thus the management of the psychiatric and behavioral concomitants of these disorders was largely ceded to behavioral psychologists. Furthermore, parents and advocates for the developmentally disabled strongly objected to the indiscriminate mixing of the developmentally disabled and the severely mentally ill in state psychiatric institutions. Thus state and federal policy, anger over stigmatization, and the lack of clinical interest on the part of psychiatry resulted in a wide gulf between psychiatry and the clinical services for the developmentally disabled.

Against this background, a number of advances commencing in the 1970s provided a climate in which academic psychiatry could reestablish its linkages to child psychiatry and to the behavioral complications of developmental disorders. The movement to utilize an atheoretical, phenomenologic strategy to construct a diagnostic schema for psychiatry (*The Diagnostic and Statistical Manual,* or DSM-III) that would provide predictability about course and treatment uncoupled diagnosis from psychodynamic theory. Clinicians began to apply these diagnostic criteria more widely, leading to the identification of psychiatric syndromes in populations such as children and the developmentally disabled, who were previously thought to be unaffected. For example, clinical studies indicated that depressed children often satisfied the diagnostic criteria for major depressive disorder; these observations, at variance with accepted theory of the time, led to the use of treatments for depression found to be effective in adults. With the advances in psychopharmacology, clinicians began to examine whether drugs effective for specific psychiatric disorders might have efficacy in the symptomatic management of psychiatric symptoms in special populations. For example, the use of the serotonin uptake inhibitor chlorimipramine, a drug effective in obsessive-compulsive disorder, was examined in developmentally disabled children with compulsive self-injurious behavior. Finally, the cytogenetic teasing out of different causes for mental retardation began to reveal behavioral phenotypes unique to specific syndromes such as Down syndrome, Prader-Willi syndrome, and Fragile X syndrome. The link between developmental brain disorders caused by specific genetic abnormalities and particular behavioral problems rekindled interest both in clinical research and psychiatric management of developmental disorders.

The rapid advances in brain research over the last two and a half decades, moreover, provided the foundation for the understanding of nervous system development and function that has now permitted the rise of a new and meaningful discipline of developmental neuropsychiatry. The application of the methods of molecular biology to developmental brain research is disclosing the laws dictating the formation of the brain and its neuronal circuitry. Furthermore, animal models to elucidate the role of specific genes through the creation of mice transgenic for normal or mutant genes now allow investigators to track the consequences of abnormal gene expression on brain development and function. At a clinical level, powerful imaging methods provide windows into the human brain to determine quantitatively abnormalities in structure and function in specific

disorders. The findings from neuroscience research have undermined the traditional classification of disorders simply on the basis of their age of symptomatic onset and have revealed that the seeds of psychopathology in disorders such as schizophrenia and Alzheimer's disease are sown early in brain development.

Against this background, Dr. Harris's two-volume work on developmental neuropsychiatry sets the agenda for this emerging clinical specialty. Written by an individual with the developmental expertise of a pediatrician, the behavioral sophistication of an adult and child psychiatrist, and a deep appreciation of neuroscience, his two books offer an integrated yet comprehensive conceptual approach to developmental neuropsychiatry. Grounded in neuroscience but enriched by clinical realities, the first volume provides the unified vision of the "new" psychiatry, which places the brain at the epicenter of psychopathology and recognizes the essential interplay between intrinsic vulnerabilities and life experience. The second volume translates this unifying neuroscientific perspective into the practical clinical issues of the diagnosis, assessment, and management of specific developmental disorders. Dr. Harris's *Developmental Neuropsychiatry* continues the tradition of Leo Kanner's *Child Psychiatry,* first published 60 years ago, in defining the field of developmental psychopathology in a way that will have significance for years to come. Thus this two-volume set will be an essential resource not only for physicians but for all professionals involved in the treatment of developmental disorders.

Joseph T. Coyle, M.D.
Eben S. Draper Professor of
Psychiatry and Neuroscience
Chairman, Consolidated
Department of Psychiatry
Harvard Medical School

PREFACE

Anomalies when rightly studied yield rare instruction; they witness and attract attention to the operation of hidden laws or of known laws under new and unknown conditions; and so set the inquirer on new and fruitful paths of research.

— H. Maudsley, 1880

An appreciation of recent advances in developmental and cognitive psychology, an understanding of basic brain mechanisms, knowledge about recent approaches to modeling in the cognitive neurosciences, and an awareness of descriptive psychopathology are essential background for professionals who are working with children and adolescents with neurodevelopmental disorders. This book provides a resource and a critical appraisal for both the student and the practitioner on the central topics related to developmental neuropsychiatry. It is an effort to bring together in one place background material in these many areas and to offer a developmental perspective that addresses maturation of the brain, the facilitating psychosocial environment, and competence in the mastery of developmental tasks by the disabled person. This approach considers that developmental impairment may magnify brain mechanisms, thereby providing a window on developmental processes that may be difficult to isolate when studied in the normally maturing person in an average expectable environment, the standard situation in which Gesell sought to establish landmarks of development.

The co-occurrence of mental events and neural events has long been recognized. For the experiencing person, subcortical events are cortically reconstructed and influence behavior; the latter is most evident in the case of traumatic life events. Developmental changes take place from infancy throughout the life span. Determining how they occur is a major challenge to current research.

The book is intended to provide a synthesis of recent developments in basic neurobiology, cognitive neuroscience, ethology, child development, and developmental psychopathology and apply them to children and adolescents with neuropsychiatric conditions. Specific conditions occurring during the developmental period are reviewed to examine the potential basis for differences among them, and methods of assessment and effective means of intervention are discussed. Included are conditions involving brain disorder or dysfunction whose origins are genetic, metabolic, traumatic, toxic, or psychosocial. Their effects on developing persons and their families are central to the discussion. Although both sexes are affected, these conditions occur most commonly in males. For convenience in reading, the pronoun "he" is used to denote both sexes throughout the text.

Developmental Neuropsychiatry: The Fundamentals is divided into three parts contain ing background information on basic neural science, cognitive neuroscience, and child developmental research, which should prove helpful to the reader in considering developmental psychopathological disorders. This information is presented to acquaint the reader with this material and is not intended to be an exhaustive review.

The overall goal of this book is to assist the professional working with developmental disorders to facilitate the mental growth and social adaptation of children and adolescents with neurodevelopmental disorders. It provides background information that will help them facilitate change in these children and their families. The intended audience includes child and adolescent psychiatrists, developmental pediatricians, child neurologists, physicians in training (fellows, residents, and medical students), nurses, educators, psychologists, and other nonmedical professionals who treat these conditions and neuroscientists who wish to learn more about child and adolescent neuropsychiatric disorders.

Baltimore, Maryland   J.C.H.
August 1995

ACKNOWLEDGMENTS

Developmental Neuropsychiatry provides a comprehensive summary of knowledge acquired and literature consulted as a result of my work with children and adolescents with developmental disorders and their families. It is the outcome of many interactions and discussions with faculty members, residents, medical students, and nonmedical professionals over the past two decades at the Johns Hopkins Medical Institutions. Dr. Paul McHugh, Chairman of the Department of Psychiatry, the Johns Hopkins University School of Medicine, was instrumental in stimulating me to consider writing a textbook and has provided ongoing guidance. Dr. Joseph Coyle, Director of the Division of Child and Adolescent Psychiatry at the Johns Hopkins University School of Medicine from 1982 to 1991, enthusiastically supported the book and offered his expertise in developmental neuroscience. Dr. Hugo Moser, Director of the Johns Hopkins Center for Research in Mental Retardation and Related Aspects of Human Development, encouraged me in the early stages of manuscript development and provided the primary setting for me, as the director of developmental neuropsychiatry, to evaluate and treat children and adolescents with developmental disorders.

Dr. Paul MacLean, Chief, Laboratory of Brain Evolution and Behavior at NIH, stimulated my interest in comparative neuroanatomy, established a position for me as guest worker in his laboratory (1978–1984), and made me as excited as he is about the prospects of evolutionary neurobiology. Dr. Edward Edinger, analytic psychologist and former Chairman of the Jung Training Center in New York, encouraged me to think about the psychology of developmental disorders and how the self system might emerge in those with disabling conditions. Dr. Edinger provided an important and greatly appreciated stimulus in looking at the developmental perspective on the pervasive developmental disorders and its interface with psychological theory.

Dr. Roland Fisher, formerly at Johns Hopkins and now Professor at the University of the Balearics in Mallorca, stimulated my interest in the brain/mind interface, particularly as to how experience may shape the brain. Ralph Harper, Adjunct Professor at Johns Hopkins in the history of ideas program, and an existential theologian, reflected with me on the nature of the life experiences of the family of the disabled person. Most important, he provided ongoing support which sustained me throughout the preparation of the manuscript and its final stage of completion. Finally, my wife, Dr. Catherine DeAngelis, reminded me of the importance of completing what I had begun and in all ways provided the environment that made this book possible. Simply put, without her this book could not have been written.

A number of colleagues have been instrumental in reading and critiquing the various parts of these books. A single-authored textbook is now uncommon, and its completion would not have been possible without the assistance of colleagues at the Johns Hopkins University School of Medicine and the NIH Laboratory of Comparative Ethology. Dr. M. Christine Zink, D.V.M., Ph.D., Associate Professor of Comparative Medicine and Pathology at the Johns Hopkins University School of Medicine, reviewed the initial chapter on molecular neurobiology and provided a comprehensive critique. The chapter on the development of neurotransmitter systems is an expansion of an earlier chapter on this subject, which I prepared with Dr. Joseph Coyle, now Professor of Psychiatry and Neuroscience and Chair of the Consolidated Department of Psychiatry at Harvard University School of Medicine. His expertise in this area was invaluable.

Dr. Paul Wender, Professor, Department of Psychiatry, University of Utah School of Medicine, reviewed the entire section on basic neural science. Dr. Wender had stimulated my interest in developmental neuropsychiatry during my child and adolescent psychiatry residency in 1973 as we discussed minimal brain dysfunction (now AD/HD), its diagnosis and treatment, each Friday morning. Drs. Stephen Suomi and Dee Higley, NIH Laboratory of Comparative Ethology, provided helpful critiques of Chapters 12 through 17 dealing with ethology and the developmental perspective. Dr. Suomi generously arranged for me to become a guest worker in the Laboratory of Comparative Ethology (1984–1992), where I conducted behavioral research on separation vocalizations in squirrel monkeys with Dr. John Newman.

The chapters of Part I, Volume II, on assessment and rating scales were reviewed by Dr. Ludwik Szymanski, Director of the Diagnostic Evaluation Clinic, the Children's Hospital Medical Center, Harvard University. I am particularly appreciative of Dr. Szymanski's help. He and I have worked closely for many years on the Mental Retardation and Developmental Disability Committee of the American Academy of Child and Adolescent Psychiatry. The chapter on neuropsychological testing was reviewed extensively with Dr. Martha Denckla, Professor of Neurology and Director of Developmental Cognitive Neurology, Kennedy Krieger Institute, the Johns Hopkins University School of Medicine. This chapter underwent multiple revisions under her guidance. The chapter on the evaluation of brain structure and functions, which deals with the various neuroimaging techniques, was reviewed by Dr. Nick Bryan, Director of Neuroradiology, Johns Hopkins University School of Medicine. Dr. Bryan provided a comprehensive critique, and his suggestions were readily incorporated into this chapter. Dr. Ludwik Szymanski was also the reviewer of Chapters 5 through 9 of Part II, Volume II, on developmental disorders, an area in which he is eminently qualified. He pointed out the relevance of these chapters to both physicians and nonphysicians who work with the developmental disorders.

Part III, Volume II, on behavioral phenotypes, was reviewed by Dr. Hugo Moser, who made many valuable comments and suggestions, particularly relating to the metabolic disorders. This section was revised extensively in keeping with his suggestions. His help was particularly appreciated in the section on adrenoleukodystrophy, an area in which he and I have worked together for many years.

Dr. Paul Wender reviewed Chapters 13 through 17 of Part IV, Volume II, on developmental psychopathology and commented on their usefulness to physicians and nonphysicians working with these types of problems. Dr. Ludwik Szymanski reviewed Chapters 18 through 21 on the treatment of children with developmental disorders as well as Chapter 22 on public law and the rights of the disabled. Final thanks are to Dr. Frank Oski, Chairman, Department of Pediatrics, the Johns Hopkins University School of Medicine, who reviewed the overall structure of the manuscript.

The works of Sir Michael Rutter, C.B.E., M.D., provided the foundation for the establishment of this specialty area. I have benefited from my contacts with him over the years and have sought to follow his lead in the further development of this specialty. Contacts with many other individuals have enriched my experiences with children with developmental disorders and contributed in great part to my thinking and perspective. Among them are Leo Kanner, Alejandro Rodriguez, Dennis Whitehouse, Arnold Capute, Sakkubai Naidu, Fred Palmer, Bruce Shapiro, Susan Hyman, Joan Gerring, Allan Reiss, Wayne Fisher, Rebecca

Landa, Richard Allen, Paula Tallal, Susan Harriman, Eileen Atkins, Jean Patz, Georgette Evler, and a host of others whose professional association has made our mutual interest in the care of children exciting and worthwhile.

Gratitude is expressed particularly to the many authors whose publications I have summarized in this textbook. Their efforts have led to a better understanding of developmental disorders. I bear full responsibility for the synthesis of their work.

Finally, I express my appreciation to the administration of the Department of Psychiatry at the Johns Hopkins University School of Medicine and the Kennedy Krieger Institute for providing support for a one-year, full-time sabbatical to allow me to integrate the disparate elements of the field of developmental neuropsychiatry and frame them into what I hope is a comprehensive and coherent textbook that may be used by both physicians and nonphysicians who devote their efforts to working with children, adolescents, and their families as they compensate and struggle with disorders of development.

Special thanks are due Joan Bossert, my editor at Oxford University Press. From our initial meeting in 1988 at the Society of Neuroscience meeting through the completion of my manuscript she has provided unfailing support, been a sounding board, offered insightful suggestions, and demonstrated her expertise in navigating these books through the production process. For all this, I am especially grateful.

Baltimore, Maryland J.C.H.
August 1995

CONTENTS

BASIC NEURAL SCIENCE

The chapters in Part I on basic neural science emphasize development from the perspectives of molecular neurobiology, neuroanatomy, the establishment of neurotransmitters and neuronal signaling, sleep, and circadian rhythms, and the influences of genetic factors on the expression of behavior. The overall goal of Part I is to provide a basic understanding of how brain development takes place, thereby providing necessary information essential for understanding neurobiological factors and genetic influences on developmental disorders.

Molecular neurobiology has emerged from molecular biology and neuroscience. Advances in molecular neurobiology include methods for the isolation and amplification of DNA fragments, leading to their replication (DNA cloning), and the development of restriction endonucleases that cleave DNA and allow analysis of DNA fragments. Other advances include the use of retroviral reverse transcriptase to copy RNA into stable complementary DNA (cDNA), which allows RNA structures to be analyzed, the development of gel systems for separation of DNA and RNA by size, and the rapid sequencing of DNA. New automated methods are available to produce polyclonal and monoclonal antibody reagents for protein identification and isolation. These developments have made it possible to introduce cloned genes into transgenic animals (mice). The value of these analytic tools for disorders involving the brain has been demonstrated in the cloning of and structural characterization of the mRNA for growth hormone, somatostatin, pro-opiomelanocortin, neurotransmitter receptors, and ion channels.

Developmental neuroanatomy benefits from refined neuroanatomical methods that have led to better delineation of the developing nervous system. This has led to a better understanding of how neural cells establish their own particular identities and how patterns of neuronal connection are established and subsequently maintained. The phases of development which lead to final organization of the brain include neurogenesis and migration of neurons, histogenesis, cell migration, cell differentiation, cell death, and myelination. Subsequently, regional brain anatomy is defined. Brain imaging techniques allow *in vivo* study of the metabolic maturation of brain during development. Refinements in techniques to study developmental neuroanatomy have important implications for investigating and understanding the developmental disorders.

Knowledge of the development of neurotransmitter systems, synaptic transmission, and methods of neuronal signaling is critical to an understanding of the developmental disorders. Neurotransmitter mechanisms have been better defined with the identification of new substances that act as neurotransmitters, the recognition of co-localization of neurotransmitters and neuropeptides, and the delineation of the structure of neurotransmitter sub-types. As the anatomical localization of the major neurotransmitter systems and their functions are better understood, so also is their potential role in human psychopathology.

Sleep and circadian rhythms may have a crucial role in the development of the brain over time. Circadian rhythms become progressively refined during development. REM sleep, in particular, may play an important role in brain development, and dreams may have an important adaptive function as experiences are integrated into long-term memory. In this regard, the ontogeny of sleep and changes in sleep and circadian rhythms during development and developmental aspects of dreaming at different ages may contribute to an understanding of the developmental disorders.

Genetics is particularly important as it pertains to developmental disorders. An understanding of genetic transmission complements findings in the new molecular genetics. Knowledge about genetics can play an important role in the prevention of developmental disorders and in their treatment. Methods of genetic assessment include twins studies, cross-fostering studies, and family genetic studies. Specific features of genetic risk apply to a variety of neuropsychiatric disorders.

CHAPTER 1

MOLECULAR NEUROBIOLOGY: THE NEW GENETICS

Advances in molecular neurobiology promise to enhance our understanding of developmental neuropsychiatric disorders in children. The most important, recently developed techniques in neurobiology allow the role played by genes in regulating neuronal development to be studied. Furthermore, the environmental factors and interactions that influence gene expression can be assessed. In normal development, new combinations of linked genes occur through crossover between their loci. Recombinations commonly occur in the human genome, which consists of over 100,000 genes distributed along each of 23 pairs of chromosomes. Major advances have been made in molecular neurobiology through the study of recombinant DNA technology, which allows manipulation of DNA to produce artificial recombinations.

This chapter reviews molecular genetic approaches that are being applied to the study of developmental disorders to establish a relationship between neuropsychiatric illness and an individual's genetic endowment. It discusses and defines important terms utilized in molecular genetics, including a basic review of Mendelian genetics; a discussion of DNA, RNA, protein synthesis, genetic structure, and DNA cloning; and how this information may be applied to psychiatric disorders.

Ultimately, understanding these cellular mechanisms may result in gene replacement therapy or gene attenuation therapies. Currently, interventions for these disorders are limited to providing medical care and psychological support to the individual and family.

CLASSICAL AND MOLECULAR GENETICS

Classical, or Mendelian, genetics focuses on the *phenotype,* a term that refers to recognizable characteristics of a specific individual. These characteristics are observable, such as height or eye color, or are more fundamental, such as products of metabolism or blood groups. The latter are referred to as *endophenotypes* in contrast to the physically observable *exophenotype.* More recently, the term "behavioral phenotype" has been introduced to designate behavioral patterns associated with identifiable syndromes that are not learned and are characteristic of that disorder. In some instances, these syndromes have a clearly identified genetic basis; in others, this is not the case.

One's genetic individuality is the result of differences in the form of the genes (designated alleles) that occupy a site or locus. Most phenotypes are not entirely determined by the genotype, the collection of genes inherited by an organism, but are the result of an interaction between the genotype or the endophenotype, which is derived from it, along with environmental interactions. In studying hereditary disorders, the genotype, the phenotype, and the relationship between them must be considered. Between genotype and the exophenotypic behavior, then, is a complex process involving multiple endophenotypes. The nature of environmental influence varies substantially among phenotypes. In neuropsychiatry, the exophenotypes, or clinical syndromes, are influenced substantially by environmental events from the molecular to the social level. On the other hand, behavioral phenotypes may be modified by the environment but remain characteristic of the syndrome. Furthermore, different etiologies, either environmental or genetic, may be present in individuals with the same diagnosis. Therefore, identical phenotypes may have heterogeneous bases. For example, there are multiple etiologies for autistic disorder.

Moreover, a number of different mutations in one gene can give rise to the same or very similar syndromes. This is referred to as *allelic heterogeneity*. The term "nonallelic" heterogeneity is used when a disorder can be caused by mutations in several different genes located at different sites in the genome. An example is tuberous sclerosis. Furthermore, a clinical syndrome may have a genetic basis in some individuals, but in others an environmental basis. In this instance, the environmentally caused syndrome is referred to as a *phenocopy*. An individual may possess a defective gene that is not expressed exophenotypically, so the gene has a penetrance of less than 100%. In situations where penetrance is low, environmental influences may be crucial. In addition, a gene may determine sensitivity to environmental factors or may influence the degree of exposure to them.

In contrast to Mendelian genetics, molecular genetics focuses on the genotype and the endophenotypic abnormality rather than the classic observations in genetics on the exophenotype (Watson et al., 1987; Lewin, 1990).

BACKGROUND OF HUMAN GENETICS

The chromosomes that carry genetic information are highly compact and reside within the cell nucleus. These chromosomes are made up of nucleic acids and proteins. In the human, there are 22 paired homologous autosomes and a pair of sex chromosomes. Along each chromosome, genes are linearly placed and function as the units of heredity.

The recognition that inherited characteristics are carried by a pair of unitary factors, one coming from each parent, is attributed to

Mendel (1865). He studied attributes of garden peas including height, seed color, and surface characteristics (e.g., smooth or wrinkled). Mendel identified seven attributes that were controlled by seven pairs of "unit characters," which acted as the physical units of heredity. The term "gene" as a description for unit inheritance was introduced by Wilhelm Johannsen, a Danish plant geneticist, in 1909 (Thompson, McInnes, and Willard, 1991).

Mendel proposed three basic laws, which established the basic principles of heredity (Thompson, McInnes, and Willard, 1991). These are *Unit Inheritance,* the *Law of Segregation,* and the *Law of Independent Assortment.* In regard to *Unit Inheritance,* Mendel stated that the blending of characteristics of parents does not occur. Parental traits may not be seen in first generation offspring but may reappear unchanged in later generations. The *Law of Segregation* states that as the gametes, the sperm or ovum, form, the pairs of identical genes separate (segregate) and do not influence one another. This law indicates that alleles (variant forms of a particular gene) segregate during each generation. Consequently, the germ cells in the formation of a sperm or ova contain one copy of each allele. Mendel recognized that in a particular mating, parents could have two identical copies of the same factor or two different copies. Therefore, if the parent were homozygous at a particular chromosomal locus, both alleles would be identical and all germ cells would contain the same form of that particular allele. In other instances, the parent might be heterozygous; that locus consequently would have two different alleles, so germ cells would contain one allele or the other. Some variations of genes will be dominant; others will be recessive. If an individual inherits a copy of a dominant and a recessive gene or two copies of a dominant gene (one from each parent), the dominant gene(s) will be expressed; i.e., the characteristics it causes will be present. For dominant inheritance, one copy of a dominant gene is needed, but for recessive inheritance, two copies of the recessive gene are required. When the rule of segregation is broken and members of a pair of chromosomes do not normally segregate, the consequence is a severe abnormality in the offspring.

The *Law of Independent Assortment* states that traits controlled by different gene pairs (e.g., hair color) pass from the parent gamete to the offspring independent of one another. There is random recombination of paternal and maternal chromosomes in the gametes. Therefore, in considering two traits that are determined by a single gene, the phenotypes that arise in the first generation and in subsequent crosses in future generations can be predicted by hypothesizing that the association between alleles that determine each phenotype is entirely random. It has been demonstrated that Mendel's *Law of Independent Assortment* is strictly true only for unlinked genes, that is, genes that are on separate chromosomes or genes that are substantially distant from one another on the same chromosome and therefore behave independently.

The practical outcome of Mendel's findings are best seen through genetic counseling. When parents mate who have autosomal recessive genes for a particular trait, the number of offspring produced with that trait is one in four. However, if a parent is homozygous for an autosomal dominant gene, all offspring will express the phenotype if there is complete penetrance. This will occur regardless of gender and will be independent of the genotype of the other parent. Sex-linked recessive and dominant traits can also be predicted by tracking a gene through multiple generations.

GENETIC DIVERSITY

The genetic code provides for a strikingly large diversity of genetic information. The proteins are polymers that comprise a linear sequence of amino acids. Their structure and their functional properties depend on their size and the amino acid sequence. For example, in a protein of 100 amino acids there are 23^{100} possible combinations when the 23 amino acids are used as building blocks. If DNA were a random mixture of polymerized nucleotides in a genome, the size found in the human (3×10^9 base pairs total length per haploid set of chromosomes), then we would expect any specific 17 base pair sequences to be represented only once in a genome by chance (Whatley and Owen, 1989). However, the genome of an organism is not a random collection of bases; the base sequence is the result of extensive evolutionary selection pressure to make it functional. The protein coding regions of DNA generally are contained in the unique class of DNA that is described in the following section.

BASIC MOLECULAR BIOLOGY

DNA Structure

Genes are made up of DNA, a polymer of deoxyribonucleotides, and consist of two chains of nucleotide bases which are wrapped around each other to form a double helix. Each of these nucleotides consists of a purine or pyrimidine base that is attached to a modified sugar, a deoxypentose phosphate. When the nucleotides are polymerized through linkages between their phosphate groups, they are referred to as *nucleic acids*.

In the nucleus of a cell, DNA exists as a paired structure that contains four bases that may be arranged in any order along a sugar-phosphate spine. The four nucleotide bases are adenylic acid (A), guanylic acid (G), cytidylic acid (C), and thymidylic acid (T). A and G are purine nucleotides, and C and T are pyrimidine nucleotides. Each DNA strand has a particular polarity. At one end of the strand there is a free 5′ phosphate group, at the other end a 3′ hydroxyl group. The polarity of each strand in nucleic acid duplex runs in opposite directions, so the two strands are antiparallel.

Two DNA strands pair with hydrogen bonding and form the double helical structure with their free 5′ phosphate and 3′ hydroxyls at opposite ends. The hydrogen atoms that form between the opposing pairs are essential to steric properties that maintain the paired structure of a DNA molecule. Base pairing is strictly aligned. The most stable hydrogen bonding occurs between A/T and G/C pairs, so A always pairs with T and G with C. Each strand contains a sequence of bases that are complementary to the other. This principle of complementarity has important consequences in that it explains why single strands of nucleic acids can form stable duplexes. Furthermore, it is a critical element for nucleic acid synthesis because one strand acts as a template, so the second strand can be copied or synthesized, using that strand. These principles of polarity and the pairing of bases offer a predictive tool in that knowledge of a sequence of bases in one strand automatically reveals the sequence of the bases in the complementary strand.

DNA Replication

To replicate themselves, cells must pass on genetic information, a complicated process because there are frequent errors in copying. A central property of DNA is the capability for self-replication. During the replication process the strands unwind and enzymes, known as *DNA polymerases,* move along the unwinding

double helix. During replication, each strand serves as a template for the complementary strand. The synthesis of a daughter strand takes place by the addition of the 5' phosphate of a deoxyribonucleotide to the free 3' hydroxyl on a growing strand. The chain growth takes place in the direction from the 5' to the 3' elements. Consequently, each parent strand gives rise to a complementary daughter strand and immedi-

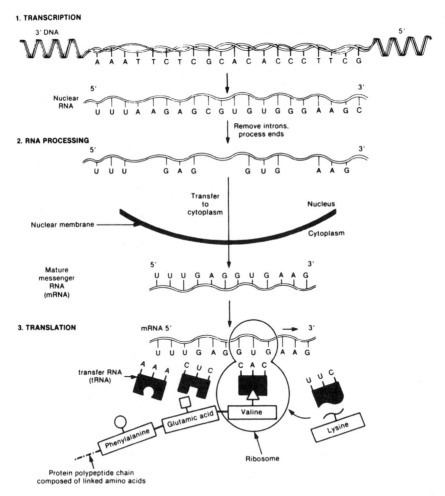

Figure 1–1. *Flow of genetic information.* This diagram shows how protein synthesis occurs following the genetic instructions in DNA. In the transcription process, a segment of DNA is transcribed into an RNA molecule. The introns are then snipped out, and the mature messenger RNA (mRNA) molecule is moved out of the cell's nucleus to a ribosome. In the translation process, transfer RNA (tRNA) molecules help translate the genetic code in the mRNA into amino acids, which are linked together to form a peptide or protein (from U.S. Congress, Office of Technology Assessment, 1986).

ately forms a new duplex structure with it, which is joined by hydrogen bonding. By the end of the cycle of replication, two new DNA duplexes have been produced, each with a parent strand and a daughter strand.

Genetic information is encoded through the sequence of bases along the DNA. To be used, it must first be read or transcribed and then decoded or translated, as shown in Figure 1–1.

The genetic information is transported from the cell nucleus to the cytoplasm by a type of RNA known as *messenger RNA (mRNA)*. This is copied directly from one strand of DNA, so each molecule of mRNA has bases in a sequence complementary to that found on the DNA molecule (gene) from which it was copied. This transfer of genetic information from the gene to mRNA is referred to as *transcription*. Having reached the cytoplasm, mRNA acts as a template to assemble protein molecules. This takes place in the ribosome, the protein synthesizing unit of the cell. Protein construction is based on the sequential reading of groups of three bases: each triplet sequence, or codon, codes for a specific amino acid, with some acting as signals to begin or terminate construction. The amino acids are then polymerized to produce a final protein product. The final result is a conversion from linear genetic information to an enzyme or structural protein.

These processes are described in more detail in the following sections.

STRUCTURE OF THE GENE

In recent years it has become apparent that the process of transferring genetic information is more complicated than previously thought, especially in higher organisms. Much of the DNA in higher organisms does not code for structural information, but may exist to regulate the expression of the coding regions (i.e., enhancer or promoter regions). Within genes that code for single proteins, there are noncoding regions (introns) which separate the coding regions (exons). During transcription of the gene, the original RNA transcript is processed by splicing out noncoding regions along with other post-transcription modifications – for example, addition of poly (A) and end capping before cytoplasmic release (see Figure 1–2). This processing is regulated by sequence information, such as particular base sequences at splice junctions (Whatley and Owen, 1989).

This promoter region is needed for activation of gene transcription. When the promoter region is absent or there is a mutation, a severe loss or attenuation of gene transcription occurs. The exact mechanisms for transcriptional activators regulating gene transcription is not fully

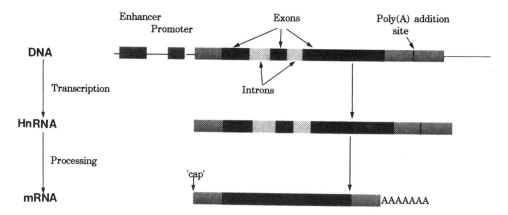

Figure 1–2. *The structure of a typical eukaryotic gene.* Genes are characterized by a promoter that is located close to the start of transcription and enhancer sequences, which may be at various sites, including within the gene itself or "downstream" of it. After transcription, specific signal sequences control processing of the mRNA precursor. These include "splicing" out of introns and addition of the poly(A) tail. The 5′ "cap" is essential for efficient translation of the mature mRNA (from Whatley, Owen, and Murray, 1989).

understood. At any given time, only a fraction of the genes are working. Many genes are selectively expressed during certain stages of development or in response to environmental signals. How genes are turned on and off remains a challenging question. Although exactly what it is that signals activation may be unknown, transcriptional activators are thought to interact physically both with DNA promoter elements and with RNA polymerase through specific binding sites for each of these. In addition, other 5' regulatory elements include consensus sequences to bind hormones and cyclic AMP to the gene. Substances such as these may play an important role in modulation of transcription.

Moreover, in the 1970s, it was shown that DNA is a dynamic molecule. Small pieces of DNA, called *jumping genes,* do sometimes move within or between chromosomes, resulting in changes in gene expression. These findings have led to the view that DNA responds to ongoing events in the cell. This dynamism of the genome has received new emphasis with the recognition that some genes do not have fixed locations on the chromosome. Genes that can change position within DNA are referred to as *transposable genes,* or *transposons.* In addition, RNA is occasionally reverse transcribed into DNA.

RNA SYNTHESIS

RNA, or ribonucleic acid, is a single-stranded polymer made of ribonucleotides. It shares some structural and chemical properties with DNA but differs in other ways and carries out different functions. RNA consists of four nucleotides: A, G, and C, which are also found in DNA, and uridylic acid (U) — instead of T, found in DNA. Polymerization of the ribophosphate during RNA synthesis occurs in the same way as in DNA synthesis, and RNA has the 5' to 3' polarity, as does DNA. However, RNA exists in the cell as a single-stranded molecule. By pairing with complementary bases, RNA strands do form hybrid duplexes with either single-stranded DNA or other RNA molecules. Furthermore, RNA strands may self-hybridize to form loops, as in transfer RNA. Messenger RNA (mRNA) is an information carrier for the genetic instructions encoded in DNA. RNA polymerases are responsible for transcription of

an mRNA copy from the DNA template in the cell nucleus. Nucleic acid strands serve as templates for synthesis of complementary strands and are not copied directly.

Before mRNA becomes a functional message and a mature transcript, the primary mRNA transcript, which is derived from genes containing introns, must be processed. The transcript at specific sites and the free ends are then joined. The mature mRNA transcript is a continuous structure made up entirely of exons as shown in Figure 1–2. It should be pointed out that a messenger RNA molecule is not complete until it has been chemically processed in several different ways. This sometimes involves a recoding or reinterpretation of the genetic message. (Ciaranello, Wong, and Rubenstein, 1990).

PROTEIN SYNTHESIS

After the primary transcript is processed, the mature mRNA moves from the cell nucleus into the cytoplasm and attaches to ribosomes. These ribosomes use the mRNA as a template and direct polypeptide synthesis. The assembly of the polypeptide chain involves transfer RNA (tRNA). This is a stable form of a single-stranded RNA. The transfer RNA, during protein synthesis, binds to the mRNA through codon–anticodon pairing. Every transfer RNA has an anticodon, and a unique transfer RNA exists for every functional codon. During the process of synthesis, the ribosome traverses the mRNA template, reads it, and directs the polypeptide synthesis. Enzymes that are specialized to complete protein synthesis link amino acids in sequence in a growing polypeptide chain. The polypeptide chain remains connected to the ribosome until the final synthesis is completed. Proteins that are synthesized possess polarity with the first amino acid in the chain having an amino group and a free carboxyl group. Numerous ribosomes can concurrently read the same mRNA, so one polypeptide may be completed at 3' end of the assembly while a new one is beginning at the 5' end.

Following synthesis, additional protein processing may occur. For example, glycosylation is frequently observed in enzymes and also in neurotransmitter receptors. Another modification in processing is the addition of a phosphate group, or *phosphorylation.* The phosphorylation process is essential for the activation of many enzymes. Furthermore, many proteins, including receptors, enzymes, and ion channel proteins undergo cyclic changes in their activity by removal or addition of phosphate groups. An important intracellular event is phosphorylation of intracellular proteins by protein kinases, which are activated when receptors are stimulated.

TYPES OF GENETIC MUTATION

A change in the sequence of bases in coding areas of DNA may have significant effects on both cell metabolism and cell structure. The simplest genetic mutations are base substitution mutations, which occur during the replication of DNA when an incorrect base is inserted into a daughter strand. This is referred to as a *point mutation,* and an example would be the substitution of an A for a G. If a base substitution occurs within an exon, then a single amino acid change may occur, which may or may not have functional consequences. A particularly severe problem may occur when base substitutions take place at exon–intron junctions, which may eliminate them. Moreover, the production of a novel stop signal may cause the premature termination of protein synthesis. Changes outside the coding region also may have an effect on gene expression (e.g., a mutation at a promoter sequence could abolish transcription of a gene, and one at a splice junction may lead to abnormal processing of mRNA).

Frame shift mutations arise from a deletion or an insertion that is not an exact multiple of three base pairs, which occurs during the DNA replication. This changes the reading frame of the gene because the stop codon formed is not normal. The result is an elongated or a truncated protein. In addition to the substitution mutation and the frame shift mutation, other types of mutations are known that include exon deletion (some or all of an exon is omitted from a gene, so the protein that results is severely truncated in size and is usually dysfunctional), exon duplication (a segment or even entire exon is repeated in tandem, so repetition of a particular segment of the protein obliterates its function), and the loss of an exon–intron boundary (the mRNA then encodes amino acid sequences not found in the protein with an associated total loss or attenuation of function).

In addition to point mutations, mutations causing deletions of large segments are being more commonly identified, as are translocations. Translocations occur where a chromosome is broken and regions go to rejoin at a different site on another chromosome. Yet not all DNA changes are damaging, and some changes may even improve the activity of an enzyme leading to a selective advantage.

THE ANALYSIS OF DNA

All cells have basically the same genotype. However, the massive amount of this genetic substance in molecular terms (approximately 10^8 base pairs of DNA/chromosome) makes analysis a formidable task. In genetics, the two characteristics of DNA that are particularly important in its analysis are first, the linear nature of the genetic information, which allows an ordering of base sequences and the sequence of genes in the chromosome; and second, that the two DNA strands are complementary, which has previously been discussed.

Above a certain temperature, DNA will denature; i.e., the two strands of the helix will separate. Yet because of the characteristics of base pairing (A-T and G-C), a particular sequence of DNA will only recognize and then hybridize to its corresponding complementary partner. Although a certain degree of mismatch may be possible, generally purified single-strand DNA sequences will recognize only the complementary DNA sequence from which they were transcribed. Likewise, a purified RNA sequence will recognize only the DNA sequence from which it was transcribed. Therefore, purified sequences can be used as detectors or probes for corresponding sequences in a mixture of nucleic acids. These DNA properties may be used effectively in the analysis of DNA. Three methods have been particularly important in this regard, namely, restriction enzymes, molecular cloning, and Southern blotting (Steel, 1984a, 1984b).

Restriction Enzymes

The discovery of restriction enzymes, or restriction endonucleases, has been a key element in approaching the analysis of DNA. These enzymes act as a kind of chemical scissors to cut DNA where specific base sequences occur in the molecule; not at random. The restriction enzymes each recognize a different sequence of bases, which results in fragments of manageable size (usually 10^3 to 10^4 base pairs). Fragments of this number of base pairs are about the size that is expected for most genes. Therefore, restriction enzyme digestion enables genes to be handled more or less in isolation instead of as part of one single, long molecule.

The Cloning of DNA

The second major discovery in DNA analysis was the ability to purify specific sections of DNA to act as probes. DNA cloning is one of the most powerful techniques in modern biology. It has provided information on protein sequences far more efficiently than traditional sequencing techniques. Ciaranello, Wong, and Rubenstein (1990) provide a description of the DNA cloning process. There are two main types of gene probe. In the first, cDNA is produced from mRNA transcripts by the action of the reverse transcriptase enzyme. This allows the isolation of DNAs that represent specifically expressed messages in a particular tissue. cDNA probes represent copies of the coding sequence of genes. In addition to this first method of cloning DNA, another method permits the gene to be cloned from genomic DNA, which is extracted and digested with restriction enzymes. Genomic or cDNA sections are inserted into the genome of vectors such as bacterial plasmids or bacteriophages (using restriction enzymes), that replicate freely within a host bacterium, such as *Escherichia coli.* Only one DNA fragment is inserted into each bacterium, which replicates in the bacteria and then may be recovered. The bacteria are grown on appropriate media and produce bacterial colonies that each contain multiple copies of the specific DNA fragment originally inserted.

This process of molecular cloning leads to biological purification and amplification of particular fragments. The collected bacterial colonies from each source are referred to as a *library.* In the library, there is a probability that any given sequence from the original DNA mixture will be found. For example, 10 to 100 copies of each message may be present in the

library. Subsequently, the library is screened using specific techniques to identify the cDNA of interest. Techniques used depend on what is previously known about the protein being evaluated prior to beginning the cloning. For example, when amino acid sequences in the protein are known, short synthetic nucleic acids (oligonucleotide probes) are used to bind all the cDNAs that contain these sequences. On the other hand, if cDNA has been purified but not sequenced, the amino acid sequences are unknown. Steps must be taken to identify the cDNAs encoding it. The success of these procedures requires that the bacteria used as a host be able to synthesize the protein being evaluated. Because some proteins are toxic to bacteria, other methods may be needed.

When a colony of bacteria that has expressed the desired cDNA is identified, the particular colony is isolated and grown into larger quantities. The bacteria are then lysed, and the cDNA insert is excised from the vector, using the appropriate restriction enzyme, as shown in Figure 1–3.

Now isolated, the cDNA can be chemically sequenced to find the primary structure of the protein which it encodes. Furthermore, the cDNA may be placed into a suitable host cell (transfection) so that an encoded protein will be produced. The properties of the encoded protein can be studied in a controlled environment. This method has been used to identify novel proteins such as neurotransmitter receptors. The purified receptor can then be used to study its effects. In a final step, the cDNA can be hybridized to form genomic DNA so that genes encoding particular target proteins can be isolated and examined for their structure.

Southern Blot Analysis

This is a fundamental technique of molecular genetics which was developed by E. M. Southern for transferring DNA fragments that have been separated by agarose gel electrophoresis to a nitrocellulose filter on which specific DNA fragments can then be detected by their hybridization to radioactive probes (Southern, 1975). The current procedure, as shown in Figure 1–4, is as follows: First, genomic DNA is cut with a restriction enzyme. A large number of different-sized DNA fragments are produced, which can be separated according to their size through elec-

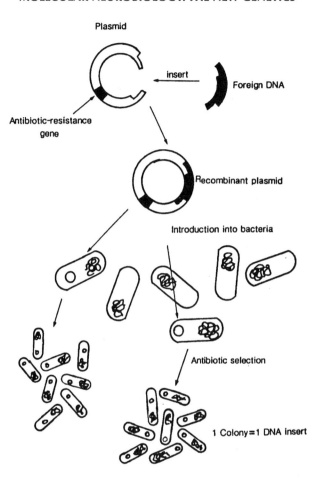

Figure 1–3. *Bacterial cloning.* Foreign DNA is inserted into a bacterial plasmid that contains an antibiotic resistance gene. Following infection, bacteria that contain plasmid are able to grow in the presence of antibiotics whereas those without plasmids cannot. When bacteria are plated on an antibiotic selection medium, this produces bacterial colonies, each of which is derived from a single bacterium and which contains a pure population of recombinant plasmid (from Whatley, Owen, and Murray, 1989).

trophoresis on an agarose gel. Due to the specificity of the restriction enzyme, only a few specific fragment sizes will contain the DNA region targeted for investigation. To detect these fragments, the DNA has to be treated with alkali to denature it into single strands of DNA. It may then be transferred to a membrane sheet of either nitrocellulose or modified nylon by a blotting procedure. The result is a copy of the gel, which is blotted onto the nitrocellulose or modified nylon, which retains the electrophoretically produced arrangement of DNA fragments. This blot is then exposed to a DNA probe radioactively labeled for detection. The applied DNA probe will bind to that part of the filter which contains its complementary sequence. Surplus DNA probe will not bind elsewhere and is washed away. The specific position on the membrane of the fragment containing the region of DNA that is to be analyzed and whose sequence corresponds to that of the probe is then determined by autoradiography.

The Southern blot analysis can be used to detect a sequence of interest in a starting sample of DNA and can also provide information in regard to the surrounding region. The information in the surrounding region in regard to the size of DNA is contained between the enzyme recognition sites on either side.

The full characterization of a section of

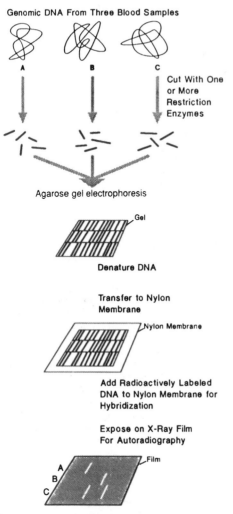

Genomic DNA From Three Blood Samples

Cut With One
or More
Restriction
Enzymes

Agarose gel electrophoresis

Gel

Denature DNA

Transfer to Nylon
Membrane

Nylon Membrane

Add Radioactively Labeled
DNA to Nylon Membrane for
Hybridization

Expose on X-Ray Film
For Autoradiography

Film

Variations in DNA sequences at particular marker sites are
observed as differences in numbers and sizes of DNA fragments among samples taken from different individuals (shown
here as samples A, B, and C).

Figure 1–4. *The Southern blot procedure for
anlayzing specific DNA sequences.* This is a technique for transferring DNA fragments that have been
separated by agarose gel electrophoresis to a notro-
cellulose filter on which specific DNA fragments
can then be detected. The detection of restriction
fragment length polymorphisms (RFLPs) is completed, using radioactively labeled DNA probes
(from U.S. Congress, Office of Technology Assessment, 1988).

DNA will require knowledge of the exact
base sequence. Techniques are now available
to determine the base sequence of purified
pieces of DNA through chemical or enzymatic means. The main factor limiting the
analysis of base sequence is that the procedures are labor-intensive and time-consum-
ing. Despite this, the Human Genome Project,
described in the appendix to this chapter, is
addressing the sequence of the full genome.
New procedures are being developed to speed
up the process of DNA sequencing by using
automated technology.

APPLICATION OF MOLECULAR GENETICS
TO NEUROPSYCHIATRIC DISORDERS

Gene Mapping

The first task in identifying a genetic disorder is
to demonstrate that a defect in a particular gene
or in the gene's expression plays a role in a
developmental or neuropsychiatric disorder. This
extension of basic neuroscience to the study of
behavior is called *behavioral genetics.* The study
of behavioral genetics requires background in
understanding gene expression and regulation.
The regulation of each gene and the role of its
product in regard to behavior must be considered.
The end point is a demonstration that particular
gene defects or their expression are specific to a
developmental or a neuropsychiatric disorder.

   After demonstrating that a defect is important in a disorder, the next approach is gene
mapping. Here, one employs variants or polymorphisms (polymorphism is the occurrence
together in a population of two or more alternative genotypes) of a particular gene in families
with the condition to determine whether or not
the variant or the polymorphism is linked to a
specific illness susceptibility gene. That is, that
the gene is cotransmitted, or transmitted along
with the specific disorder.

   Because a gene is inherited as part of a
chromosome region that is millions of base
pairs in length, an identified polymorphism
that is traced through a pedigree will be a
marker for an entire chromosomal region. This
would include the gene itself and adjacent regulatory sequences as shown in Figure 1–2.

When there is no linkage demonstrated, no abnormality is found in the structure of the genetically coded protein or any other aspect of the gene that can be linked to inheritance of a particular disorder.

These pedigree linkage studies include some genes that are at a distance from the marker, which are physiologically unrelated to it in that area of the chromosome. The entire human genome can be scanned with approximately 150 evenly spaced polymorphisms. A major limitation of these linkage methods is that although a linkage marker may be valid for clinical predictions and for mapping gene deficits, the mapping at best identifies a large area. Consequently, the demonstration of disease linkage does not specifically prove which gene is involved. Other methods are required to move along the chromosome and study the expression of a gene within the linked region. These linkage methods apply only to disorders in which a single locus plays an essential role in disease transmission. Although this should be established before doing linkage studies, in practice, this question may not be resolved without the linkage studies. The detection of the presence of a single locus that results in susceptibility to a disorder is clearly important and the linkage process is an important first step in looking for disorders where there may be a single gene locus.

The field of psychiatric genetics includes the sciences of psychiatry, molecular biology, and genetics. One approach to psychiatric genetics is to use modern molecular human genetic approaches to identify and clone genes for genetic disorders, such as Fragile X syndrome. This approach has been referred to as *reverse genetics* or *positional cloning*. There are two approaches to cloning a gene. The original biochemical approach begins with the known gene product, whereas the genetic approach starts with the known location in the genome. In the past, researchers would study the biochemistry of the disorder, find the missing gene or defective protein, and eventually identify the gene and clone it. This approach is inadequate for disorders of unknown etiology. For such conditions, the genetic approach uses the fact that a gene can be mapped. Once its position is known, then molecular biological techniques to clone the gene may be used to discover which protein it makes. This leads to an understanding of both normal function and the pathophysiology leading to the genetic abnormality. In complex human disorders, establishing knowledge of both normal function and pathophysiology is necessary before intervention to prevent the disorder is possible.

Linkage mapping is possible because of the organization of DNA into long strands within the chromosomes and the behavior of that DNA during meiosis. Meiosis is the genetically relevant part of gamete formation. During gamete formation, there are recombinational events when parts of a paternal chromatid actually interchange and connect with sections of the homologous maternal chromatid. As a result, a block of genes from the individual's mother and a block from the individual's father are produced. This is a precise process, so the recombined chromosome continues to have exactly one copy of all the genes. However, the ancestral origins of these specific genes are shuffled around.

If there is normal genetic variation in some part of the DNA, we are able to use that variation to follow transmission of a specific ancestral copy. Those positions, or loci that show such variation are referred to as *markers*. Currently, enough markers have been identified on most chromosomes to utilize them in arrays along a chromosome. If they are close enough together, a whole group of markers may be transmitted intact. On other occasions, we may find that there has been a crossover event in which the sperm cell from the father has genes in one region that come from his own father's chromosome and in the adjacent region from his mother's chromosome. Information of this kind demonstrates the precise order of genes and thus offers a means to measure the distances between them. Genes ordinarily are transferred in blocks, yet these recombination events lead to shuffling in a "probabilistic" way.

As a result, if a gene is located somewhere on the chromosome, its pattern of transmission can be traced through families if there are markers. The normal variation would flag nearby positions on the chromosome. If those markers are close enough to the disease gene, the pattern of transmission through families of the disease and the marker would be essentially identical.

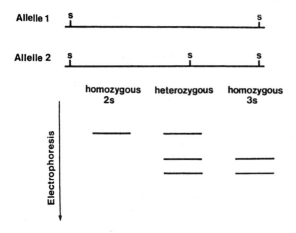

Allelle 1

Allelle 2

homozygous
2s

heterozygous

homozygous
3s

Electrophoresis

Figure 1–5. *Restriction fragment length polymorphisms.* Random alterations in the base sequence on this piece of DNA has resulted in the formation of two alleles: Allele 1 contains two recognition sites (S) for a particular restriction enzyme; allele 2 has an additional recognition site. The electrophoresis profile shows the pattern of fragments produced following digestion by restriction enzyme of DNA from individuals representing the three possible combinations of genotype. This fragment pattern can therefore be used to analyze the genotype of a particular individual at this specific locus (from Whatley, Owen, and Murray, 1989).

In 1978 the first DNA polymorphism (the simultaneous occurrence of many alleles) to be identified directly in the DNA molecules was discovered (Kan and Dozy, 1978). Although this was a restriction-fragment-length polymorphism (RFLP), there are now additional techniques to detect DNA polymorphisms (Botstein et al., 1980). As a result of the discovery of these polymorphisms, geneticists today can follow through families essentially any part of any chromosome to observe exactly what has been transmitted: for example, questions such as which grandchildren inherit which genes from which grandparent. These molecular biological techniques have been particularly useful in understanding genetic diseases (Kidd, 1991).

Disorders with Known Genetic Locus

In those instances of disease where a specific genetic locus has been identified, the characterization of the molecular abnormality is relatively simple. For example, a gross deletion may be identified by Southern blotting techniques from alterations in the size of a band, which are detected by a disease gene probe. In addition, point mutations may be detected through the use of DNA sequencing or the use of oligomer probes that are specific for that mutation. The Southern blotting techniques also may be used to detect carriers and for prenatal diagnoses without more detailed analysis of molecular pathology. This screening has been made possible through the discovery of restriction-fragment-length polymorphisms (RFLPs).

Restriction enzymes cleave DNA at specific base sequences. However, the locations of these restriction sites vary from one individual to another except in the case of identical twins. The variability in restriction sites is due almost completely to random base substitutions in DNA sequences. These substitutions have no phenotypic effect, but can result in the loss or gain of a recognition site for a particular enzyme. As a result, the fragments produced by digestion of one individual's DNA with a restriction enzyme will not be the same as those produced from another person's DNA. RFLPs, as shown in Figure 1–5, may be detected by Southern blotting as variations in size of specific restriction fragments, which are labeled with a specific probe.

In these cases, the polymorphic site may be within or, more commonly, close to the sequence that is recognized by the probe. Because they ordinarily are inherited in simple Mendelian fashion, the RFLPs can be used as genetic markers to distinguish between different alleles and subsequently to trace inheritance through families. Collecting DNA from large numbers of family members may make the identification of a disease allele in that family feasible. This procedure will result in determining whether the allele has been inherited by a particular individual in the family.

Disorders in Which the Genetic Locus Is Not Known

For many inherited diseases, including most psychiatric disorders, a specific biochemical abnormality which is responsible for symptoms is not known. Therefore, it cannot be used as a starting point to identify the molecular defect. In these instances, a different approach is necessary, beginning with the knowledge that a disease is genetic as well as information on its mode of transmission. With this information, it may be possible to locate a genetic abnormality. The procedure used is referred to as positional cloning. Here, the molecular cloning of a gene is carried out on the basis of the knowledge of its gene map position without prior knowledge of the gene product. Because this procedure is the reverse of the initial genetic approaches, it is sometimes referred to as *reverse genetics*. The key to this approach is in the use of RFLPs as genetic markers.

Basically, there are three approaches that may be employed to find linkage using RFLPs. The first is a *random search* strategy. Here, unknown pieces of DNA, which are selected at random, are used as probes to detect and follow polymorphisms in families in which multiple family members are affected. The identity and location in the genome of these anonymous markers is then determined only if linkage is established. This is the method that was used to localize the gene for Huntington's disease to chromosome 4. This approach has since become more systematic, so it is now possible to utilize systematically constructed linkage maps of the human genome in the search process. These linkage maps contain collections of primarily autonomous markers whose positions on a chromosome have been mapped. They are highly polymorphic and have been assembled so that they are approximately evenly spaced throughout the genome. Such probes are separated at distances that allow detection of linkage between them and any intervening marker. The availability of the maps provides an opportunity to systematically search for linkage.

A second approach involves the use of a *candidate gene,* which is suspected to be involved in the disorder and may be used as a probe. In psychiatric disorders, genes coding for particular enzymes involved in the biosynthesis and metabolism of monoamine neurotransmitters might be utilized as candidate genes. Although considerable guesswork is involved in this approach, the involvement of a particular neurotransmitter in the disorder can be assessed using this method. The assessment issue is whether a mutation of this particular neurotransmitter gene is responsible for the disease.

A third approach is focused on *probes that label a particular part of the genome,* such as a particular chromosomal region. For example, an association between Down syndrome and Alzheimer's disease resulted in a successful search for the linkage of familial Alzheimer's disease to chromosome 21.

COMPLEX INHERITANCE

The techniques of linkage analysis focus on diseases that show Mendelian transmission. Because the major psychiatric disorders may be more complicated and have multifactorial etiologies, the question has been raised about the validity of this approach for complex disorders that may be heterogeneous. However, in some instances of these conditions, such as schizophrenia or bipolar disorder, Mendelian transmission may be taking place. Just as there is a familial form of Alzheimer's disease, there are also pedigrees of individuals with major psychiatric disorders where multiple family members are affected. Populations where single genes have a major effect may be involved in some families, so linkage analysis may be useful. Still, the validity of this approach can only be established by unequivocal demonstration of linkage, because there are many possible explanations other than single gene defects for familial clustering of psychiatric disorders in selected families.

If linkage is established for a major psychiatric disorder, the next step is the definition of the molecular defect. When this has occurred, it may be possible to determine the biochemical consequences of the deficit. The next step is to follow the sequence of changes that result in the phenotype. Insights gained from the study of possible atypical cases with strong family loading may serve as a starting point to look at cases that may have more complex etiology.

MOVING FROM LINKAGE TO GENETIC DEFECT

The recognition of DNA polymorphisms that are tightly associated with a disease allows prenatal and presymptomatic diagnoses. Yet these benefits are not the major ones resulting from the discovery of linkage. The more important issue in demonstrating linkage is that it is the first step in identifying a defective gene itself.

From the linkage marker, there are a series

of steps essential to move to the gene. The next step is further genetic mapping, using linkage analysis of families with multiple members who are affected. The issue is to develop probes that recognize loci close to the disease gene. New markers may be generated from the chromosome being evaluated, using somatic cell hybrids (see the glossary at the end of this chapter), or specifically sorted chromosome libraries. Eventually, markers on either side of the gene locus are identified, and additional genetic mapping leads to reduction in the size of the region known to contain the disease locus. The procedure is complicated because RFLPs are not informative in every family, although the situation is improving as the number of markers increases. Moreover, human pedigrees also contain few meioses because breeding occurs slowly. In common genetic diseases, it is fortunate to identify a disease locus with a resolution of one centimeter. Initial approaches, using cloning sequencing and Southern blotting with agarose gel electrophoresis, analyze distances up to 100 kilobase pairs (kbp). In the human chromosome, 1,000 kbp, or one megabase pair (Mbp), occupy approximately one meter. Therefore, there is a substantial resolution gap that must be addressed. This gap is particularly complicated in psychiatric illness, where conditions are relatively rare, penetrance may be age-dependent, diagnostic uncertainty may be evident, and there may be variability in phenotypic expression. In addition, nonallelic heterogeneity may reduce the accuracy of the mapping procedure. Consequently, if linkage is established, it is possible to estimate the position to within only several million base pairs by these methods.

Recently, newer techniques have made the resolution gap easier to breach. Techniques of chromosome jumping, which allow distances up to one Mbp to be covered in a single step are now available, and new vectors, which clone fragments up to 500,00 kbp, have been developed. In addition, physical mapping is improving through the use of special techniques, such as pulsed field gel electrophoresis, which may be used to separate very large as well as very small DNA fragments. In this approach, DNA is subjected to two alternative pulsed fields at 90 degree angles. This approach allows the generation of very large fragments of DNA by using restriction enzymes that recognize rate sites in the human genome.

The development of these techniques and newer ones is enabling molecular analysis to cover the same order of genomic distance as classic genetic techniques (Whatley and Owen, 1989). New approaches allow increasingly refined analysis, and new strategies allow the detection of genes among the noncoding sequences, which make up most of the DNA.

Once linkage is established, the search for a disease gene within a linked region is more complex than the original search for linkage. Consequently, affected individuals who have more easily identifiable genetic lesions (such as deletions, duplications, or chromosomal translocations) are needed to further define the location of a disease gene. This approach has been successful in several disorders, such as Duchenne Muscular Dystrophy. With the establishment of the Human Genome Project, molecular techniques are increasingly advancing to allow rapid identification of genes within large regions of the genome.

In summary, the positional cloning, or reverse genetic, approach attempts to identify genetic defects without reference to prior knowledge of a disease process itself. These approaches should be combined with efforts to identify candidate genes, the more functional approach. Continued efforts to study the biological basis of neuropsychiatric disorders must continue in parallel with genetic studies so that information from both may be shared. In addition to the investigation of functional systems, such as neurotransmitter-related enzymes and receptors, molecular biology may enable us to identify new candidates through the analysis of the expression of a genome in disorders that are identified with genetic components.

INVESTIGATIONS OF GENE EXPRESSION

The study of gene expression through identification of endophenotypes also may shed light on pathological processes. Disorders with complex genetic components or disorders in which the gene environment interaction is suspected highlight the importance of characterizing endophenotypes. Knowledge of the endophenotype is essential in psychiatric disorders, where definition of exophenotypes may be difficult to establish. In disorders with genetic components, analysis of genes expressed in the condition may provide leads to endophenotypic characterization. Through gene expression, functional aspects of a genome are studied rather than the purely structural aspects described through the positional cloning approach.

The approach used to identify genes whose expression may be altered in the disease state is carried out through comparing their relative quantity in control subjects and affected individuals. Still, it may be found that a mutation causing a condition may completely block the readout of the affected gene. As a result, there is an absence of that particular mRNA in the cell. On the other hand, genes underexpressed or overexpressed in a diseased tissue may lead to genetic defects. It may not always be apparent how structural changes in DNA result in functional changes. Yet studies of gene expression may be valuable to complement purely genetic approaches, and ultimately may serve to identify the causal gene in a specific chromosome region.

Either a random search method or the expression of the candidate gene for the illness may be utilized. For example, study of the dopamine D_4 receptor in schizophrenia using the candidate gene approach is a consideration. mRNA exists in the cytoplasm of a cell as a mixture of many sequences, each of which may be translated into an individual protein and may be extracted from brain tissue postmortem or through surgical excision. Just as with DNA, the complex mRNA mixture may be purified using molecular cloning techniques. As a result, many mRNA species may be evaluated simultaneously, using these techniques. This allows the search for a gene's expression without prior assumption about what the gene is. Here, the gene expression, through the production of its mRNA, is being utilized in analyses.

The random search method is an analysis of the relative amounts of several mRNAs in the brain. Here, mRNAs are used as templates to produce cDNA libraries that are specific to different regions of the brain. This allows comparison to libraries from control subjects and affected individuals. If a clone is expressed at different levels or times during the illness, it may be used as a candidate gene probe in later DNA studies. mRNA mixtures also may be

analyzed by first utilizing them to direct protein synthesis. Such protein products may be analyzed themselves. With these strategies, it may be possible to characterize a protein involved in the pathogenesis of a disease.

Another approach is to use candidate genes. Here one relies on hybridization of a probe for that gene with the mRNA mixture to allow evaluation of the amount of its complementary mRNA. This approach may give a quick answer to whether the relative expression of a particular gene is altered. These quantitative hybridization experiments may be done in solution, or they may be carried out with the mRNA bound to a filter after size separation in the gel, using the northern blot procedure. Moreover, the technique of *in situ* hybridization allows the quantity of a particular mRNA to be evaluated in a fixed preparation such as a tissue slice. In this instance, hybridization of a gene probe occurs to mRNA molecules, which are immobilized in the preparation in a way similar to RNA fragments bound to a northern blot (see Appendix). In *in situ* hybridization, the gene probes may be radiolabeled to demonstrate fine resolution of the label following autoradiography. In these ways, gene probes can be used as cytochemical markers, i.e., markers within cells, in a way similar to the use of probes in immunohistochemistry. These approaches increase the amount and degree of information that can be established about gene expression, and offer the ability to find changes in gene expression in very small anatomical regions or in groups of cells. This approach has been used to study the expression of the gene for the brain amyloid precursor in several brain regions in Alzheimer's disease.

On the one hand, there are disadvantages to an approach that studies gene expression. The clearest disadvantage is that mRNA populations reflect or show the pattern of gene expression only at the specific time that the RNA was extracted. It is possible that some psychiatric disorders are the result of abnormalities of gene expression that occur only at certain stages in development. On the other hand, there are advantages because it is theoretically possible that a disease may have a complex genetic basis that might involve several regulator genes at different and separate loci, but the disorder may be expressed more simply. In addition, an evaluation of an endophenotype may allow the identification of state as well as trait markers and, in this way, afford insight into the biological basis of a condition that is relapsing or remitting. Using these approaches, it may be possible to identify groups of genes that are coordinately controlled or genes that have effects on specific cellular functions and nerves. In this way, it may be possible to link genes functionally from different chromosomal loci.

In summary, the techniques of molecular genetics are applicable and relevant to the study of developmental neuropsychiatric disorders. It is possible to analyze the structure of human genes directly to determine their underlying molecular pathology, especially for single-gene disorders. In addition, molecular genetic analysis provides us with a series of DNA markers that are scattered throughout the human genome. These markers can be used to link genes for disorders of unknown etiology. One of the advantages of the new techniques is that they allow the investigation of neuropsychiatric and neurological diseases at the level of the gene in the absence of prior knowledge about brain mechanisms, through the use of positional cloning techniques. These investigations may provide new starting points to study disturbed brain function. However, establishing a simple genetic component is only one aspect of etiology, and there may be multiple steps between the genetic change and the expression of the disease itself. Consequently, the evaluation of cellular endophenotypes that are associated with neuropsychiatric disorders and gene expression and function may be just as fruitful as genetic studies to understand these conditions and may help us to understand the more pure genetic data.

MOLECULAR ASSESSMENT OF LESCH-NYHAN DISEASE

The molecular techniques that are described in this chapter have been useful in facilitating our understanding of genetic diseases. Lesch-Nyhan disease results from a complete deficiency of the purine salvage enzyme, hypoxanthine-guanine phosphoribosyltransferase (HPRT), leading to hyperuricemia, neurological disorder, and a particular behavioral phenotype. Patients with partial enzyme deficiency of HPRT have hyperuricemia and gouty arthritis.

The degree of enzyme deficiency may be related to the occurrence of neurological, behavioral, and cognitive deficits.

The cDNA that encodes human HPRT has been isolated, and a full-length clone of this enzyme has been produced. The clone has been used to characterize the HPRT gene, HPRT-specific mRNA, and the steps involved in processing mRNA. The structural gene for HPRT covers 34 kb; however, the mature messenger mRNA is only 1.6 kb in length. The difference in size between the gene and messenger mRNA comes from the eight introns, which range in length from 0.1 to 10.8 kb.

Functional HPRT is a 217 amino acid protein and is encoded by a single gene on the X chromosome (Xq26–27). The gene is divided into nine exons, which are dispersed over the 44 kb of genomic DNA. The coding sequences range from 77 to 593 bp. Four autosomal pseudogenes are present within the human genome. One three-allele restriction fragment length polymorphism has been described for this X-linked gene. The genetic lesions that result in HPRT deficiency are heterogeneous and include point mutations, complete gene deletions, partial deletions, insertions, and endoduplication of exons. Subfragments of HPRT cDNA representing coding regions have been used to probe DNA restriction fragments. Davidson et al. (1991) have identified 17 independent mutations responsible for human hypoxanthine-guanine phosphoribosyltransferase (HPRT) deficiency. The majority of mutations (85%) do not represent major gene alterations and are probably the result of point mutations or single deletions. Affected hemizygous males inherit the mutant allele from asymptomatic carrier females or as the result of *de novo* germ line mutation. Carrier detection is possible through fibroblast, lymphoblast, or hair follicle tests. HPRT activity is normal in erythrocytes from carrier females. Prenatal diagnosis by enzyme assay or DNA samples is with amniocytes or chorionic villus samples. Similar approaches in analysis have been utilized in other metabolic disorders.

FUTURE DIRECTIONS

This new molecular basis for understanding gene function in relation to a disease may help to establish biological mechanisms in many neuropsychiatric disorders. Ultimately, these efforts are made so that in some specific syndromes the genetic abnormality can be potentially reversed. For example, gene therapy has been tried for an immune disorder, a lethal cholesterol defect, and several types of cancer. A viral vector has recently been developed to replace a missing gene in lung cells in cystic fibrosis. In the future, analogous approaches may become available for neuropsychiatric disorders.

APPENDIX

HUMAN GENOME PROJECT

The Human Genome Project is an international effort to compile a complete map of the entire human genetic code. The genome is defined as all the genetic information of a particular species, which creates the variety that we see among individuals. The purpose of the Genome Project is to identify and to locate all the genes and all the chromosomes in the human species. This will be done by creating maps of the genome of all the 100,000 genes. An initial step in developing a map is to look at distances between genes in the genome. Ordinarily, we consider the distances between two points as measured in increments such as miles or inches. The distances between genes are measured differently. One approach would be to count the base pairs between genes; however, this is not feasible because we know the existence and location of only 0.5% of the human genes. Another way to approach mapping is to use units of probability, which are called centiMorgans (cM), named after Thomas Hunt Morgan, a well-known geneticist. A centiMorgan represents a 1% chance that two genes will separate when chromosomes recombine during cell division, or meiosis. This measure is obtained from study of crossover frequency. For example, if a known genetic marker that has previously been identified is inherited along with the gene for a particular disease 96% of the time, then this marker and the gene become separated or crossover during cell division about 4% of the time. This means that a genetic signpost for that disease (e.g., Huntington's disease) is 4 cM from the gene. This mea-sure of probability can be translated into units of physical length to some extent. For example, the average chromosome has approximately 120 million base pairs. If genetic sites are separated by one cM and have a 1% chance of a break taking place between them, then a centiMorgan must be 1% of the 120 million base pairs, or approximately 1.2 million base pairs. Because the probability of a break does not always depend only on the distance between the genes, the correspondence between the number of base pairs and the measurement in centiMorgans will never be exact. Still, it is close enough. However, in a genome with 3 billion base pairs, a gene distance of a million base pairs is a long distance.

Genetic Maps

There are two types of genetic maps: genetic linkage maps and physical maps. The genetic linkage map shows the location of a gene or a group of genes relative to a second genetic locus based on how often they are inherited together. The genetic locus may be the gene itself or a piece of DNA with no known function whose inheritance pattern can be determined. The genetic linkage map uses the centiMorgan as its primary unit of measurement.

On the other hand, a physical map represents the physical location of identifiable landmarks on the DNA segment. Here, the major unit of measurement may be banding patterns on the chromosome or other aspects, such as actual base pair counts.

Within these two general types, there are specific kinds of maps. Among these are the cytogenetic map, the restriction map, the cosmid map, and the sequence map. The cytogenetic map shows physical locations of banding patterns created with specific chemical stains. The resolution of the cytogenetic map is coarse because chromosome staining produces about ten bands per chromosome. Since the average chromosome has 120 million base pairs, then a band includes about 10 to 12 million base pairs. Using a cytogenetic map, gross chromosomal abnormalities may be located to within 10 million base pairs.

The restriction map is a genetic linkage map that uses genetic markers called *restriction-fragment-length-polymorphisms (RFLPs)* to demonstrate the probability of genetic markers being close together. The RFLPs are fragments of DNA that are cut from the same place in the same chromosome but in different people. The cutting is done with a restriction enzyme and consequently is called a *restriction map*. Restriction maps that use RFLPs take information gathered from the genetic inheritance patterns from large multigenerational families. These maps have a resolution that is approximately ten times higher than a cytogenetic map. For example, one can identify a base pair location to within a million base pairs.

The cosmid map is a physical map that gives the distance between genes and base pairs proportional to a number of bases. The cosmid map uses overlapping segments of DNA about 40,000 base pairs long that are referred to as *cosmids*. The resolution of the cosmid map is substantially greater than that of a linkage map. It is ten to a hundred times greater than a linkage map and a thousand times greater than a cytogenetic map. These maps can pinpoint the location of genes to within 10,000 to 100,000 base pairs of one another.

Finally, sequence maps are the ultimate goal in mapping. In a sequence map, the actual physical sequence of the 3 billion base pairs of the human genome of all 46 chromosomes would be available. The sequence of the human genome has not been created, but sequences have been demonstrated in specific chromosomes.

The goals of the Human Genome Project are to create a genetic linkage map with 1-cm resolution. A physical map for each chromosome is to be developed along with a clone repositor and a reconstruction cook book, which will enable other researchers to duplicate the physical map. Another goal of the project is to improve the technology for sequencing segments of DNA and to obtain the actual sequences of large areas of the human genome. Finally, the project aims to develop new and more effective computer data bases.

In the Human Genome Project, it must be kept in mind that there is considerable variability among the genetic codes of individuals, as much as one base pair per thousand. Because the human genome contains up to 3 billion base pairs, genetic differences among individuals may vary by as much as 3 million base pairs of DNA. Consequently, actual genetic maps will not be of a particular person; rather, specific chromosomes or parts of chromosomes from many different individuals will be mapped, and the map will be a synthesis of many individuals.

In addition to the human genome, bacterial maps, yeast maps, and maps of mice chromosomes are also included in the Genome Project.

REFERENCES

Botstein, D., White, R.L., Skolnick, M., and Davis, R.W. (1980). Construction of a genetic linkage map in man using restriction fragment length polymorphisms. *American Journal of Human Genetics,* 32:314–331.

Ciaranello, R.D., Wong, D.L., and Rubenstein, J.L.R. (1990). Molecular neurobiology and disorders of brain development. In S.I. Deutsch, A. Weizman and R. Weizman (eds), *Application of basic neuroscience to child psychiatry.* Plenum Medical Book Company, New York.

Davidson, B.L., Tarle, S.A., Van Antwerp, M., Gibbs, D.A., Watts, R.W.E., Kelley, W.N., and Palella, T.D. (1991). Identification of 17 independent mutations responsible for human hypoxanthine-guanine phosphoribosyltransferase (HPRT) deficiency. *American Journal of Human Genetics,* 48:951–958.

Kan, Y.W. and Dozy, A.M. (1978). Polymorphism of DNA sequence adjacent to the human β-globulin structural gene: Relationship to sickle mutation. *Proceedings of the National Academy of Sciences,* 75:5631–5635.

Kidd, K.K. (1991). Progress toward completing the human linkage map. *Current Opinion in Genetic Development,* 1:99–105.

Lewin, B. (1990). *Genes IV.* Oxford University Press, New York.

Mendel, G. 1865 (published in 1866). Versuche über Pflanzen-hybriden. *Verh. Naturf. Verein Brünn,* 4:3–47. Royal Horticultural Society (1901) translation reprinted by Harvard University Press (1948). Translation appears in Stern, C. and Sherwood, E.R. (1966). *The origin of genetics: A Mendel source book.* W.H. Freeman, New York and London.

Ptashne, M. (1988). How eukaryotic transcriptional activators work. *Nature (London),* 335:683–689.

Southern, E.M. (1975). Detection of specific sequences among DNA fragments separated by gel electrophoresis. *Journal of Molecular Biology,* 98:503–517.

Steel, C.M. (1984a). DNA in medicine, the tools, Part I. *Lancet, ii,* pp. 908–911.

_____. (1984b). DNA in medicine, the tools, Part II. *Lancet, ii,* pp. 966–968.

Thompson, M.W., McInnes, R.R., and Willard, H.F. (1991). *Genetics in medicine,* 5th ed., pp. 53–95. W.B. Saunders Co., Philadelphia.

U.S. Congress, Office of Technology Assessment, "Technologies for detecting heritable mutations in human beings" OTA-H-298 (U.S. Government Printing Office, Washington, DC, September 1986).

_____. "Mapping our genes—The Genome Project: How big, how fast?" OTA-BA-373 (U.S. Government Printing Office, Washington, DC, April 1988).

Watson, J.D., Hopkins, N.H., Roberts, J.W., Steitz, J.A., and Weiner, A.M. (1987). *Molecular biology of the gene,* 4th ed. Benjamin-Cummings, Menlo Park, CA.

Whatley, S.A. and Owen, M.J. (1989). Molecular genetics and its application to the study of psychiatric disorders. *International Review of Psychiatry,* 1:219–230.

_____, _____, and Murray, R.M. (1989). The new genetics and neuropsychiatric disorders. In E.H. Reynolds and M.R. Trimble (eds), *The bridge between neurology and psychiatry,* pp. 353–379. Churchill Livingstone, Edinburgh, Scotland.

GLOSSARY

(Modified from Thompson, M.W., McInnes, R.R., and Willard, H.F., 1991 *Genetics in Medicine.* W.B. Saunders Co., Philadelphia.)

Allele One of the alternative versions of a gene that may occupy a given locus.

Allelic heterogeneity The presence of different mutant alleles at the same locus, each of which may produce an abnormal phenotype.

Amplification The production of multiple copies of a DNA sequence.

Anticipation The progressively earlier appearance of and increased severity of a disease in successive generations.

Autosome Any nuclear chromosome other than the sex chromosome. There are 22 pairs in the human karyotype.

Bacteriophage A virus that infects bacteria, used in molecular biology as a vector for cloning.

Base pair (bp) A pair of complementary nucleotide bases, e.g., in double-stranded DNA; a unit used in the measurement of the length of a DNA sequence.

Candidate gene In the search for a disease gene, a candidate gene is one that is known to be located in the region of interest. Its gene product has properties that suggest it may be the gene being sought.

Carrier An individual who is heterozygous for a specific, frequently mutant, allele; used for heterozygotes for autosomal recessive alleles, for females heterozygous for X-linked alleles. The term may be used for an individual who is heterozygous for an autosomal dominant allele but is not expressing it (e.g., a heterozygote for the ALD disease allele who is presymptomatic).

cDNA Complementary or copy DNA, a synthetic DNA transcribed from a specific RNA through the action of the enzyme reverse transcriptase. It is distinguished from genomic DNA.

CentiMorgan (cM) The unit of linkage, named for Thomas Hunt Morgan. Two loci are said to be 1cM apart if recombination is detected between them in 1% of meioses.

Chain termination mutation A mutation that generates a stop codon, thus preventing further synthesis of the polypeptide chain.

Chromatid After DNA synthesis in a dividing cell, a chromosome is composed of two identical parallel strands, the sister chromatids, connected at the centromere. The chromatids separate at anaphase, when each becomes a chromosome of a daughter cell.

Chromosomal disorder A clinical condition caused by an abnormal chromosome constitution where there is extra or missing chromosome material.

Chromosome walking The standard method of trying to locate a specific gene within a defined region.

Clinical heterogeneity The production of clinically different phenotypes from mutations in the same gene.

Clone In molecular biology, a copy of DNA sequences created by recombinant DNA techniques.

Coding strand In double-stranded DNA, the strand has the same 5′-to-3′ sense (and the same sequence, except that T substitutes for U in mRNA) as does mRNA. The coding strand, or sense strand, is not transcribed by RNA polymerase.

Codominant If both alleles of a pair are expressed in the heterozygous state, then the alleles (the traits determined by them, or both) are codominant.

Codon A triplet of three bases in a DNA or RNA molecule that specifies a single amino acid.

Complementarity The complementary nature of base pairing in DNA.

Complementary DNA DNA synthesized from a

messenger RNA template, through the enzyme reverse transcriptase. See also *genomic DNA*.

Crossover or **crossing over** The reciprocal exchange of segments between chromatids of homologous chromosomes, a characteristic of the prophase of the first meiotic division.

Cytogenetics The study of the microscopic appearance of chromosomes and their behavior during cell division to the genotype and phenotype of the individual. It also refers to the study of human chromosomes and their abnormalities.

Concordant In human genetics, a twin pair in which both members exhibit a certain trait.

Deletion The loss of a sequence of DNA from a chromosome. The deleted DNA may be of any length from a single base pair to a large part of a chromosome.

Discordant In human genetics, a twin pair of which one member shows a certain trait and the other does not. See *concordant*.

DNA (deoxyribonucleic acid) The molecule that encodes the genes responsible for the structure and function of living organisms and allows the transmission of genetic information from generation to generation.

DNA polymerase An enzyme that can synthesize a new DNA strand, using a previously synthesized DNA strand as a template.

Dominant A trait is dominant if it is phenotypically expressed in heterozygotes.

Ecogenetic disorder A disorder resulting from the interaction of a genetic predisposition to a specific disease with an environmental factor.

Empiric risk The probability that a trait will occur or recur in a family, based on past experience rather than on knowledge of the causative mechanism.

Enhancer A DNA sequence that acts on the same chromosome to increase transcription of a nearby gene. The enhancer may be upstream or downstream to the gene and may be in the same or the reverse orientation.

Epigenetic The term that refers to any factor that can affect the phenotype without change in the genotype.

Eukaryote A unicellular or multicellular organism in which the cells have a nucleus with a nuclear membrane and other specialized characteristics. See also *prokaryote*.

Exon A transcribed region of a gene that is present in mature messenger RNA.

Expressivity The extent to which a genetic defect is expressed. If there is variable expressivity, the trait may vary in expression from mild to severe but is never completely unexpressed in individuals who have the corresponding genotype.

Frameshift mutation A mutation involving a deletion or insertion that is not an exact multiple of 3 base pairs and thus changes the reading frame of the gene. The stop codon thus formed will not be the normal one, and in almost all cases a truncated or elongated protein will be made.

G bands The dark and light cross-bands seen in chromosomes after treatment with trypsin and Glemsa stain.

Gamete A reproductive cell (ovum or sperm) with the haploid chromosome number.

Gene A hereditary unit; in molecular terms, a sequence of chromosomal DNA that is required for production of a functional product.

Gene map A representation of chromosomal locations of mapped genes.

Genetic code The base triplets that specify the 20 amino acids found in proteins.

Genetic marker A locus that has readily classifiable alleles and can be used in genetic studies. It may be a gene, a restriction enzyme site, or any characteristic of DNA that allows different versions of a locus (or its product) to be distinguished from each other and followed through families. See *polymorphism*.

Genome The complete DNA sequence, containing the entire genetic information of a gamete, an individual, a population, or a species.

Genotype (1) The genetic constitution (genome); (2) more specifically, the alleles present at one locus.

Heterozygote (heterozygous) An individual or genotype with two different alleles at a given locus on a pair of homologous chromosomes. Typically, one allele is the normal form and the other is mutant, but the term is also used to refer to heterozygosity for different normal alleles.

Homologous chromosomes (homologs) A pair of chromosomes of one type, one inherited from each parent, having the same gene loci in the same order. (Exception: see *uniparental disomy*.)

Human Genome Project A major current research project, international in scope, that aims to map and sequence the entire human genome.

Hybridization The pairing of complementary RNA and DNA strands to produce an RNA/DNA hybrid or of two different DNA strands (reannealing). Hybridization may be performed *in situ,* i.e., on a tissue, such that denatured DNA of cells react with RNA or DNA in single strands. The added preparation is radioactively labeled, once hybridized, and followed by autoradiography.

The radioactive probe represents a gene (nucleic acid), most often a labeled cDNA clone derived from the mRNA. It is hybridized with denatured DNA *in situ* (in the cell itself). The position of the gene is then determined. See *in situ hybridization.*

Imprinting The differential expression of genetic material, at either a chromosomal or an allelic level, depending on whether the genetic material has been inherited from the male or female parent.

Insertion A chromosomal abnormality in which a DNA segment from one chromosome is inserted into a nonhomologous chromosome.

In situ **hybridization** Mapping a gene by molecular hybridization of a cloned DNA sequence, labeled by radioactivity or fluorescence, to a chromosome spread on a slide.

Intron A segment of a gene that is initially transcribed but is then removed from within the primary RNA transcript by splicing together the sequences (exons) on either side of it.

Karyotype The chromosome constitution of an individual. The term is also used for a photomicrograph of the chromosomes of an individual arranged in the standard classification and for the process of preparing such a photomicrograph.

Karyotyping Chromosomes in a cell arranged and analyzed according to size and banding patterns.

Linkage Genes on the same chromosome show linkage if they have a tendency to be transmitted together through meiosis. Contrast with *synteny.*

Linkage disequilibrium The tendency of specific combinations of alleles at two or more linked loci to occur together on the same chromosome more frequently than would be expected by chance.

Linkage map A chromosome map showing the relative positions of genes and other DNA markers on the chromosomes, as determined by linkage studies.

Locus The position of a gene on a chromosome. Different forms of the gene (alleles) may occupy the locus.

Lod score A statistical method that tests genetic marker data in families to determine whether two loci are linked. The lod score is the logarithm to base 10 of the odds in favor of linkage. By convention, a lod score of 3 (odds of 1000:1 in favor) is taken as proof of linkage, and a lod score of -1 (100:1 against) as proof that the loci are unlinked.

Meiosis The special type of cell division occurring in the germ cells by which gametes containing the haploid chromosome number are produced from diploid cells. Two meiotic divisions occur: meiosis I and meiosis II. Reduction in number takes place during meiosis I.

Messenger RNA (mRNA) An RNA, transcribed from the DNA of a gene, that directs the sequence of amino acids of the encoded polypeptide.

Microdeletion A chromosomal deletion too small to be seen under the microscope.

Missense mutation Mutation that changes a codon specific for one amino acid to specify another amino acid.

Mitochondrial DNA (mtDNA) The DNA in the circular chromosome of the mitochondria. Mitochondria are cytoplasmic organelles that possess their own unique DNA. Mitochondrial DNA is present in many copies/cell. It is maternally inherited and evolves 5 to 10 times as rapidly as genomic DNA. This is in contrast with the behavior of Mendelian genetics, in which reciprocal crosses show the contributions of both parents to be equally inherited.

Mitochondrial DNA has been completely sequenced. It is known to code for two types of ribosomal RNA, for 22 transfer RNAs, and for 13 polypeptides. The mtDNA replicates within the mitochondria which divide by simple fission. Human evolution has been traced from mitochondrial DNA sequences.

Mitochondrial inheritance The inheritance of a disorder encoded in the mitochondrial genome.

Nondisjunction The failure of two members of a chromosome pair to disjoin during meiosis I, or two chromatids of a chromosome to disjoin during meiosis II, so that both pass to one daughter cell and the other daughter cell receives neither.

Nonsense mutation A single-base substitution in DNA resulting in a chain-termination codon.

Northern blot A blotting technique, named for its analogy to Southern blotting, for detection of RNA molecules by hybridization to a complementary DNA probe.

Nucleotide A molecule composed of a nitrogenous base, a 5-carbon sugar, and a phosphate group. A nucleic acid is a polymer of many nucleotides.

Pedigree In medical genetics, a diagram of a family history indicating the family members, their relationship to the proband, and their status with respect to a particular hereditary condition.

Penetrance Concept referring to the all-or-none expression of a mutant genotype. Usually refers to dominant traits in heterozygotes. If a condition is expressed in less than 100% of persons who carry the responsible allele, it is said to have *reduced penetrance;* if, for example, only 70% of persons with the allele express the trait, it is 70% penetrant. Contrast with *expressivity.*

Plasmid Independently replicating, extrachromosomal circular DNA molecules in bacteria, used in molecular biology as vectors for cloned segments of DNA.

Point mutation A single nucleotide base pair change in DNA.

Polygenic Inheritance determined by many genes at different loci, with small additive effects. Also termed *quantitative.* Not to be confused with *multifactorial,* in which environmental as well as genetic factors may be involved.

Polymerase chain reaction (PCR) A technique in which a short DNA or RNA sequence can be amplified $>10^6$ times by means of two flanking oligonucleotide primers and repeated cycles of amplification with DNA polymerase. Permits analysis of a short sequence from very small quantities of DNA or RNA without the necessity of cloning it first.

Polymorphism The occurrence together in a population of two or more alternative genotypes, each at a frequency greater than that which could be maintained by recurrent mutation alone. A locus is arbitrarily considered to be polymorphic if the rarer allele has a frequency of .01, so that the heterozygote frequency is at least .02.

Positional cloning The molecular cloning of a gene on the basis of knowledge of its map position, without prior knowledge of the gene product. Sometimes called *reverse genetics.*

Prokaryote A simple unicellular organism, such as a bacterium, lacking a separate nucleus and simpler than eukaryotic cells in other ways. See *eukaryote.*

Promoter DNA sequences located in the 5' end of a gene that determine the site of initiation of transcription and the quantity and sometimes the tissue distribution of mRNA.

Recessive A trait or gene that is expressed only in homozygotes or hemizygotes.

Reciprocal translocation Chromosomal rearrangement involving exchange of segments between nonhomologous chromosomes.

Recombinant An individual who has a new combination of genes not found together in either parent. Usually applied to linkage analysis.

Recombinant DNA A DNA molecule constructed from segments from more than one parental DNA molecule.

Recombination The formation of new combinations of linked genes by crossing over between their loci.

Regulatory gene A gene that codes for an RNA or protein molecule that regulates the expression of other genes.

Restriction endonuclease An enzyme, derived from bacteria, that can recognize a specific sequence of DNA and cut the (usually double-stranded) DNA molecule within the recognition site or at some nearby site.

Restriction-fragment-length polymorphism (RFLP) A polymorphic difference in DNA sequence between individuals that can be recognized by restriction endonucleases. See *polymorphism.*

Retrovirus A virus, with an RNA genome, that propagates by conversion of the RNA into DNA by the enzyme reverse transcriptase.

Reverse genetics The molecular approach to identifying genes on the basis of their location in the genome, without knowledge of the gene product. See *positional cloning.*

Reverse transcriptase An enzyme that catalyzes the synthesis of DNA on an RNA template.

RNA (ribonucleic acid) A nucleic acid formed upon a DNA template, containing ribose instead of deoxyribose. Messenger RNA (mRNA) is the template on which polypeptides are synthesized. Transfer RNA (tRNA), in cooperation with the ribosomes, brings activated amino acids into position along the mRNA template. Ribosomal RNA (rRNA), a component of the ribosomes, functions as a nonspecific site of polypeptide synthesis.

Southern blot A technique, devised by E.M. Southern, for transferring DNA fragments that have been separated by agarose gel electrophoresis to a nitrocellulose filter, on which specific DNA fragments can then be detected by their hybridization to radioactive probes.

Splicing The splicing out of introns and splicing together of exons in the generation of mature mRNA from the primary transcript.

Structural gene A gene coding for any RNA or protein product.

Synteny The physical presence together on the same chromosome of two or more gene loci, whether or not they are close enough together for linkage to be demonstrated.

Tandem repeats Two or more copies of the same

(or very similar) DNA sequence arranged in a direct head-to-tail succession along a chromosome.

Telomere The end of each chromosome arm. Human telomeres end with tandem copies of the sequence $(TTAGGG)_n$, which is required for the proper replication of chromosome ends.

Transcription The synthesis of a single-stranded RNA molecule from a DNA template in the cell nucleus, catalyzed by RNA polymerase.

Transfection Transfer of a gene, or cDNA (next to a promoter), into a cell, enabling the transfected cell to form a new gene product.

Transgenes Foreign genes introduced directly into the nucleus of a fertilized egg, integrated into nuclear DNA, and expressed in the phenotype. These are genetic chimera.

Transgenic mice Mice that carry a foreign gene (transgene) in their genome, produced by injection of oocytes with the foreign DNA. DNA that is integrated into the mouse genome may be expressed. If the transgene has been incorporated into the germline, it may also be transmitted to the progeny.

Translocation The transfer of a segment of one chromosome to another chromosome. If two nonhomologous chromosomes exchange pieces, the translocation is reciprocal.

Uniparental disomy The presence in a karyotype of two chromosomes of a pair both inherited from one parent, with no representative of that chromosome from the other parent.

Western blot Technique analogous to Southern blotting, used for detection of proteins, usually by immunological methods.

Zygosity Twins may be either monozygotic (MZ) or dizygotic (DZ). To determine whether a certain twin pair is MZ or DZ is to determine their zygosity.

CHAPTER 2

DEVELOPMENTAL NEUROANATOMY

The human brain contains 10^{11} nerve cells with at least a thousand times that number of interconnections. It is several magnitudes more complex than the most powerful computer now available. We are only beginning to understand its functions. We do not yet know how many categories of cells there are in the brain, yet the features of individual cells are better known than most other cell types. Knowledge of the molecular function of neurons provides the key to the biochemistry of brain functions and a beginning to better treatment of mental illnesses. As a communication system, the brain governs responses to stimuli, processes information, and generates the control of complex behavior. These brain functions may occur without conscious intentionality. Identity theory suggests that mind functions may accompany the activation of these complex interconnections as a "change in quality" producing a qualitatively different system. In this view, self-perspective becomes self-referential and self-observing; the whole establishes awareness in reference to its parts.

The total genetic information available (10^5 genes in mammals) is not adequate to specify the estimated 10^{15} neuronal interconnections. Consequently, development relies on epigenetic processes, which may activate subsets of genes, in combination, periodically during development. Epigenesis refers to changes that influence the phenotype without altering the genotype. These influences originate within the developing embryo and from the external envi-

ronment. The internal factors include intercellular signals, such as nerve growth factor, and cell surface molecules. The external factors are nutritive factors, sensory experience, social interactions, and learning. All of these express their effects via changes in neuronal activity. These internal regulative processes are essential to construct the immature brain; however, the environmental influences lead to the more specific anatomical changes, which are involved in the distribution and in the function of synapses and essentially shape the brain.

Because of the multiplicity of these influences, there is considerable vulnerability as changes in form and in function take place during development; for example, the biochemical and biophysical processes that are under genetic regulation may be affected by toxins and infection.

This chapter reviews the phases of neuronal development, development of regional brain anatomy, development of the cerebral cortex, functional anatomy of the cerebral cortex, and development of other brain regions (e.g., basal ganglia, cerebellum), and concludes with a review of the metabolic maturation of the brain, using positron emission tomography (PET) scanning procedures.

OVERVIEW

An understanding of the emergence of behavior begins with the development of the brain. Particularly important is an appreciation of the roles of individual classes of specialized nerve cells and the formation of specific connections between them. A representative neuron is depicted in Figure 2–1, which shows dendrites, cell bodies, axons, and axon terminals. The specialized cells found in various brain regions are shown on the right.

The basic question is; How do neural cells establish specific identities, and how are patterns of neuronal connections established and then maintained? Development follows in a series of orderly steps, with precise timing for each neural structure.

As the brain develops, an overall pattern emerges that is periodically punctuated by brief neuronal events that establish the final organization. Prenatal brain development may be divided into two major phases (Lyon and Gadisseux, 1991). The first phase occurs in the first 20 weeks of fetal life, the period of organogenesis, neuronogenesis, and neuronal migration. In this first phase, the neural tube closes and the basic morphology of the brain is

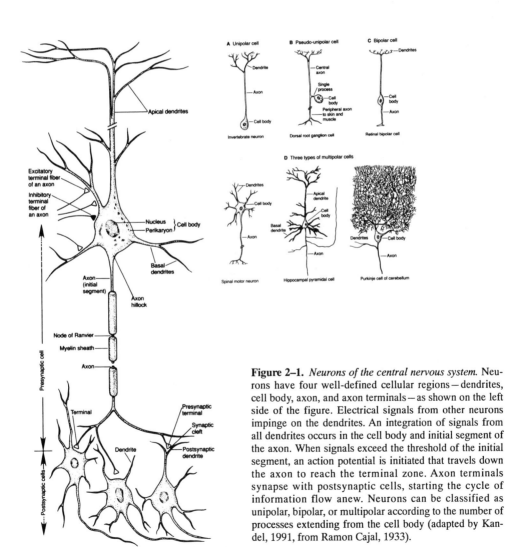

Figure 2–1. *Neurons of the central nervous system.* Neurons have four well-defined cellular regions—dendrites, cell body, axon, and axon terminals—as shown on the left side of the figure. Electrical signals from other neurons impinge on the dendrites. An integration of signals from all dendrites occurs in the cell body and initial segment of the axon. When signals exceed the threshold of the initial segment, an action potential is initiated that travels down the axon to reach the terminal zone. Axon terminals synapse with postsynaptic cells, starting the cycle of information flow anew. Neurons can be classified as unipolar, bipolar, or multipolar according to the number of processes extending from the cell body (adapted by Kandel, 1991, from Ramon Cajal, 1933).

established. During this first phase, neuroblasts are formed (neuronogenesis) in proliferative zones and migrate to definitive sites along radial glial fibers. The dividing neuroblasts produce the immature postmitotic neurons that make up the nervous system during this initial phase of histogenesis. These originate as nests of epidermal germinal cells that lie within the center of the primordial brain, which provide the source for the immature postmitotic neurons that finally generate component regions of the brain. However, neuroblast cell division is not continuous, but entails locally discrete and synchronized phases of cell multiplication. The formation of brain regions is precisely timed with the most primitive and caudal part of the brain, the brainstem, which is formed before the more complex and evolved structures such as the cerebral cortex.

The second phase of development takes place from 20 to 40 weeks, with neuronal growth and maturation. A remarkable cellular precision in the formation of axonal contacts has been demonstrated. Factors that control the arborization of the axonal processes are the subject of investigation. For example, in the frog following the transsection of the optic nerve, rotation of the eye following a critical period of development results in a regrowth of axons to the original and appropriate neurons in the geniculate nuclei (Jacobson, 1991). Studies in the rodent indicate that disruption of the normal laminar distribution of cortical neurons does not prevent the final development of appropriate synaptic connections between the thalamus and the relocated cortical pyramidal cells (Caviness and Rakic, 1978).

The next process of brain development requires the elaboration of the receptive portion of neurons, the dendrite, and the communicating portion of the neurons, the axon, which ultimately meet to form the synaptic contacts. Gliogenesis, myelination, and cerebral angiogenesis occur during this phase. Concurrently, there is a natural loss of synaptic connections and cell death, as neuronal circuitry is modified and as trophic factors and neurotransmitters are elaborated.

These developments occur primarily during the early stages of brain development, (i.e., before 2 years of age in humans). The elaboration and modification of axonal-dendritic synaptic contacts continues, but to a much more limited extent, throughout maturation. A critical characteristic of old age may be the loss of the ability to develop new synaptic contacts. The length of axonal projections varies from a few millimeters or less, as in local circuit GABAergic neurons in the cerebral cortex, to up to a meter in the noradrenergic and serotonergic pathways innervating the spinal cord.

THE PHASES OF NEURONAL DEVELOPMENT

The complex functions of the nervous system (i.e., perception, motor coordination, motivation and memory) involve specific interconnections among neural cells. The process of maturation of the brain follows a gradual sequence of anatomic and physiologic events, as outlined earlier, which may be listed in seven steps: neurogenesis with production of neuroblasts (immature neurons and glial cells), neuronal migration, cell differentiation and axonal and dendritic growth, synaptogenesis, synthesis of neurotransmitters, myelination of axons, and final modulation of neuronal circuitry. Axons establish contact by forming synaptic contact with selected target cells. Initial synaptic contacts are modified to produce the final mature pattern of neuronal connections. These phases of development ordinarily overlap in time, but may occur simultaneously. For example, synaptogenesis may occur immediately before the biosynthesis of neurotransmitters. Further neuronal migration may occur before or after synaptogenesis. In a specific brain region, all of these events are timed and follow the same sequence from one person to the next. These developmental processes result in an immature brain, which assimilates environmental input and responds. Sensory systems begin to operate *in utero,* so environmental processes may affect the brain prior to birth. Extrinsic input affects anatomic changes related to the distribution and function of synapses. These processes are described in more detail in the following sections.

NEUROGENESIS AND MIGRATION OF NEURONS

The primary events that establish brain morphology occur in the first 20 weeks of intrauterine life. During that time, neurons (stem cells for both neurons and glia) migrate to and proliferate in germinal zones, which surround the cerebral cavities, and subsequently migrate to final sites (Jacobson, 1991). There is a remarkable conservation in evolutionary neurobiology. For example, a gene coding sequence involved in developmental regulation, the homeobox domain, is expressed in an invertebrate, *Drosophila*. This homeobox domain is a 60 amino acid sequence contained in *Drosophila* regulatory proteins that bind to DNA and activate the transcription of downstream genes, some of which act as transcriptional regulatory factors. In vertebrates, there are similar homeobox domain sequences in a transcription factor that function on prolactin and growth hormone genes in mammalian pituitary. Moreover, some of these genes, like those in *Drosophila,* function developmentally as regulators of other gene expression. They also regulate some cell surface features that affect neuronal cell migration and are encoded and expressed sequentially.

Future neurons aggregate together in the brainstem regions to form functional nuclei. These include the locus coeruleus, the serotonergic raphe nucleus, and the dopaminergic substantia nigra. At the telencephalic level of brain, the migration occurs along radial glial fibers to the cortex, as previously noted. Neurons that appear earlier in development occupy deeper layers than those that are generated later, so a laminar order is established in regard to the time of neuronal production (Jacobson, 1991).

HISTOGENESIS

Histogenesis, or cytogenesis, refers to the production of different types of neurons and nerve cells. Most of the neurons of the cerebral cortex are produced by 20 weeks of gestation. DNA measurement of DNA concentrations in brain tissue has been used as a marker of cell number (Dobbing and Sands, 1973; Smart, 1991). Postmortem studies of brain tissue demonstrate that the primary acceleration in the increase of the number of cell bodies in the central nervous system takes place between 25 and 40 weeks of gestational age and subsequently in the first months of life after birth. Most of the neurons of the cerebral cortex, however, are generated by 20 weeks of gestation. The increase in DNA

between 20 and 40 weeks, the second phase of development, is largely the result of glial cell proliferation. During this time frame, there are regional differences in human brain growth. By 40 weeks of gestational age, the growth of the spinal column, the brainstem, and much of the forebrain is complete. Other brain regions, such as the neocerebellum, which initiates its primary growth at the time of birth and during the first year, are not complete. Brain growth varies in different regions of the brain, and when those regions are most rapidly growing, they are most vulnerable. The major developmental insults that occur in the developmental period result in cerebral palsy and mental retardation. Cerebral palsy is expected from antenatal injury in the mid-phases of gestation or the early trimesters (Lyon and Gadisseux, 1991). On the other hand, later injuries around the perinatal or birth period may lead to disorders in coordination of temporal and spatial sequencing movements, for example, neocerebellar functions, such as fine movements of fingers or in speech.

CELL MIGRATION

The glial cells and neurons of the cerebrum are produced in a small region near the inner side of the neural tube or, later, near the lateral ventricular system. During early phases of development, the rapid and almost synchronous migration of neurons that are formed together results in a radial alignment of cells expanding through the full thickness of the cortical plate (Jacobson, 1991). In later phases of histogenesis of the cortex, a very fine network of radially organized glial cells guides the migrating neurons. These glial cells are connected to the inner side of the germinal zone and the outer side of the cortical zone. These newly formed neurons glide along glial fibers from the germinal layer out to the cortex (Rakic, 1972).

Consequently, the formation of the cortical layers is the result of an inward–outward migration. The first of these migrations forms layer 1 and the deepest cortical layer, layer 7. Subsequent populations of neurons move through the deepest cortical layer to form a second zone, and a third group moves through the two previous zones and continues until eventually six cortical layers are formed. The last cells to migrate form layer 2. (The development of the cortex is described in greater detail later in this chapter.) In the cerebellum, on the other hand, migration results from two germinal zones. One of these is close to the fourth ventricle; the other appears later in development and is located externally under the pia mater. Consequently, cells in the cerebellum move both outward and inward to their final destinations.

During development neurons are in close contact with one another, and in their migration surface molecules interact and form a base for later synaptic connections and cytoarchitectural organization. A series of molecules regulate neurite extension and adhesion (Dodd and Jessel, 1988; Smith, 1988). These include the neural cell adhesion molecule (N-CAM), laminin, and glycoprotein, and integrin, which acts as a surface receptor.

Cell migration is vulnerable to genetic disturbances (Lyon and Gadisseux, 1991). Yet acquired disorders of migration might also occur. For example, viral infections and disruptions of vascular circulation of the brain during a specific period in development may interfere with migration or destroy a zone which has already migrated.

CELL DIFFERENTIATION

Once neurons reach their destination, they begin to grow and differentiate. The differentiation is expressed as dendritic arborization, with various cells developing particular kinds of arborized, treelike structures. In the cerebellum, the Purkinje cell (see Fig. 2–1) is the basic cytoarchitectural unit for complex neuronal circuits that allow the cerebellum to compare specific input with nonspecific input. These comparisons lead to programs for initiating well-coordinated motor behavior in time and space.

The exact timetable for differentiation of various cell groups is still not available. However, in the cerebral cortex, and particularly in the primary visual cortex, specific Golgi staining techniques demonstrate some changes that occur between the 25th and 32nd week of gestation. In the cerebellum, on the other hand, differentiation of the Purkinje cells and other local cerebellar units does not come until much later and lasts until the end of the second year of life. With arborization of cells, the surface area is enlarged

to allow multiple synaptic contacts to occur at specific sites and in a particular sequence.

In development, the synaptic density is initially quite high. Redundancy in synaptic connections during this early phase of brain development produces a large number of complex short- and long-distance connections. When the final connections are made, redundant synaptic connections will disappear.

CELL DEATH

Not only do redundant synaptic connections disappear, but large numbers of cells that provide their synaptic connections also are eliminated during development. There may be a 10% to 50% reduction, for example, in neurons of the lateral motor column in the lumbar spinal system. Similar phenomena have been seen in visual pathways. This cell death is programmed and genetically determined, although it may be influenced by environmental input, such as motor activity or inactivity. One of the factors involved is the retrograde axonal transport of nerve growth factor (NGF) from a target cell back to a cell body. NGF may then play a role in the survival or death of cells that may or may not have been successful in reaching their targets. The model of cell death has been applied in the study of a number of disorders in childhood, where it has been considered that there is a genetically determined imbalance between those programs sustaining cells and those causing cell death. These processes of synaptogenesis and cell death allow considerable plasticity and adaptation in the developing brain.

Programmed cell death, or apoptosis, is a critical aspect of development and is essential because many more neurons are produced by the nervous system than are required. Their death is necessary for the sculpting of the brain. Some neurons die that are no longer needed after serving a transient function; others die that have migrated to the wrong place. The majority of death seems related to "size matching." In many parts of the nervous system, over 50% of the neurons die before embryonic development is complete. Genes do not establish how many cells of a specific type will be produced.

In the sympathetic nervous system, developing neurons seem to compete for nerve growth factor (NGF) produced by target tissues.

Recently emphasis has shifted from competition for growth factors to the study of genes whose expression may produce neuronal death. Although such genes have not been identified for higher organisms, there has been progress with simple organisms. Key findings have been reported in the round worm *(Caenonhabditis elegans)* whose 1090 embryonic cells have been identified. Of these, 131 undergo programmed cell death as the organism matures. Two genes (ced-3 and ced-4) produce protein products that trigger programmed cell death. Another gene, ced-9, may do the opposite and save those cells that express it from programmed extinction. This genetic approach has been extended from the round worm to vertebrate neurons through work on one gene, the oncogene bcl-2, which has been found to prevent lymphocytes from undergoing programmed cell death. The bcl-2 oncogene, which shares 23% of its DNA sequences with ced-9, is effective in keeping *C. elegans* cells from dying in the absence of NGF in cultured neurons. This sequence, then, seems common in multiple cell types. The fact that it is found in both simple organisms and more complex ones, suggests that programmed cell death may be as fundamental a process as cell proliferation. Knowledge of the mechanisms of programmed cell death may lead to understanding how cells are chosen to survive during embryonic development. bcl-2 is expressed in neurons in developing brains of embryonic and young mice (Korsmeyer, 1993). Investigation of the gene has led to increased focus on identifying cell death genes like ced-3 and ced-4, which have not been identified yet in mammals.

Substances like bcl-2 might be useful in treatment of neurodevelopmental disorders or in neurodegenerative disease because bcl-2 blocks neuronal death triggered by calcium ion influx into cultured neurons. The understanding of the mechanisms involved in cell maintenance and death is critical in the developmental disorders.

MYELINATION

Myelination proceeds through the enclosure of naked axons by glial cell membranes (see Figure 2–1). The chemical composition of the myelin sheet shows significant changes in its lipid and protein structure during development (Van der Knapp, 1990). Myelination is essential to facilitate nerve conduction velocity, the speed of information transport along an axon. As an axon becomes myelinated, nerve conduction velocity increases from 2 mps (meters per second) to 50 mps. Consequently, nerve conduction velocities in peripheral nerves are slower in younger children than in older children and in adults. Furthermore, myelination is critical in the establishment of latency times for acoustic, visual, and somatosensory evoked responses during development.

The most extensive studies of myelination of the central nervous system were carried out by Yakovlev and Lecours (1967) who presented a myelination timetable that is widely recognized. Yet it is not myelination per se but whether brain regions receive fast signal conduction that is most important. The myelination of nerve cells is analogous to the development of pathways that connect brain regions that are rapidly growing.

The myelination cycle can be correlated with developmental milestones. For example, the vestibular and spinal tracts, which are essential to postural control, are myelinated by 40 weeks' gestation. On the other hand, the midbrain corticovisual pathways, which are necessary for the visual-smile response, are myelinated in infants by 2 to 3 months of age. As fine motor control develops toward the end of the first year of life, myelination is seen in the descending lateral corticospinal tracts. During the second year of life, myelination of the cerebello-cerebral connections is seen after a spurt in cerebellar cell growth has come to an end. Yet, by school age, the reticular tracts are still maturing, and those tracts that connect specific and associative neocortical areas continue their maturation during adult life. Recently, studies of myelination *in vivo* have been enhanced with the availability of nuclear magnetic resonance imaging and spectroscopy. Using these methods, a noninvasive longitudinal approach to the study of myelination during normal and abnormal development has become possible.

NEUROTRANSMISSION

The presence of networks in the brain involving specific neurotransmitters is establishing a chemical neuroanatomy (Bjorklund, Hokfelt, and Tohyama, 1992). In regard to brain development, it has been noted that small concentrations of most neurotransmitters are detectable in the first weeks of gestation, but the early presence of transmitters does not necessarily imply early neurotransmission. It also has recently been demonstrated that neurotransmitters may function as trophic factors in the earlier stages of brain development. Moreover, receptor sites may be present before their neurotransmitters are detected. The fact that external influences may influence the brain when neurotransmitters are still trophic messengers may help to explain some of the long-lasting effects of medications or toxic substances that reach the embryo, fetus, or child on their later neurologic and psychosocial development (Schwaab, 1991). In the chapter on neurotransmitters, these questions will be addressed in greater detail.

MICROCIRCULATION AND NEURONAL ACTIVITY

In studying the effects of drugs and toxins on the developing brain, the development of the blood-brain barrier and its role in early prenatal and postnatal life needs to be considered. The basic structure of the blood-brain barrier provides the interface between endothelium cells and neurons with glial cells in between. Certain structures, such as the choroid plexus and the outer arachnoid membrane, are also part of this blood-brain barrier system. A restraint on movements of molecules and ions at this barrier is largely governed by lipid solubility. In addition to the passive barrier system, these interfaces also involve transport proteins, which may move electrolytes, sugars, amino acids and nonelectrolytes between blood and the cerebral spinal fluid. This is often an active transport against existing concentration gradients. Furthermore, enzymes in blood and enzymes bound to cerebral endothelium may degrade these molecules. The development of the blood-brain barrier is the result of a fine structural development involving blood vessels, glial cells, and neurons.

DEVELOPMENT OF REGIONAL BRAIN ANATOMY

The phases of brain development in the first 20 weeks are accompanied by morphological changes in the pattern of the brain. Early in development, regional brain anatomy begins simply, but it becomes complex through the folding of segments and by differentiation of neural cells. As a result, structures that belong to systems that are ultimately unrelated may be located next to one another. Due to this contiguous anatomical arrangement, local insults may affect more than one functional system. An *in vivo* understanding of these functional relationships in regional brain anatomy is being established through brain imaging studies.

The brain begins embryonically as a neural tube that gives rise to six brain regions. The neurons and glial cells are derived from a specialized section of ectoderm, the neural plate. Through signals sent to the dorsal ectoderm from the mesoderm (especially the notochord), neural induction takes place (see Table 2–1).

The neural plate, embryonic day 18 (E18), folds and through the process of neurulation forms the neural tube (E21). The cavity of the neural tube produces the ventricular system of the central nervous system. The neuroepithelium, epithelial cells that line the neural tube, produces the neurons and glial cells. Neuroblasts derived from these early neuroepithelial cells become the cells of the brain and spinal cord. Neural crest cells from the dorsal region of the neural tube emigrate to form peripheral tissues, including sensory and autonomic neurons and the adrenal medulla. The caudal, or back, part of the neural tube, gives rise to the spinal cord, and the dorsal (front) part gives rise to the brain. Three brain vesicles — the forebrain, midbrain, and hindbrain form by E28. This early tube brain bends twice — at the junction of the spinal cord and hindbrain, and at the junction of the hindbrain and midbrain.

This is followed by a third flexure, the pontine flexure. By E35, the forebrain and hindbrain have subdivided. With this final division, the six major regions of the mature nervous system are complete, i.e., five brain regions and the spinal cord (see Fig. 2–2).

During the next six weeks, the forebrain gives rise to (1) the end brain (telencephalon), from which is derived the cerebral neocortex (dorsolateral wall), the basal ganglia (ventral wall), the hippocampal formation (medial wall), and the amygdala (region lateral to basal

Table 2–1. Chronology of Human Brain Development

Time of gestation	Anatomical structure
15 days	Primitive streak is present.
16 days	Notochord is present.
18–21 days	Neural plate is present.
20 days	Somites begin to form, and neural folds begin to fuse.
	Neural crest forms at the side of neural fold fusion. Neural tube made up of a roof plate, a floor plate, and two alar and two base plates.
22 days	Optic grooves and otic placode are present.
24 days	Rostral neuropore closes.
26 days	Caudal neuropore closes.
28 days	Forebrain, midbrain, and hindbrain vesicles form. Spinal ganglia are present.
32 days	Optic cup and otocyst are present.
33 days	Thalamic anlage is present.
35 days	Forebrain divides into telencephalon and diencephalon.
	Hindbrain divides into metencephalon and myelencephalon. Cerebellum begins to develop.
6 weeks	First cerebral cortical neurons are born.
	Lateral geniculate nucleus (LGN) begins to develop. Pituitary develops. Anlage of striatum is present.
7 weeks	Primordial plexiform layer is present in the cerebral cortex.
	Ganglion cell axons reach LGN.
8 weeks	Cerebellar external granular layer begins to form. Lips begin to move reflexively.
10 weeks	Cerebellar Purkinje cell layer forms. Intrahemispheric commissures begin to form. Longitudinal sulcus is present.
11 weeks	Layers 7, 1, and undifferentiated cortical plate are present in cerebral cortex.
12 weeks	Amygdala nuclei are present. Myelination begins in the spinal cord. Swallowing reflex is present.
15–16 weeks	Layers 7, 6, 5, 1, and undifferentiated cortical plate are present in cerebral cortex.
18–20 weeks	Layers 7, 6, 5, 4, 1, and undifferentiated cortical plate are present in cerebral cortex. LGN layers are present. Central sulcus present.
24–26 weeks	Layers 7, 6, 5, 4, 3c, 1, and undifferentiated cortical plate are present in cerebral cortex. Sucking reflex is present.
26 weeks	Central sulcus and lateral fissure are present.
28–30 weeks	Layers 7, 6, 5, 4, 3c, 3b, 1, and undifferentiated cortical plate are present in cerebral cortex.
26–34 weeks	Dendritic spines and branches form on the pyramidal cells of the visual cortex.
38–40 weeks	Layers 7, 6, 5, 4, 3, 2b, 1, and undifferentiated cortical plate present in cerebral cortex.
Third trimester and postnatally	Synaptic maturation, granule cell migration, and axon myelination take place.

From Rubenstein, Lotspeich, and Ciaranello, 1990.

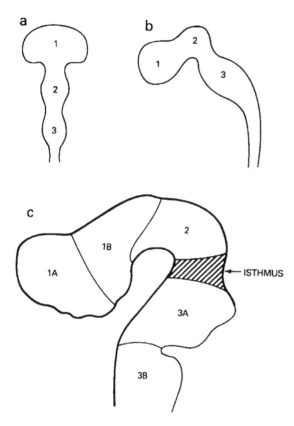

Figure 2–2. *Compartmentation of the brain early in ontogeny.* Diagrams in (a) and (b) show dorsal and lateral views of the three initial swellings (vesicles) of the brain. The three vesicles are identified as the (1) prosencephalon, (2) mesencephalon, and (3) rhombencephalon. In the human embryo, the swellings are evident at 4 weeks. As shown in (c), shortly thereafter (2 weeks in the case of the human embryo) the prosencephalon subdivides into the telencephalon (1A) and diencephalon (1B) while the rhombencephalon becomes apportioned into the metencephalon (3A) (pons and cerebellum) and myelencephalon (3B) (medulla) (drawings adapted by MacLean, 1990, from ones appearing in His (1904) and in Villiger (1931).

ganglia); and (2) the between brain (diencephalon), which lies between the two hemispheres. This is composed of the thalamus, subthalamus, and hypothalamus as well as the optic cup (retina). The midbrain (mesencephalon) remains undivided and forms the midbrain of the mature nervous system. Finally, the hindbrain gives rise to the afterbrain (metencephalon), made up of the pons and cerebellum, and the myelencephalon, which forms the medulla. The most caudal portion gives rise to the spinal cord. The cerebral hemispheres eventually grow to cover most of the diencephalon and midbrain. The embryonic subdivisions and mature forms are listed in Table 2–2.

The cells of the cerebral hemispheres undergo a major proliferation beginning at 11 to 12 weeks of embryonic life. The cortex first expands ros-

trally to form the frontal lobes. Next, it expands dorsally to form the parietal lobes and, finally, posteriorly and inferiorly to form the temporal and occipital lobes. This expansion forces the cortex and the immediately underlying structures (i.e., the caudate, hippocampal formation, and neocortical gyri of the limbic system) into a C shape. The lateral ventricles are anatomically related to the latter structures, so the now C-shaped caudate nucleus roughly parallels the shape of the lateral ventricle. The caudate is incompletely separated from the putamen by the internal capsule. Near the end of the caudate lies the amygdala. The head of the caudate is an important anatomic landmark in studying the normal brain and is affected in certain compulsive behavior disorders and movement disorders. It ordinarily sticks out into the anterior horn of the lateral ventricle and may be visualized by CT,

Table 2–2. The Major Subdivisions of the Central Nervous System

Three-vesicle stage	Five-vesicle stage	Major mature derivatives	Related cavity
1. Forebrain (prosencephalon)	1a. Telencephalon (endbrain)	1. Cerebral cortex, basal ganglia, hippocampal formation, amygdala, olfactory bulb	Lateral ventricles
	lb. Diencephalon	2. Thalamus, hypothalamus, subthalamus, epithalamus, retinae optic nerves and tracts	Third ventricle
2. Midbrain (mesencephalon)	2. Mesencephalon (midbrain)	3. Midbrain	Cerebral aqueduct
3. Hindbrain (rhomben- cephalon)	3a. Metencephalon (afterbrain) 3b. Myelencephalon	4. Pons and cerebellum 5. Medulla oblongata (medullary brain)	Fourth ventricle Fourth ventricle
4. Caudal part of neural tube	4. Caudal part of neural tube	6. Spinal cord	Central canal

From Kandel, 1991.

MRI, and PET imaging techniques. The other subcortical regions that fold into a C shape with the expansion of the cortex make up the major parts of the limbic system, which is involved in emotions, learning, and memory (see Fig. 2–3).

Its four major parts form two C-shaped structures. The first of these is made up of the fornix (anterior) and the hippocampus (posterior). The other is formed by the cingulate gyrus and parahippocampal gyrus (see Fig. 2–4).

DEVELOPMENT OF THE CEREBRAL CORTEX

The surface of the neocortex is greatly expanded in humans, so the surface of the human neocortex is ten times greater than that of a rhesus macaque monkey. The cortex is divided into distinct regions, each of which shows different anatomy and function, as described previously. This regional specialization is a cornerstone of modern brain study. These regions are referred to as *cytoarchitectonic areas*. That regional specialization occurs was not recognized for many years because of the parallel processing that goes on in the nervous system.

Many sensorimotor and other mental functions utilize more than one neural pathway. When a region is damaged, others are able to compensate partly for the loss. This capacity for compensation makes it more difficult to obtain

behavioral evidence for localization of function. Moreover, functions that are localized to discrete regions in the brain are not the complex faculties of mind, but rather more elementary brain operations. The complex faculties are constructed from serial and parallel (distributed) connections among several brain regions. Consequently, damage to a single area does not result in the disappearance of a specific mental function as early locationists had suggested. Furthermore, even when a function does disappear, partial return may occur because undamaged parts of the brain may reorganize sufficiently to perform the function that was lost. This leads to the conclusion that interrelated local brain functions are not a series of links in a single chain. If they were, related functions would all be disrupted if the single link were destroyed. Instead, interrelated functions are processed through many neuronal pathways, which are distributed and parallel. Consequently, the destruction of a single link may disrupt only one pathway and may not permanently interfere with the full performance of the whole system. Those parts of the system that remain may modify their performance to compensate for the loss of a particular elementary operation.

Advances in the brain sciences and in neuropsychological testing have resulted in a better appreciation that complex mental functions may be divided into subfunctions. Each of

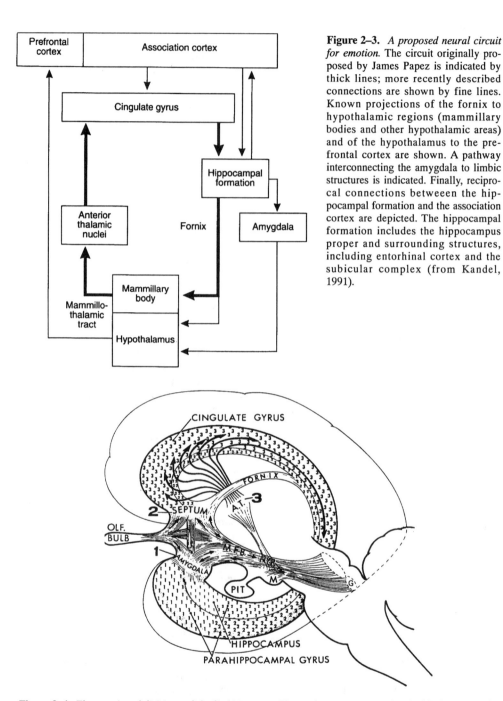

Figure 2–3. *A proposed neural circuit for emotion.* The circuit originally proposed by James Papez is indicated by thick lines; more recently described connections are shown by fine lines. Known projections of the fornix to hypothalamic regions (mammillary bodies and other hypothalamic areas) and of the hypothalamus to the prefrontal cortex are shown. A pathway interconnecting the amygdala to limbic structures is indicated. Finally, reciprocal connections betweeen the hippocampal formation and the association cortex are depicted. The hippocampal formation includes the hippocampus proper and surrounding structures, including entorhinal cortex and the subicular complex (from Kandel, 1991).

Figure 2–4. *Three main subdivisions of the limbic system.* The nuclear groups associated with the amygdalar, septal, and thalamocingulate divisions are respectively labeled with the large numerals 1, 2, and 3, and the cortical sectors primarily associated with them are overlain with the smaller corresponding numerals. The numerals overlying the archicortical areas are somewhat smaller than those identifying the rest of the limbic cortex. Abbreviations: A.T., anterior thalamic nuclei; G, dorsal and ventral tegmental nuclei of Gudden; HYP., hypothalamus; M, mammillary bodies; M.F.B., medial forebrain bundle; PIT, pituitary; OLF., olfactory (from MacLean, 1990).

these functions, i.e., perception, new learning, and remembering, seems continuous to the person, yet each process is composed of several information processing components that are independent. As a result, the simplest cognitive task is the result of integrated and coordinated activity from several distinct brain regions. Moreover, information is not stored as a general representation such that a particular person is remembered, but rather is subdivided into specific categories. In the cortex, these categories are distributed in the various anatomically distinct lobes, that is, frontal, parietal, occipital, and temporal.

Probably the most striking example of the divisibility of mental processes was demonstrated in split brain studies. Sperry (1968), and later Gazzaniga (1988), investigated mental unity following surgical disconnection of the cerebral hemispheres. In these studies, epileptic patients whose two cerebral hemispheres were surgically separated by dividing the corpus callosum, the fiber tract that connects the two hemispheres, demonstrated that each hemisphere represents an independent sense of self-awareness. In these studies it was demonstrated that each hemisphere demonstrates awareness of tactile stimuli applied to the contralateral hand, (the hand opposite that hemisphere) but is not aware of stimuli to the same side. Consequently, if identical objects are placed in both hands, the object in the left hand may be identified by the right hemisphere, but due to the sectioning of the corpus callosum, this object cannot be compared with the same object placed in the right hand. That other object can only be identified by the left hemisphere, which is no longer connected and therefore no longer communicating with the right. Moreover, in most instances in split brain subjects, the right hemisphere cannot understand language, which is understood well by the isolated left hemisphere. This has been demonstrated through studies where opposing commands have been selectively given to each hemisphere. These split brain studies demonstrate that in assessing mental activities, we are addressing the most essential questions in biology that have to do with the representation of self-awareness and consciousness (Chapter 11).

We are only beginning to understand the representation of complex behavior in the brain. The section that follows describes the development of the cerebral cortex that makes possible these abilities.

EMBRYONIC DEVELOPMENT

The cerebral cortex initially makes up only about 3% of the endbrain, or telencephalon. Yet by the time of birth, it comprises 80% of the endbrain and about two thirds of the entire brain (Rakic, 1988a). As indicated earlier, the surface of the neocortex in the human is ten times that of the rhesus macaque.

The adult neocortex is about 2 mm in thickness and covers over one square foot of surface area (Hubel, 1988). Through development, the neocortex becomes a six-layered structure, each layer providing a different function. The top layers, layers 5 and 6, send their output to noncortical regions of the brain. Layer 4 beneath them receives input from the thalamus, and layers 2 and 3 receive input from layer 4. These layers (2, 3, and 4) then send output to other cortical brain regions. The different layers contain different types of neurons and neurotransmitters. The lower layers (2 and 3) are made up of small and medium-size pyramidal cells, whereas layer 4 contains small granular stellate cells, and layer 5 medium-size pyramidal cells. In layer 6 are both pyramidal and fusiform cells. The distribution of neurotransmitters in the cortex is described in Chapter 3.

As previously described, the early neural tube contains a single layer of epithelial cells. These neuroblasts divide approximately every 6 hours to increase the thickness of the neural tube wall. Cell division leads to variability in thickness, depending on which brain region is destined to receive those particular cells. All neurons destined for the neocortex are produced in the proliferative zone near the cerebral ventricle. In the fetus, this zone is organized as a pseudostratified epithelium where cells divide asynchronously; that is, their nuclei move away from the ventricular surface to synthesize DNA and then move back to the surface to undergo another mitotic cycle (Sidman and Rakic, 1973). Anatomical studies show that neuronal and glial cells coexist in the ventricular zone from the time of onset of corticogenesis. The ventricular zone is divided by glial septa into well-demarcated columns of stem or precursor cells, which Rakic defines as "proliferative units." At about E42 in human fetal brain, these proliferative units begin producing postmitotic neurons, which migrate to prespecified positions in the cortex. In humans, the first cortical neurons are generated around E40, and their production lasts until about E125. Neocortical neurons are not produced for the remainder of gestation; the full complement of cortical neurons is established during the middle third of gestation. Rakic (1985) suggests that the stability of this neuronal population (i.e., no additional neurons are produced) is essential to allow cognitive experience to be preserved as information in assembled synapses throughout the life span. The proliferative units initially contain 3 to 5 cells, but later may include as many as 12.

Following its formation from a precursor cell, the neuron begins to migrate from the proliferative unit to its final position within the cortex. This massive migration, which occurs in the middle of gestation, coincides with the concurrent growth of the cerebral wall and the establishment of sulci and gyri on its surface. The outer margins of the cerebral wall are established below the pia mater. The young neurons pass through the various cellular zones by following extended shafts of radial glial cells. The radial glial cells are nonneuronal bipolar cells whose processes extend across the fetal cerebral wall from the beginnings of the genesis of the cortex, but appear most prominently during mid-gestation. Moreover, groups of postmitotic cells follow these radial pathways, which consist of single or multiple glial fibers. As the cells move along the glial surface, they pass axonal and dendritic processes and most likely utilize adhesion molecules in their journey. Rakic (1988a) suggests that a single pair of binding, complementary molecules that relate to the glial cells may account for the radial migration. A better understanding of the mechanisms of neuronal migration is of particular importance in understanding several congenital and acquired malformations of the cortex. Several adhesion molecules are being evaluated in this regard.

The first group of cells which begin their migration in the seventh embryonic week form a subplate zone (layer 7) and also the molecular layer, or layer 1 of the cortex. The next set of migrating neurons move to cortical layer 6 and are present there by embryonic week 15 to 16. These newly migrating neurons are established in the middle of the first cell layer and split

these cells into the subplate zone and the molecular, or marginal, zone. During this same period, layer 5 is formed, layer 4 being established in the 18th week, layer 3 in the 24th week, and layer 2 by the 38th week. All cells in each layer begin their migration at about the same time. Moreover, the oldest layers are deepest in the cortex. For this to occur, cells that make up the younger layers must migrate past the older layers, so the cells that make up layer 5 must pass layer 6 cells. All the cortical layers are constructed largely during the first half of gestation.

The migrational pattern from a given proliferative unit in the ventricular zone results in the formation of columns of related cells in the mature cortex. These vertical arrangements of related cells are referred as *ontogenetic columns.* Each column spans the width of the cerebral cortex; a column varies in its neuronal composition from approximately 80 cells in the anterior cingulate cortex to more than 120 in the primary visual cortex.

Rakic (1988a, 1991) postulates that neurons become "committed" to differentiate into particular mature phenotypes soon after their birth and before their migration to the cortex is completed. As evidence of commitment, he notes that irradiation in rat embryos will inhibit normal neuronal migration but not prevent the neurons from acquiring their normal morphology and making connections. Moreover, the transplantation of ventricular layer cells from an embryonic ferret into the endbrain, or telencephalon, of a newborn ferret led to the transplanted cells migrating to the cortical areas appropriate for the donor cells. Furthermore, Schwartz and Goldman-Rakic (1986) demonstrated that some neurons send off their axons across the corpus callosum even while in the process of migrating. There is also evidence in transgenic mice of abnormal migrations of neurons. Caviness, Crandall, and Edwards (1988) found that despite abnormal migrations of neurons in reeler mice, their neurons form structures and connections that are appropriate for the time of birth. Each of these approaches provides additional evidence that neuronal identity may be determined before migration to the cortex and that environmental change does not specifically affect the differentiation.

Overall, the established adult cerebral cortex is an assembly of repeating units made up of ontogenetic columns (Rakic, 1988a). The original recognition that the cortex is functionally organized in vertical columns comes from Mountcastle (1957, 1979). With this organization, neurons within a single column in a primary sensory-cortical area respond to similar characteristics. These include receptive field modality input, such as orientation to light. Cells within a specific ontogenetic column are developmentally and functionally related to one another. Unlike the neocortex, the older parts of brain, such as the hippocampal formation and primary olfactory cortex, contain only two layers of cells. Adjacent to these limbic, or allocortical, regions are the paralimbic or mesocortical domains. In them, there is a transition in the number of cell layers from the two-layered allocortex through the mesocortex (progressively with 3, 4, and 5 layers) to the six-layered neocortex.

FUNCTIONAL ANATOMY OF THE CEREBRAL CORTEX

Although anatomically the cerebral cortex would appear to be a uniform 6-layered structure made up of repeating ontogenetic columns, functionally there are discrete domains, which show anatomical differences. Mesulam (1986) refers to these domains as architectonic areas.

The mechanism of control of structure and the functional identity of the various cortical regions is under investigation. Rakic (1988a, 1991) suggests that two models be considered. The first model proposes that specification of cortical areas is under genetic control; the second suggests that the function of an area is molded by synaptic input, which is received from other parts of a brain. The genetic mechanism is supported by findings that the correct topographic connections are found in the visual cortex of mice without eyes. Furthermore, ocular dominance columns develop prenatally in monkeys (Hubel, 1988). These studies of the development of the eye suggest that a differentiated visual cortex may develop without visual input. Furthermore, the divisions of the telencephalon begin before synapses have started to form. This would suggest that there is a genetically encoded map to establish this sequence.

Such coding would require sets of controlling genes, one of which might influence the number of ontogenetic columns in a specific domain, another of which would control the identity of the neurons that are produced within a particular column (Rakic, 1988a). The second model is that all cortical neurons are equipotential. If this were the case, then the afferent axons would instruct the neuron on the type of cortex to form. Evidence supporting this second approach comes from work with retinoganglion cells. If retinoganglion cell afferents are rerouted to the auditory thalamus, the thalamic afferents will then innervate the auditory cortex (Sur, Garraghty, and Roe, 1988). In this experiment the primary auditory cortex was demonstrated to detect visual stimuli, although many of the electropsyiological properties of the cortex could not be distinguished in the primary visual cortex. Other rerouting experiments of visual afferents into the somato-sensory thalamus have been carried out. Results have demonstrated that various sensory cortices can function interchangeably. Yet it is not known whether more complex aspects of vision, such as color recognition and movement, can be decoded by these auditory and somato-sensory cortices.

Another kind of experiment that reports the importance of the local milieu on cortical differentiation involves the transport of fetal occipital neurons into the motor cortex of newborn rats. Ordinarily, occipital neurons elaborate axons, which transiently enter pyramidal tracts, but later these axons degenerate. In contrast, neurons in the motor cortex produce axons that permanently make up the pyramidal tract. When fetal occipital neurons were transplanted into the motor cortex, the occipital neurons elaborated axons that became a stable part of the pyramidal tract. These results suggest that the local environment of transplanted occipital neurons modified them. Still, it is not known which aspects of the environment induced changes in the transplanted cells.

Moreover, Rakic (1988b) carried out experiments in which he decreased the number of thalamic afferents to the visual cortex by enucleating embryonic cats. With the loss of the eye, significant neuronal death occurs in thalamic regions involved in vision. As a result, thalamic neurons that project to the visual cortex are reduced in number. Rakic found that there was a corresponding decrease in the number of ontogenetic columns that the thalamic afferents innervated. He also demonstrated that the visual cortex appeared normal based on various criteria. From this, he concluded the cortex can develop independent of input from the thalamus; however, the parcellation of the various cytoarchitectonic domains is affected by thalamic input.

DEVELOPMENT OF OTHER BRAIN REGIONS

The cerebral cortex is of particular importance for complex functions, including language and thought. These brain regions are disturbed in children with neurodevelopmental cognitive disorders. In addition, subcortical regions, such as the cerebullum and basal ganglia, may also be involved. Therefore, the development of subcortical structures is also important to understand.

Like the cerebral cortex, most of the subcortical structures also develop from progenitor cells, or stem cells, in the ventricular zone. Cellular division leads to thickenings in the ventricular region and to cell migration just as occurs for cortical cells. However, the subcortical cells that form nuclei do not migrate all the way to the surface, but remain deep in the brain. Furthermore, many subcortical structures are not layered, as is the cerebral cortex. Most brainstem nuclei, the basal ganglia, and the amygdala do not have apparent cell layers. Some subcortical structures are layered, such as parts of the thalamic nuclei, superior collicus, and the cerebellum. Those regions that are layered may perform more complex functions.

Basal Ganglia

The basal ganglia provide a neural system through which behavior is affected by the cortex. The most striking effects are those that involve voluntary movement, which may be expressed in movement disorders and, as recent evidence suggests, in compulsive forms of behavior. These behaviors are produced through a balanced opposition in cortically driven activity of striatopallidal and striatonigral

pathways. The compartmental organization of the striatum provides the cellular and molecular mechanisms that are essential to regulate this balance (Gerfen, 1984). Even though all striatal neurons utilize GABA as a neurotransmitter, the majority of striatopallidal neurons express the D_2 dopamine receptor and enkephalin. On the other hand, the majority of striatonigral neurons express the D_1 dopamine receptor, dynorphin, and Substance P. Gerfen (1992) points out that, in the dopamine-depleted striata, D_2 agonists decrease and D_1 agonists increase peptide expression in striatopallidal and striatonigral neurons. These findings suggest that the direct action of dopamine may be to oppositely modulate output pathways. In the normal arrangement for the striatum, intra- and intercellular interactions occur that lead to more complex regulation of these striatonigral and striatopallidal outputs. The fundamental activity of the basal ganglia may be to select from many possibilities a specific behavioral action. The balanced opposition in activity of the striatonigral and striatopallidal neurons may provide a mechanism whereby a specific behavior is facilitated or not facilitated. Further research is needed to examine the subpopulations of the striatal output neurons to better understand the cellular and molecular mechanisms involved.

Of interest is the organization of the caudate putamen complex of the basal ganglia. The neurons are not organized into layers, but they show a different kind of order. The caudoputamen is first noted at E35 to be made up of two sets of cellular components, the patch and matrix systems. Both patch and matrix include groups of cells that differ in their neurotransmitters, neurotransmitter receptors, their afferent and efferent connections, and the time during development when they appear.

Amygdaloid Nucleus

In the lateral amygdaloid nucleus there are developmental changes. The adult nucleus is homogeneous in its cellular distribution, but the embryonic nucleus seen at 12 weeks of gestation contains 7 to 11 columnar cell clusters. With development, these columns coalesce and establish the homogeneous adult form (Nikolic and Kostovis, 1986).

Subpopulations of Striatal Neurons

The coordination of subpopulations of striatal neurons depends on the integrative action of the corticostriatal system, which interacts with intrastriatal organization to regulate the balanced opposition between output systems.

Overall, the corticostriatal system is described in terms of parallel processing mechanisms (Alexander, DeLong, and Strick, 1986). Here, segregated but parallel circuits connect limbic, prefrontal, ocular-motor, and motor-cortical areas through subregions of the basal ganglia with thalamic nuclei that feed back to the same cortical areas (see Fig. 2–5). This inhibition has been suggested as the basic mechanism by which these basal ganglia systems affect behavior. Basal ganglia output nuclei (i.e., the internal segment of the globus pallidus and the substantia nigra pars reticulata) provide tonic inhibition of ventral thalamic nuclei and of the superior colliculus. The inhibition of these inhibitory pathways results from cortical excitation of inhibitory striatal projections. As a result, movements are initiated in response to sensory activity, memory, or motivational cues. Cues are correlated with pauses in the tonic activity of substantia nigra output neurons (Hikosaka and Wurtz, 1983a, 1983b). The opposed tonic activity of these neurons is regulated in part by striatal outputs to the external segment of the globus pallidus. Balanced opposition of cortically driven striatal output systems apparently is responsible for the generation of normal movements.

Anatomically, even though the striatum lacks cytoarchitectural definition, subpopulations of neurons are organized into functional compartments. The compartmental organization involves at least two levels. The first of these is defined by segregation of the striatal output neurons into patch and matrix compartments (see Fig. 2–6). These are related to laminar and regional aspects of cortical organization. The second level of compartmental organization involves the separation of projections to the external segment of the globus pallidus into the substantia nigra.

The striatal patch and matrix compartments are defined by their specific neurochemical

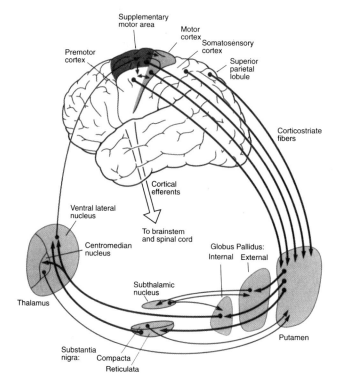

Figure 2–5. *Basal ganglia motor circuit.* The motor circuit of the basal ganglia is a subcortical feedback loop from the motor and somatosensory areas of the cortex, through restricted portions of the basal ganglia and thalamus, and back to the premotor cortex, supplementary motor area, and motor cortex (from Kandel, 1991).

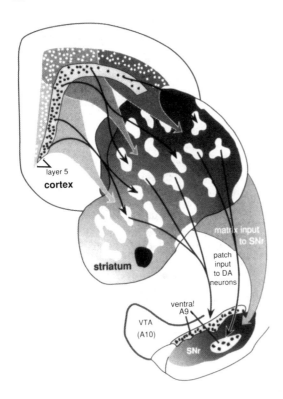

Figure 2–6. Patch-matrix compartmental organization of the basal ganglia depicting the corticostriatal and striatonigral pathways. Corticostriatal neurons in the deep parts of layer 5 provide inputs to the striatal patch compartment, whereas superficial layer 5 neurons provide inputs to the striatal matrix. Patch neurons provide inputs to the location of dopaminergic neurons in the ventral aspect of the substantia nigra pars compacta and islands of dopamine neurons in the pars reticulata. Striatal matrix neurons provide inputs to the location of GABAergic neurons in the substantia nigra pars reticulata (SNr) (from Gerfen, 1992).

markers and the connections of the underlying neurons. The striatal patch compartment is defined by areas of μ-opiate receptor binding and areas of low acetylcholinesterase labeling, which have been referred to as *striosomes* (Graybiel and Ragsdale, 1978). The striatal matrix compartment, which is complementary to the patches, is made up of neurons that contain a calcium binding protein and a plexus of somatostatin immunoreactive fibers (Gerfen, 1985). Other neurochemical markers, (e.g., enkephalin and Substance P) and the sum of the input and output connections show heterogeneity in the striatum, which may or may not be consistent with the patch and matrix compartment. Consequently, when these markers are taken into account, there are multiple levels of compartmental organization, some of them related to patch-matrix compartments.

Cerebellum

The development of the cerebellar cortex requires emphasis in that it shows another pat-

tern of morphogenesis (Altman and Bayer, 1985). The cerebellum has two germinal zones: the ventricular layer and the external granular layer. The cerebellum begins its development at E28, when rapid cellular division of stem cells in the ventricular layer occurs before neuronal migrations. These migrations follow pathways that again are elaborated by radial glial cells, called *Bergmann astrocytes.* Neuronal migration takes place toward the pial surface and forms the Purkinje cell layer by E70. This cerebellar cortical development shows similarities to cerebral cortical development.

A portion of the cerebellar cortex also comes from a germinal zone that temporarily covers the outer surface of the cortex. These cells have also originated in the ventricular zone but have migrated along the outer surface of the cerebellum to form its external granular layer. This section is apparent about E60, and from these cells are produced three cell types, the basket and stellate cells (interneurons in the cerebellar cortex's most superficial layer, the molecular layer) and granule cells. These granule cells migrate from the cerebellar surface to the substance of the cerebellum. In doing so, they pass the Purkinje cell layer and form an internal cell layer. The external granular layer begins to decrease in size by about E210 and completely disappears after 2 postnatal years. This granular layer has been used as a marker in the study of developmental disorders, such as autism, where its persistence has been noted. Furthermore, the internal granular layer continues to form during postnatal life. It is the only part of the mammalian brain that produces new cells after birth.

In the brainstem, a transient germinal zone is also produced. This structure, the corpus pontobulbare, forms a lateral recess in the fourth ventricle. Cells in this region migrate to form pontine olivary, and arcuate nuclei.

Many regions of the brain, including the cerebral cortex, are noted for different parts of structures developing at different times. There are spatial gradients in the dates of birth of brain structures. These spatial gradients may have complex patterns. For example, gradients may involve ventrolateral or dorsomedial development. In these instances, ventrolateral neurons might be produced before dorsomedial ones.

Consequently, different parts of the brain show different patterns of development, demonstrating the complex origin of the brain.

METABOLIC MATURATION OF THE BRAIN

Patterns of Cerebral Glucose Metabolism

The development of the neonatal brain has recently been studied using functional neuroimaging techniques. These include positron emission tomography (PET) and single photon emission tomography (SPECT). Using these techniques, ontogenetic changes in local cerebral metabolic rates for glucose (LCMRglc) have been obtained through PET imaging procedures with 2-[^{18}F] fluoro-2-deoxy-D-glucose (FDG). The pattern of local cerebral metabolic rates for glucose in the human neonate is strikingly different from that seen in healthy adults. In newborns, four brain regions are metabolically prominent on PET scanning. These are the primary sensorimotor cortex, thalamic nuclei, brainstem, and cerebellar vermis. Each of these structures is old phylogenetically. Behavioral correlations in the neonate may be apparent because neonates show a limited behavioral repertoire that is dominated by subcortical brain structures. Early behaviors are primarily reflexive behaviors, such as the Moro, along with rooting and grasping reflexes. Integration of visual-motor performance, such as eye-hand coordination, is limited for neonates. Overall, newborns show limited evidence for higher cortical behaviors. This limited newborn function is consistent with their cerebral glucose metabolic activity.

During the first year of life, PET imaging shows glucose metabolic patterns proceeding with functional maturation of older anatomical structures occurring before that of newer areas. The sequence of functional development correlates with the maturation of neurophysiologic-neuroanatomic events and changes in behavior as shown in Table 2–3 (Chugani, 1992). For example, the visuospatial integrative functions are acquired in the second or third month of life as primitive reflex patterns become reorganized. Concurrently, increases in local cerebral glucose utilization are observed in the parietal, temporal, and primary visual cortex, the basal ganglia, and the cerebellar hemispheres. Glucose metabolic activity in most of the frontal lobe is relatively low during the period from 2 to 4 months of age.

During the second and third months of life, when metabolic maturation of cortical regions (encephalization) is noted, there is a concurrent maturation in the electroencephalogram activity. Certain patterns, such as frontal rhythmic delta waves and frontal transients, disappear, and the precursors of the alpha rhythm become apparent for the first time.

The last region to show a maturational increase in local glucose metabolism is the frontal cortex. Maturation of the lateral part of the prefrontal cortex occurs at 6 to 8 months before that of the phylogenetically newer dorsal frontal region, which occurs at 8 to 12 months. The maturation of the frontal cortical regions coincides with the appearance of higher cortical and cognitive abilities. During this maturational period in the last third of the first year of life, the infant begins to show attachment behavior

Table 2–3. Local Cerebral Glucose Metabolism and
Behavioral Landmarks in the First Year of Life

Age	Glucose Metabolic Pattern	Behavior
<1 month	Active sensorimotor cortical and subcorticalregions, midbrain/brain stem, paleo-cerebellum	Predominantly subcortical and primitive sensorimotor level of function; intrinsic brainstem reflexes.
2–3 months	Increasing glucose metabolic activity in basal ganglia, cerebral cortex (except frontal and association regions), cerebellar hemispheres	Suppression of intrinsic subcortical reflexes. Visuo-sensorimotor integration. Electroencephalogram: Disappearance of neonatal patterns (trace alternans, frontal sharp transients, frontal rhythmic delta). Sleep spindles and precursor of alpha rhythm appear.
8–9 months	Increasing glucose metabolic activity in frontal and association cortices	Cognitive or hypothesis-forming development. Stranger anxiety. More meaningful interaction with surroundings.

From Chugani, 1992.

and to demonstrate stranger anxiety. Further-more, performance on the delayed response task, a neuropsychological paradigm for frontal lobe integrity, improves during this period of frontal lobe metabolic maturation. Anatomically, there is an expansion of dendritic fields and an increase in capillary density in the frontal cortex during this time period.

In summary, by one year of age, local glucose metabolic patterns qualitatively are similar to those seen in the normal adult. The pattern of glucose metabolic maturation during the first year of life follows a developmental progression. However, metabolic maturation of the brain is not fully completed. In investigating normal control children during their development, Chugani (1992) has found that most brain areas, specifically the neocortex, continue to undergo maturational changes throughout their development. These findings, which are shown in Figure 2–7, are of considerable interest, but are still preliminary, although they are intriguing in regard to brain development (Chugani, 1992).

The neonatal values are about 30% lower than adult rates, but gradually increase until adult metabolic rates are reached by the second year of life. After that time, LCMRglc values

increase and by the third postnatal year exceed adult values. The plateau is reached around age 4 and extends until age 9. Subsequently, a gradual decline to adult values is noted by the end of the second decade (Chugani, Phelps, and Mazziotta, 1987). The peak in LCMRglc above the adult value is seen primarily in neocortical regions, which reach a peak that is twice that of adult values. The oldest structures of the brain (e.g., the brainstem and the cerebellum) demonstrate metabolic maturity at birth. Subcortical structures, such as the basal ganglia and the thalamus, show intermediate levels of change. Overall, it is the evolutionarily most recent brain regions that show the most metabolic change during development. Similar changes have been noted in increased average cerebral blood flow in 3- to 11-year-olds and in increased oxygen utilization in children (Kennedy and Sokoloff, 1957).

Chugani (1992) suggests that the rapid increase in LCMRglc seen in development corresponds to the period of rapid overproduction of synapses and nerve terminals which occurs in the developing brain as described by Huttenlocher (1979, 1982, 1987). The plateau between ages 4 and 9, when LCMRglc is greater than adult values might correspond to the increased cerebral energy needed because of transient

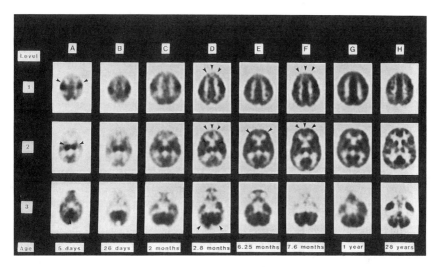

Figure 2–7. *Developmental changes in local cerebral metabolic rates for glucose.* These positron emission tomography images illustrate developmental changes in local cerebral metabolic rates for glucose (LCMRglc) in the normal human infant with increasing age, as compared with the adult (image size not on same scale). Level 1 is a superior section, at the level of the cingulate gyrus. Level 2 is more inferior, at the level of the putamen, and thalamus. Level 3 is an inferior section of the brain, at the level of the cerebellum and inferior portion of the temporal lobes. The gray scale is proportional to LCMRglc, with black being highest. Images from all subjects are not shown on the same absolute gray scale of LCMRglc; instead, images of each subject are shown with the full gray scale to maximize gray scale display of LCMRglc at each age. In each image, the anterior portion of the brain is at the top of the image, and the left side of the brain is at the right of the image. *A,* In the 5-day-old patient, LCMRglc is highest in the sensorimotor cortex, thalamus, cerebellar vermis *(arrows),* and brainstem (not shown). *B–D,* LCMRglc gradually increases in parietal, temporal, and calcarine cortices; basal ganglia; and cerebellar cortex *(arrows),* particularly during the second and third months. *E,* In the frontal cortex, LCMRglc increases first in the lateral prefrontal regions by approximately 6 months. *F,* By approximately 8 months, LCMRglc increases in the medial aspects of the frontal cortex *(arrows)* as well as the dorsolateral occipital cortex. *G,* By 1 year, the LCMRglc pattern resembles that of adults *(H)* (from Chugani, 1992).

amounts of high cerebral connectivity. The subsequent metabolic maturational decline may correspond to the later period of "pruning," or selective elimination of the excessive connections.

Brain Plasticity and Local Metabolic Activity

It is well known that younger children, unlike adults, may show little functional deficit following brain damage. This finding is generally thought to be related to the developmental reorganizational ability in the brain. Recent findings on local brain metabolism suggest that the period between 8 and 10 years, when the LCMRglc for a number of cortical regions begins to decrease, corresponds to the time when brain plasticity following injury is lessened. In regard

to plasticity, the example of Genie (see Chapter 8) is pertinent. Children who have been isolated from language exposure are most successful in acquiring language if intervention is initiated in early childhood. Language acquisition decreases markedly if attempts are begun after 10 years of age (Curtiss, 1981). This age cut-off may also apply for language recovery following brain injury. This has been studied in children who have received hemispherectomy (Basser, 1962). Lenneberg (1967) hypothesized that there is a critical period of language acquisition, which ends around age 10, after which the ability to acquire language is more limited, although language acquisition is still possible (Newport and Supalla, 1990).

Furthermore, changes in LCMRglc are noted in the visual cortex at approximately 8 to 10 years of age and here also correspond to a time when plasticity begins to decrease. For example, clinically significant deprivation of stimulus to one eye in young children, caused by occlusion of an eye due to cataracts or for treatment of certain kinds of strabismus, leads to a reduction in general visual acuity (i.e., amblyopia). This is a sensitive period because proper stimulation of the eye, combined with a patch over the other eye, can markedly reduce or eliminate amblyopia. (However, in some instances, amblyopia, may be induced in the eye that is patched.) Plasticity is reported to end at age 8 to 10 years (Awaya, 1987). Furthermore, similar findings have been reported for the development of depth perception.

These findings suggest that maturational trends in both the human brain and in animal subjects may be carried out noninvasively through the use of metabolic studies involving PET scanning. These techniques may productively be utilized in children who have surgery for refractory epilepsy. Following surgery, functional deficits involving sensory or motor systems may occur. The extent of these deficits may be related to the age when the insult to the brain occurred, the age at surgery, and other factors. A better understanding of windows of developmental plasticity may provide an improved rationale for the timing or avoidance of such surgery. Additional areas where metabolic imaging may be of help are in the study of inborn errors of metabolism, cerebral palsy, and hypoxic-ischemic encephalopathy, as well as other childhood onset neuropsychiatric disorders.

PATHOLOGICAL PROCESSES DURING THE DEVELOPMENTAL PERIOD

The maturation of the nervous system is a complicated process that involves an interplay between precisely timed developmental events coordinated by genetically determined programming. However, the cellular DNA contains a limited amount of information, so all developmental events cannot be regarded as directly controlled by the genes. Cell–cell interactions also play a part. The neurotransmitters may themselves be specially involved in the intercellular communication that regulates the development of neuronal systems (Black, 1982).

In humans, the period of neurogenesis occurs during the first 20 weeks. Pathological events, such as the use of drugs (alcohol), during this time will give rise to abnormalities during the phases of organ development. These early insults in development will cause deficits in the production or migration of neurons, or may lead to a disturbance in the normal arrangements of neurons, so structural deficits may occur in brain development. For example, abnormal neuronal migration is a consideration in the genesis of autistic disorders. Pathological insults later in development produce more subtle effects on neuronal growth, synapse formation, and other neuronal functions. These later insults may be responsible for deficits that are functional rather than clearly structural, possibly related to the emerging neuronal connectivity in the brain (Evrard et al., 1988).

REFERENCES

Alexander, G.E., DeLong, M.R., and Strick, P.L. (1986). Parallel organization of functionally segregated circuits linking basal ganglia and cortex. *Annual Review of Neuroscience,* 9:357–381.

Altman, J. and Bayer, S.A. (1985). Embryonic development of the rat cerebellum: 3. Regional differences in the time of origin, migration, and settling of purkinje cells. *Journal of Comparative Neurology,* 231:42–65.

Awaya, S. (1987). Stimulus vision deprivation amblyopia in humans. In R. D. Reinecke (ed), *Strabismus,* p. 31. Grune and Stratton, New York.

Basser, L.S. (1962). Hemiplegia of early onset and the faculty of speech with special reference to the effects of hemispherectomy. *Brain,* 85:427.

Bjorklund, A., Hokfelt, T., and Tohyama, M. (1992). *Handbook of chemical neuroanatomy.* Elsevier Science Publishers, Holland.

Black, I.B. (1982). Stages of neurotransmitter development in autonomic neurons. *Science,* 215:1198–1204.

Caviness, V.S.J. and Rakic, P. (1978). Mechanisms of cortical development: A view from mutations in mice. *Annual Review of Neuroscience,* 1:297–326.

Caviness, V.S.J, Crandall, J.E., and Edwards, M.A. (1988). The reeler malformation: Implications for neocortical histogenesis. In A. Peters and E.G. Jones (eds.), *Cerebral cortex,* pp. 59–90. Plenum Press, New York.

Chugani, H.T. (1992). Functional brain imaging in

pediatrics. *Pediatric Clinics of North America*, 39–4:777–796.

_____, Phelps, M.E., and Mazziotta, J.C. (1987). Positron emission tomography study of human brain functional development. *Annals of Neurology*, 22:487.

Curtiss, S. (1981). Feral children. In J. Wortis (ed), *Mental retardation and developmental disabilities XII*, p. 129. Brunner/Mazel, New York.

Dobbing, J. and Sands, J. (1973). The quantitative growth and development of the human brain. *Archives of Disease in Childhood*, 48:757–767.

Dodd, J. and Jessel, J.M. (1988). Axon guidance and the patterning of neuronal projections in vertebrates. *Science*, 242:692–699.

Evrard, P., de Saint-Georges, P., Kadhim, H.J. and Gadisseux, J.F. (1988). Pathology of prenatal encephalopathies. In J.H. French, S. Harel, and P. Casaer (eds), *Child neurology and developmental disabilities*. Paul Brookes, Baltimore.

Gazzaniga, M. S. (1988). *Mind matters: How mind and brain interact to create our conscious lives*. Houghton Mifflin, Boston.

Gerfen, C.R. (1984). The neostriatal mosaic: Compartmentalization of corticostriatal input and striatonigral output systems. *Nature*, 311:461–464.

_____. (1985). The neostriatal mosaic: I. Compartmental organization of projections from the striatum to the substantia nigra in the rat. *Journal of Comparative Neurology*, 236:454–476.

_____. (1992). The neostriatal mosaic: Multiple levels of compartmental organization in the basal ganglia. *Annual Review of Neuroscience*, 15: 285–320.

Graybiel, A.M. and Ragsdale, J.C.W. (1978). Histochemically distinct compartments in the striatum of human, monkey and cat demonstrated by acetylcholinesterase staining. *Proceedings of the National Academy of Sciences USA*, 75:5723–5726.

Hikosaka, O. and Wurtz, R.H. (1983a). Visual and oculomotor functions of monkey substantia nigra pars reticulata. III. Memory contingent visual and saccade responses. *Journal of Neurophysiology*, 49:1268–1284.

_____ and _____. (1983b). Visual and oculomotor functions of monkey substantia nigra pars reticulata. IV. Relation of substantia nigra to superior colliculus. *Journal of Neurophysiology*, 49:1285–1301.

His, W. von (1904). *Die Entwickelung des menschlichen gehirns*. Hirzel, Leipzig, Germany.

Hubel, D.H. (1988). *Eye, brain and vision*. W.H. Freeman, New York.

Huttenlocher, P.R. (1979). Synaptic density in human frontal cortex — Developmental changes and effects of aging. *Brain Research*, 163:195.

_____ and de Courten, C. (1987). The development of synapses in striate cortex of man. *Human Neurobiology*, 6:1–9.

_____, _____, and Gary, L.J. (1982). Synaptogenesis in human visual cortex — Evidence for synapse elimination during normal development. *Neuroscience Letters*, 33:247.

Jacobson, M. (1991). *Developmental neurobiology*, 3rd ed. Plenum Press, New York.

Kandel, E.R. (1991). Nerve cells and behavior. In E. R. Kandel, J. H. Schwartz, and T. J. Jessell (eds), *Principles of neural science*, 3rd ed. pp. 18–32. Elsevier Science Publishing Co., Inc., New York.

_____, and Jessell T.M. (eds) (1991). *Principles of neural science*, 3rd ed. Elsevier Science Publishing Co., Inc., New York.

Kennedy, C. and Sokoloff, L. (1957). An adaptation of the nitrous oxide method to the study of the cerebral circulation in children: Normal values for cerebral blood flow and cerebral metabolic rates in childhood. *Journal of Clinical Investigation*, 36:1130.

Korsmeyer, S.J. (1993). Programmed cell death: Bcl-2 (Review). *Important Advances in Oncology*, 19–28.

Lenneberg, E. (1967). *Biological foundations of language*, p. 125. John Wiley & Sons, New York.

Lyon, G. and Gadisseux, J.F. (1991). Structural abnormalities of the brain in developmental disorders. In M. Rutter and P. Casaer (eds), *Biological risk factors for psychosocial disorders*, pp. 1–19. Cambridge University Press, Cambridge.

MacLean, P. (1990). *The truine brain in evolution: Role of paleocerebral functions*, pp. 269–277. Plenum Press, New York.

Mesulam, M.M. (1986). Patterns in behavioral neuroanatomy: Association areas, the limbic system, and hemispheric specialization. In M.M. Mesulam (ed.), *Principles of behavioral neurology*. F.A. Davis, Philadelphia.

Mountcastle, V.B. (1957). Modality and topographic properties of single neurons of cat's somatic sensory cortex. *Journal of Neurophysiology*, 20:408–434.

_____. (1979). An organizing principle for cerebral function: The unit module and the distributed system. In F.O. Schmitt, and F.G. Worden (eds), *The neurosciences: Fourth study program*, pp. 21–42. MIT Press, Cambridge, MA.

Newport, E.L. and Supalla, T. (1990). Maturational constraints on language learning. *Cognition Science*, 14:11.

Nikolic, I. and Kostovis, K. (1986). Development of the lateral amygdaloid nucleus in the human fetus: Transient presence of discrete cytoarchitectonic units. *Anatomical Embryology*, 174:355–360.

Rakic, P. (1972). Mode of cell migration to the superficial layers of fetal monkey neocortex. *Journal of Comparative Neurology,* 145:61–84.

———. (1985). Limits of neurogenesis in primates. *Science,* 227:154–156.

———. (1988a). Specification of cerebral cortical areas. *Science,* 241:170–176.

———. (1988b). Defects of neuronal migration and pathogenesis of cortical malformations. *Progress in Brain Research,* 73:15–37.

———. (1991). Development of the primate cerebral cortex. In M. Lewis (ed), *Child and adolescent psychiatry: A comprehensive textbook,* pp. 11–28. Williams and Wilkins, Baltimore, MD.

Ramon y Cajal (1933). *Histology,* 10th ed., Wood, Baltimore, MD.

Rubenstein, J.L.R., Lotspeich, L., and Ciaranello, R.D. (1990). The neurobiology of developmental disorders. In B.B. Lahey and A.E. Kazdin (eds), *Advances in clinical child psychology,* Vol. 13. Plenum Press, New York.

Schwaab, D.F. (1991). Relation between maturation of neurotransmitter systems in the human brain and psychosocial disorders. In M. Rutter and P. Casaer (eds), *Biological risk factors for psychosocial disorders,* pp. 50–66. Cambridge University Press, Cambridge, UK.

Schwartz, M.L. and Goldman-Rakic, P.S. (1986). Some callosal neurons of the fetal monkey frontal cortex have axons in the contralateral hemisphere prior to the completion of migra-tion. *Society for Neuroscience Abstracts,* 12:1211.

Sidman, R.L. and Rakic, P. (1973). Neuronal migration with special reference to developing human brain: A review. *Brain Research,* 62:1–35.

Smart, J.L. (1991). Critical periods in brain development. In G.R. Bock and J. Whelan (eds), *The childhood environment and adult disease.* (Ciba Foundation Symposium 156, pp. 109–124). John Wiley & Sons, New York.

Smith, S.J. (1988). Neuronal cytomechanics: The action-based motility of growth cones. *Science,* 242:708–715.

Sperry, R.W. (1968). Mental unity following surgical disconnection of the cerebral hemispheres. *Harvey Lectures,* 62:293–323.

Sur, M., Garraghty, P.E., and Roe, A.W. (1988). Experimentally induced visual projections into auditory thalamus and cortex. *Science,* 242:1434–1441.

Van der Knapp, M.S. (1990). MR imaging of the various stages of normal myelinization during the first year of life. *Neuroradiology,* 31:459–470.

Villiger, E. (1931). *Brain and spinal cord.* W.H.F. Addison, ed. Lippincott, Philadelphia, PA.

Yakovlev, P.I. and Lecours, A.R. (1967). The myelogenetic cycles of regional maturation of the brain. In A. Minkowski (ed), *Regional development of the brain in early life,* pp. 3–64. Blackwell, Oxford.

CHAPTER 3

DEVELOPMENT OF NEUROTRANSMITTER SYSTEMS AND NEURONAL SIGNALING MECHANISMS

As the brain develops, an overall pattern emerges that is periodically punctuated by brief neuronal events that establish its final organization (Coyle and Harris, 1987; Jacobson, 1991). At the cellular level, brain development can be divided into four primary events: neuroblast cell division, neuronal migration, transmitter-specific differentiation, and synaptogenesis, as described in the previous chapter. This chapter considers neurotransmitter development, synaptic transmission, and neuronal signaling mechanisms. Definitive evidence of the involvement of these specific neurotransmitter systems in major mental disorders has yet to be established. However, in several neuropsychiatric disorders, a clear role is played by neurotransmitters in the mechanism of action of psychotropic drugs. These potential roles will be outlined following the description of each neurotransmitter system.

DEVELOPMENTAL ASPECTS OF NEUROTRANSMISSION

Biochemical differentiation appears to be involved in the migration of immature neurons to their ultimate resting place. The type of chemical messenger or neurotransmitter that the neuron will utilize may be a factor in the migration process. However, the specialized biochemical mechanisms responsible for neurotransmitter synthesis generally occur after the immature neuron has reached its final destination. Immature neurons may temporarily demonstrate the biochemical characteristics typical for an alternative neurotransmitter before assuming the definitive neurotransmitter characteristics, which they will retain when mature (Katz et al., 1983).

Epigenetic factors also may be involved in the expression of a neurotransmitter. For example, when individual ganglion cells were grown in tissue culture, changing the culture medium led to the conversion of individual adrenergic neurons to cholinergic neurons (Furshpan et al., 1976). Moreover, neurotransmitters may have trophic effects or toxic effects on the production of neurons and in the establishment of their interconnections. Neuronal growth cone extension is regulated by local intracellular calcium ion levels (Ca^{++}) (Lipton and Kater, 1989). If calcium is low, the growth cone is inactive. With increasing calcium ion levels, the cone begins to move, but if calcium is too high, they retract. Some neurotransmitters (e.g., glutamate, an excitatory neurotransmitter) can regulate neuronal process growth through controlling Ca^{++} influx. This effect may be blocked by inhibitory neurotransmitters or by the provision of trophic factors. Excitatory neurotransmitters may produce excitotoxicity, which in itself may play a role in regulating cell number and intercellular connectivity. Nonetheless, excitotoxicity may also be a factor pathologically in neuronal damage (Kater, Mattson, and Guthrie, 1989). In addition, neurotransmitter receptors may affect the growth cone—e.g., D_1 dopamine receptors may inhibit the motility of growth cones through the activation of adenylate cyclase by increasing intracellular cAMP concentration (Lankford, DeMello, and Klein, 1988).

The factors that control the ultimate phenotypic expression of neurotransmitter characteristics are still not fully characterized. However, a super family of neurotrophic factors, which include nerve growth factor (NGF), brain-derived neurotrophic factor (BDNF), and neurotrophin-3, have been reported. In less complex systems, such as the peripheral nervous system, local interactions with neighboring neurons and neurotrophic cues, such as the hormone nerve growth factor (NGF), are thought to play important roles in the specification of neurotransmitters (Black, 1982; Patterson, 1978). In the central nervous system, BDNF may, for example, support the survival of dopaminergic cells in the substantia nigra (Hyman, Hofer, and Barde, 1991).

NEUROTRANSMISSION AT THE SYNAPTIC LEVEL

The transmission of information from the receptive dendritic extensions from their cell bodies down the axon to the nerve terminals takes place by means of an electrochemical wave of excitation that leads to membrane depolarization (Figure 3–1).

These action potentials are generated through the influx of ions through channel-linked receptors that open with the waves of depolarization at the nerve terminal for rapid neurotransmission, or through a non-channel-linked system with slower transmission, which is tied to a binding site that is functionally coupled to an enzyme (Kandel, Siegelbaum, and Schwartz, 1991). The nerve cell, like other secretory cells, secretes a substance that regulates the communication between neuronal cells. These neurotransmitters are released through exocytosis from the nerve terminals when a wave of depolarization reaches them.

The various neurotransmitters are divided into different classes based on their mode of synthesis and their neurophysiologic effects. The mode of synthesis is different for the neuropeptides and the nonpeptide neurotransmitters. Synthesis of the neuropeptides occurs

through a messenger RNA–dependent process within the neuronal cell body itself. The neuropeptide is then transported down the axon to the nerve terminal, where the active neuropeptide is released following specific stimulation (Coyle, 1985). Here neurotransmitter synthesis is closely tied to the translational events within the neuronal cell body. A second class, the nonpeptide neurotransmitters, which includes biogenic amines, amino acids, and certain other substances, are synthesized within the nerve terminal through processes regulated by enzymes contained within that terminal. In this case, neurotransmitter synthesis is not closely tied to translational events within the neuronal cell body; instead, it is controlled at the nerve terminal. Finally, the newest group of proposed neurotransmitters, nitric oxide and carbon monoxide, are an exception to this pattern in that they neither are stored in synaptic vesicles nor released by exocytosis; rather, they diffuse out from the cell. Through these mechanisms, the neuron is able to respond to rapid changes in neurotransmitter demand.

There are three broad categories of postsynaptic responses to neurotransmitters: excitatory, inhibitory, and modulatory. However, this simple three-way division does not adequately depict the subtle relations among the neurotransmitter receptors, various ion channels, G-proteins, and enzymatic processes that mediate the neuronal effects of the neurotransmitters, as described later in this chapter. An excitatory or inhibitory response represents information communicated within the brain in regard to whether a receptive neuron fires or not. On the other hand, a neuromodulator, such as a biogenic amine transmitter, appears to alter neuronal responsiveness to these excitatory or inhibitory inputs. The neurotransmitter receptors, which are located on the postsynaptic neurons, translate the message encoded by the neurotransmitter. The precision of this highly specific interaction historically has been likened to the relationship between a key (the neurotransmitter) and a lock (receptor-transducer) (Ehrlich, 1900).

A neurotransmitter released by a particular neuron is produced throughout all its axonal extensions and nerve terminal contacts, thus providing it a biochemical identity. The neuron contains the biochemical processes necessary

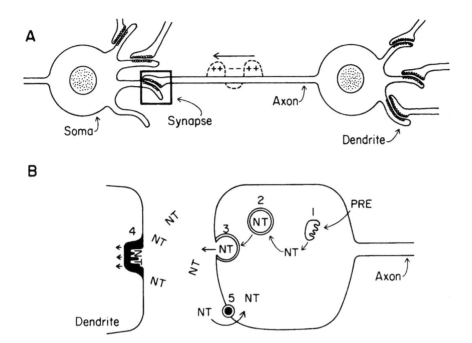

Figure 3–1. *Representation of typical synaptic transmission. Part A.* The structural components of the neuron include the soma (cell body), the dendrites, the axon, and the synapse. *Part B.* The processes involved in chemical synaptic transmission at the synapse are illustrated. Precursors for the neurotransmitter are taken up into the terminal and converted by enzymes to the neurotransmitter (1). The neurotransmitter is stored in vesicles (2) for release (3) into the synaptic cleft, where it interacts with receptors (4) on the dendrite. In many cases the neurotransmitter is inactivated by reuptake (5) at transporter sites into the nerve terminal (from Coyle and Harris, 1987).

for synthesis, storage, release, and inactivation of its specific neurotransmitter (see Table 3–1).

However, the neuron does not possess the biochemical means to utilize or dispose of other neurotransmitters. Moreover, there is evidence for colocalization of more than one neurotransmitter in the same nerve terminal area (Hokfelt et al., 1980). This colocalization generally involves both a neuropeptide (e.g., cholecystokinin) and a nonpeptide neurotransmitter, such as a biogenic amine. Neurons that use specific neurotransmitters tend to be grouped together in clumps of cell bodies known as "nuclei" or to have specific laminar distributions, as in the cerebral cortex.

Over a hundred neurotransmitters have been identified, and the number is increasing rapidly, yet those implicated in the pathophysiology of psychiatric disorders or in the mechanism of action of psychotropic drugs are far more restricted, evidencing our lack of understanding about the roles most of these neurotransmitters perform in normal and abnormal behavior.

DEVELOPMENT OF BRAIN NEUROTRANSMITTERS

The best-known neurotransmitters are those most often associated with psychiatric disorders. Extensive investigations of the development of specific neurotransmitter systems in the brain have been carried out in subprimate species, most commonly in the laboratory rat. So far, the information available from studies on the developing human and nonhuman primate brain is limited but does suggest that findings in the rat are applicable to man (Goldman-Rakic and Brown, 1982).

The noradrenergic, dopaminergic, serotonergic, and cholinergic neuronal systems are

Table 3–1. Neurotransmitter Metabolic and Receptor Characteristics

	Dopamine	Norepinephrine	Serotonin
Precursors	Phenylalanine, tyrosine	Phenylalanine, tyrosine	Tryptophan
Synthetic enzymes (rate limiting)	Tyrosine hydroxylase	Tyrosine hydroxylase Dopamine- β-hydroxylase	Tryptophan hydroxylase
Storage	Synaptic vesicles	Synaptic vesicles	Synaptic vesicles
Catabolic enzymes			
Intracellular	MAO	MAO	MAO
Extracellular	COMT	COMT	
Receptors			
Presynaptic	D_2, D_3	α_2	$5HT_{1A}$, $5HT_{1D}$
Postsynaptic	D_1, D_2, D_3, D_4, D_5	α_1, α_2, β_1, β_2	$5HT_{1A}$, $5HT_{1C}$, $5H_{1D}$, $5H_{T2}$,
Ion channel			$5HT_3$
Second messengers	cAMP, Ca^{++}, DAG, IP3, K^+	cAMP, Ca^+, IP3, arachadonic acid, phosphatidic acid	cAMP, Ca^{++}, IP3, DAG, K^+

	Nitric Oxide	Carbon Monoxide	Exogenous Opioid Peptides
Precursors	Argenine	Heme	POMC, proenkephalin, prodynorphin, (inactive precursors)
Synthesizing enzymes	Nitric oxide synthase (NOS)	Heme oxygenase-2	Ribosomal synthesis from mRNA, active forms by selective proteolytic enzymes
Storage	Not stored	Not stored	Vesicles in smooth endoplasmic reticulum
Catabolic enzymes	NOS is regulated by Ca^{+2} and calmodulin		
Receptors	Does not act on membrane associated receptors. NO mediates glutamate stimulation of cGMP by NMDA receptors.	Does not act on membrane associated receptors; may act via nonglutamatergic synapses	Mu (μ), delta (δ), kappa (κ), sigma (σ), epsilon (ε)
Mode of action	Activates guanylyl cyclase; regulates cGMP	Activates guanylyl cyclase; regulates cGMP	Mu (μ) and delta (δ) are G-protein linked.

cAMP = adenosine 3', 5'-cyclic phosphate, COMT = erthrocyte catechol-O-methyltransferase,
MAO = monoamine oxidase.
Modified from Rogeness, Javors, and Pliszka, 1992.

located in the brainstem in the reticular core. They are among the neuronal systems formed earliest in development. On the other hand, the GABAergic intraneurons within the cerebral cortex are established much later in brain development as part of the genesis of the cerebral cortex. Other neurotransmitters, such as the excitatory amino acid system, are widely distributed in the CNS but found in the greatest amount in the hippocampus and cerebral cortex.

Groups of neurons located in the reticular core of the brain are involved in the mechanism of action of several classes of psychotropic drugs. The cell bodies of the reticular core neurons are widely distributed throughout the midbrain and brainstem. They have diffuse and arborized axonal projections that project extensively into large areas of the nervous system, especially into the forebrain. Their cell bodies' localization in the reticular core guarantees that

Table 3–1. *continued*

	Acetylcholine	GABA	Glutamate
Precursors	Choline	Glucose L-Glutamic acid	Glucose, glutamine, -2 oxyglutarate, aspartate
Synthesizing enzymes (Rate limiting or end product inhibition)	Choline acetyltransferase	Glutamic acid decarboxylase (GAD-l)	Glutaminase, aspartate aminotransferase, ornithine-aminotransferase
Storage	Presynaptic vesicles (release cytoplasmic)	Presynaptic vesicles (?)	Presynaptic vesicles
Catabolic enzymes	Acetyltransferase	GABA-transaminase	Multiple paths
Receptors	Muscarinic (M$_1$–M$_5$) M$_2$ Presynaptic Nicotinic (4 types)	GABA$_A$ (2 subtypes) GABA$_B$(presynaptic)	NMDA, kainic, AMPA, L-AP4 (pres- synaptic), APCD
Mode of action	Second messenger G-protein Nicotinic Ach is ionotrophic.	Ionotrophic (transmitter gated) (GABA$_A$) GABA$_B$ is G-protein linked.	Ionotrophic APCD is G-protein linked.

they receive highly diverse inputs coming both from neuronal systems in the periphery and also from neuronal systems projecting from the forebrain to lower brain regions. This anatomic organization suggests an integrative role for the reticular core. Through these interconnections the reticular core serves to regulate the activity of neurons located in the cerebral cortex, the corpus striatum, and the limbic system. Furthermore, in keeping with this anatomic organization, neurophysiologic studies suggest that the reticular core neuronal systems "modulate" neuronal activity in the cortex and related structures instead of conveying excitatory or inhibitory data to discrete neurons within these regions.

CATECHOLAMINE, SEROTONIN, AND CHOLINERGIC SYSTEMS

Neurons of the Noradrenergic System

It has been known since the 1960s that the primary source of noradrenergic innervation of the cerebral cortex, limbic system, midbrain, and cerebellum is the locus coeruleus. This nucleus is made up of a small group of pigmented neurons situated on both sides of the floor of the fourth ventricle under the cerebellum (Figure 3–2). The norepinephrine neurotransmitter is synthesized within their nerve terminals from the amino acid, tyrosine. Post-

synaptic effects of norepinephrine are mediated through α- and β-adrenergic receptors. These noradrenergic neuronal cell bodies send axons from the locus coeruleus to innervate essentially all of the neurons in the cerebral cortex and limbic system. An individual noradrenergic neuron may contact more than ten other neurons (Black, 1982).

Because the noradrenergic neurons are formed very early in brain development, they are located in the most caudal aspects of the reticular core. The locus coeruleus is produced during a brief period of intense cellular division lasting approximately 36 hours in the rodent (Lauder and Bloom, 1974). This nucleus develops in the rodent at a time when the brain has reached less than 1% of its adult weight. In humans, this is equivalent to the middle of the first trimester of pregnancy. With the coalescence of this nucleus, the neurons begin to express all the biochemical processes required for the synthesis, storage, and release of the norepinephrine neurotransmitter. Even the nascent axons that grow out from the newly formed noradrenergic neurons contain the neurotransmitter. The noradrenergic axons appear in the primordial cerebral cortex during the earliest process of its formation. Although in adult life their terminals comprise a very small percentage of the total number of synaptic contacts in the cerebral cortex, at an early stage in development of the immature cortex up to 30%

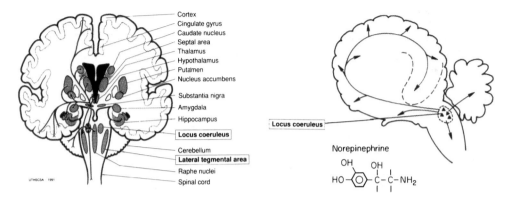

Figure 3–2. *Norepinephrine neuronal system.* The norepinephrine neuronal system is depicted in coronal section (left) showing brain structures. Solid lines represent axonal projections from cell bodies to specific brain areas. On the right, a schematic drawing is shown in sagittal section (left figure from Rogeness, Javors, and Plisza, 1992; right figure from Coyle and Harris, 1987).

of the synapses may be noradrenergic in origin (Coyle and Molliver, 1977).

This early and short-term predominance of noradrenergic terminals in the cerebral cortex suggests that noradrenergic innervation may play a critical role in cortical development. This has been demonstrated because lesions of the noradrenergic system early in development do affect synaptic plasticity in the cortex (Kasamatsu and Pettigrew, 1976). Subsequently, with the elaboration of the rich synaptic arbors of neurons intrinsic to the cortex and when other cortical inputs such as the thalamo-cortical pathways arrive, this noradrenergic predominance in the primordial cortex is relatively reduced.

A distinction must be made between the relative contribution of early developmental noradrenergic input and the full elaboration of noradrenergic processes throughout the brain with later maturation. Early in development the noradrenergic input to the cortex is relatively large, but the total volume of the cortex is still small. Maturation is accompanied by progressive increases in cortical volume, so the noradrenergic terminal arbor expands extensively. As a result, the small group of noradrenergic neuronal cell bodies in the locus coeruleus eventually produce an extensively arborized group of axons and terminals that develop in step with the brain regions that they innervate.

Noradrenergic Receptors

Both presynaptic (α_2) and postsynaptic receptors (α_1, α_2, β_1, β_2) and the second messengers have been identified, as shown in Table 3–1.

Functions of the Noradrenergic System

These noradrenergic neurons and their synaptic connections have been proposed to have many functions. Among these are an important role in mood disorders, in learning and memory, in reinforcement, in sleep-wake cycle regulation, and in anxiety. Furthermore, a major function may be to regulate cerebral blood flow and metabolism. Overall, the basic function of this system may be to establish one's global orientation toward events in the external environment and the internal milieu.

Role in Human Psychopathology

Developmentally, the noradrenergic neuronal system, which mediates arousal and anxiety, two primitive defenses necessary for survival, appears at the earliest stages of brain development. As noted, in the first year of life, increased arousal, fear of strangers, and separation anxiety emerge and may involve this system. In addition, cortical noradrenergic input may modulate synaptic plasticity and modifiability early in development (Kasamatsu and Pettigrew, 1976). This neuromodulatory function provides a basis for an hypothesized relationship between affect-laden experiences in infancy and the establishment of the synaptic organization of the cerebral cortex. Therefore, this system appears to be important in early life in interaction and regulation of behavior with the external environment. Higher levels may be associated with better concentration and selective attention, but also with anxiety and overinhibition. Conversely, low levels may be related to inattention, reduced anxiety, and lack of inhibition. Moreover, norepinephrine may be linked to a behavioral facilitatory system, which mobilizes behavior, and an opposing system, which may inhibit behavior that has no contextual match in past experiences.

The noradrenergic system has also been implicated in the pathophysiology of mood disorders through the action of antidepressant drugs. The last decade has witnessed mounting evidence of the occurrence of major depressive disorder, not only in adolescents, but also in prepubertal children (Kovacs et al., 1984; Puig-Antich and Weston, 1983). These depressive episodes have the same cognitive and physiologic features as those in adults, including anhedonia and suicidal preoccupation (Puig-Antich and Weston, 1983). Furthermore, mood disorders in children may respond to antide-

pressant treatment in a manner similar to that in adults, although this issue is not yet clearly established.

NEURONS OF THE SEROTONIN SYSTEM

The serotonergic neurons (Fig. 3–3) are located in the reticular core in the raphe nuclei in the midbrain anterior to the locus coeruleus. Serotonin neurons are formed later in brain development than those of the noradrenergic system and also send axons to virtually all areas of the fetal nervous system (Lauder and Krebs, 1976). Like the noradrenergic neurons, the serotonergic neurons provide an extremely diffuse innervation to the cerebral cortex, corpus striatum, and limbic system. These neurons utilize the indolamine, serotonin, as their neurotransmitter. It is synthesized from the essential amino acid, tryptophan, by enzymes contained in the nerve terminal (see Table 3–1). In contrast to the noradrenergic input, the serotonergic input to the cerebral cortex develops more gradually (Lidov and Molliver, 1982). The early innervation of the primordial cortex by serotonergic neurons apparently plays a role in modulating neuronal development, because disruption of the serotonergic nervous system alters the rate of cell division in the fetal cerebral cortex. The

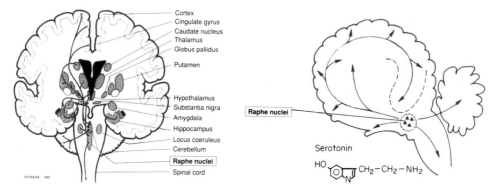

Figure 3–3. *Serotonin neuronal system.* The serotonin neuronal system is depicted in coronal section (left) showing brain structures. Solid lines represent axonal projections from cell bodies to specific brain areas. On the right, a schematic drawing is shown in saggital section (left figure from Rogeness, Javors, and Plisza, 1992; right figure from Coyle and Harris, 1987).

dual input by noradrenergic and serotonergic neurons may interact in modulating neuronal activity in the various brain regions.

Serotonin Receptors

Multiple presynaptic ($5HT_{1A}$, $5HT_{1D}$) and post-synaptic receptors ($5HT_{1A}$, $5HT_{1C}$, $5HT_{1D}$, $5HT_2$, $5HT_3$) have been identified. Receptors and second messengers are shown in Table 3–1.

Functions of the Serotonin System

The serotonin system is widely distributed and has been shown to establish a pacemaker pattern on activity (Cooper, Bloom, and Roth, 1991). By modulating effects on neuronal excitability in widely diverse brain regions and the spinal cord, the serotonin system can coordinate complex motor and sensory patterns of behavior. In animal studies, serotonin activity is greatest during waking arousal, reduced when quietly awake, substantially reduced in slow wave sleep, and fully absent in REM sleep. Increased tonic activity during waking arousal would enhance motor neuron excitability, whereas cessation of activity during REM sleep would inhibit motor movement, as is observed during this sleep state.

Role in Human Psychopathology

The serotonergic system has a potential role in the regulation of mood (Murphy, Campbell, and Costa, 1978), and may be involved in inhibiting irritable, aggressive behavior. Higher serotonin levels may be associated with better impulse control and with reduced aggression. On the other hand, low levels have been associated with poor impulse control and increased aggression. Moreover, there is clinical evidence of altered serotonin function in mood disorders (Van Praag, 1982), overly aggressive states, suicide, and schizophrenia. The serotonergic system has long been implicated in the pathophysiology of infantile autism. Consistent with the early innervation of cortical and limbic structures by the serotonergic system, the symptoms of infantile autism appear within the first 18 months of life. Over the last decade, in a significant portion of individuals suffering from infantile autism, there have been several reports of elevated levels of serotonin in whole blood (Young et al., 1982).

Neurons of the Dopamine System

The dopamine neurons in the substantia nigra lie even more anteriorly in the midbrain and, in man, are formed during a brief period of cell division in the late first trimester. The dopaminergic neurons utilize dopamine as their neurotransmitter (Fig. 3–4). Dopamine is synthesized by enzymes contained within nerve terminals from the amino acid tyrosine (see Table 3–1). Soon after their formation, dopaminergic neurons from the substantia nigra send axons to the primordial striatum. Moreover, the initial input to the striatum involves localized islands of dopaminergic innervation (Graybiel et al., 1981). These islands seem to be important developmental organizational points for the striatum, because their distribution correlates with both the ingrowth of other inputs to the striatum as well as cell divisional activity of intrinsic striatal neurons. With maturation, these initial outposts of striatal dopaminergic innervation soon spread to achieve the confluent pattern observed in the adult striatum. Quantitative neurochemical studies indicate that, in rats as well as in man, striatal dopaminergic innervation develops very gradually until puberty.

This system is more complex than the adrenergic system, because not only are there more dopamine containing cells, there are several major nuclei containing dopamine neurons and also more localized cell groups. Cooper, Bloom, and Roth (1991) suggest these be categorized according to the length of the efferent dopamine fibers (e.g., ultrashort, intermediate length, and long length). The long-length systems, which extend from the ventral tegmentum and substantia nigra, are of most importance in regard to psychiatric conditions. The targets of these long neurons are the neostriatum, i.e., the caudate and putamen (nigrostriatal system); the limbic cortex, i.e., the cingulate, medial prefrontal, and entorhinal areas (mesocortical system); and other limbic structures, i.e., the amygdala, nucleus accumbens, and septum (mesolimbic system).

The dopaminergic neurons in the substantia nigra provide a very diffuse and massive innervation to the corpus striatum (i.e., the caudate and putamen). It is estimated that 15% of the nerve ter-

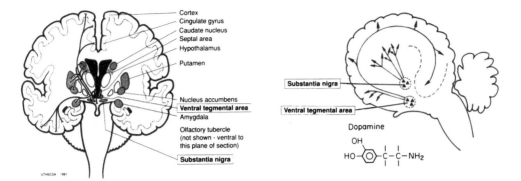

Figure 3–4. *Dopamine neuronal system.* The dopamine neuronal system is depicted in coronal section (left) showing brain structures. Solid lines represent axonal projections from cell bodies to specific brain areas. On the right, a schematic drawing is shown in saggital section (left figure from Rogeness, Javors, and Plisza, 1992; right figure from Coyle and Harris, 1987).

minal synapses in the corpus striatum are dopaminergic. This system plays a critical role in modulating motor activity, as evidenced by the the symptoms of Parkinson's disease, a disorder that involves the nigrostriatal dopamine system and results from a selective degeneration of dopaminergic neurons (Hornykiewicz, 1966). The more medially located dopamine neurons in the ventral tegmentum area (VTA) innervate the limbic system and the frontal cortex, thus providing the origins of the mesolimbic and mesocortical dopamine systems. These systems also develop gradually through late childhood into adolescence.

Dopamine Receptors

Presynaptic (D_2, D_3) and postsynaptic (D_1 to D_5) receptors have been cloned and localized to chromosome sites. A variety of second messengers are used, as shown in Table 3–1. Seeman et al. (1987) have followed the developmental course of dopamine receptors, D_1 and D_2, in human brain from autopsied tissue in children and adolescents and documented reductions in receptor number with advancing age, particularly in males. Similar findings have been confirmed *in vivo* by Wong et al. (1984), using positron emission tomography (PET).

Functions of the Dopamine System

There is indirect evidence demonstrating that dopamine neurons play a role in reward sys-

tems, attentional mechanisms, cognitive integration (Moral-Maroger, 1977; Wise, 1982), and in working memory (Goldman-Rakic and Brown, 1982). Studies on the levels of biogenic amine metabolites in cerebrospinal fluid provide an indirect assessment of neurotransmitter metabolism in developing neurons. Cerebrospinal fluid levels of monoamine metabolites change with age from infancy throughout childhood until adulthood. Interestingly, levels are highest in infants and decline with age. These changes may provide indirect evidence of reduction in neurotransmitter turnover with age, but they may also indicate reduced clearance of the metabolites from the younger child's brain. Seifert, Fox, and Butler (1980) measured dopamine and serotonin metabolites in patients ranging in age from 1 week to 45 years. There was a strong inverse correlation in children between dopamine and serotonin metabolite concentrations and age. The decline in these metabolites with age was reported to be exponential. No similar significant age effect was observed for norepinephrine metabolites. In addition, Shaywitz et al. (1980) noted a difference in the ratio of serotonin to dopamine metabolites (5-HIAA/HVA ratio) between a group of boys and girls with neurological disorders. Compared with boys, girls had a lower accumulation of the dopamine metabolites and higher accumulation of the serotonin metabolites. The researchers question whether these differences may relate to the increased prevalence of neuropsychiatric disorders such as Tourette's syndrome, attention deficit disorder, and autism in boys in comparison to girls during middle childhood. In this regard, it is noteworthy that a decline in dopamine receptor density in males is found with advancing age as assessed through PET scan studies (Wong et al., 1984).

Role in Human Psychopathology

The dopaminergic system has long been considered a factor in the pathophysiology of attention deficit disorder with hyperactivity (Wender, 1976). High dopaminergic levels are associated with increased motor activity, aggression, and stimulus-seeking behavior. Conversely, decreased motor activity, reduced aggression, poor motivation, and lack of interest in others is associated with low levels.

Stimulants, such as D-amphetamine and methylphenidate, reputedly enhance central dopaminergic neurotransmission; clinically, they reduce activity and increase attention span in affected children. Paradoxically, neuroleptics, which block dopamine receptors, can also reduce the hyperactivity (although their potential effects on cognition and movement must be considered in treatment decisions) (Werry and Aman, 1975). Shaywitz and his colleagues (1976) have demonstrated similar effects in experimental animals. They destroyed the dopaminergic neurons innervating the forebrain of newborn rats, whereupon these pubescent rats exhibited increased motoric activity. Moreover, these investigators demonstrated that this hyperactivity can be reduced by administration of stimulants. However, Hunt, Minderaa, and Cohen (1985) have reported improvements in behavior with clonidine, an α_2-adrenergic receptor agonist, suggesting that the role of dopamine systems may not be as specific as previously suggested.

The gradual development of striatal-limbic dopaminergic pathways may account for the age-related emergence of two disorders thought to involve enhanced dopaminergic neurotransmission: Tourette's syndrome and schizophrenia. In the case of Tourette's syndrome, symptoms typically emerge between 5 and 12 years of age with the appearance of hyperactivity, motor tics, and vocal tics, which evolve over

time. It is well known that the symptoms of the disorder are exacerbated by stimulants, which enhance dopaminergic neurotransmission, and are attenuated by neuroleptics, which block dopamine receptors; hence, the emergence of such symptoms would likely result from the development of altered dopaminergic neurotransmission (Singer et al., 1982). Tourette's symptoms appear to be the result of dysregulation of the dopaminergic system. Moreover, evidence has now accumulated of decreased levels of the dopamine metabolite, homovanillic acid, in the cerebral spinal fluid of Tourette patients. In light of that, there is reason to believe that the syndrome involves an increased postsynaptic response to dopamine, possibly due to a supersensitivity of the dopamine receptors (Singer et al., 1982). With the recent, more restrictive definition of schizophrenia in childhood, it is apparent that this disorder represents an earlier age of onset of a condition that is phenomenologically identical to the schizophrenic illness that typically has its onset in mid-to-late adolescence. Thus, the appearance of positive symptoms of schizophrenia, the symptoms most responsive to neuroleptic medications, occur on an age-related continuum — beginning in childhood, but peaking in late adolescence when dopamine levels in the forebrain have reached their highest levels.

Neurons of the Cholinergic System

The most anterior components of the reticular core are the cholinergic neurons of the basal forebrain complex (Fig. 3–5). Cholinergic cell bodies are scattered from the base of the midbrain overlying the hypothalamus anteriorally to the medial septum. Acetylcholine which is utilized by cholinergic neurons, as the neurotransmitter, is synthesized within the nerve terminals from choline. These neurons provide a diffuse innervation to all areas of the cerebral cortex, hippocampus, and limbic system. Studies of Alzheimer's disease, a disorder involving a striking degeneration of these cholinergic neurons, indicate that this cholinergic pathway plays an important role in memory and perhaps in other higher cognitive functions (Coyle, Price, and DeLong, 1983).

Because of the size and anterior–posterior extent of this complex, the neurons that extend

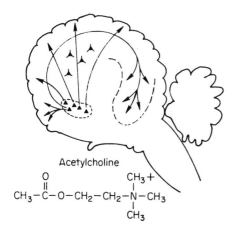

Acetylcholine

$$CH_3-\overset{\overset{O}{\|}}{C}-O-CH_2-CH_2-\overset{\overset{CH_3}{|}}{\underset{\underset{CH_3}{|}}{N}}-CH_3^+$$

Figure 3–5. *Cholinergic neuronal system.* Schematic drawing of cholinergic neuronal pathways shown in sagittal section (from Coyle and Harris, 1987).

from it undergo division over a prolonged period of time; in addition, this occurs later in development than is true for the more caudally located components of the reticular core. Nevertheless, the cholinergic basal forebrain complex is formed well in advance of the development of its target areas of innervation in the cortex, hippocampus, and limbic system. In contrast to the early appearance of noradrenergic and serotonergic fibers in the primordial cortex, invasion by cholinergic axons occurs much later. In the rodent, cholinergic innervation to the cortex does not occur until a full week after birth, and the limited information from studies with primate cortex suggests that the peak development of cholinergic innervation of cortex occurs during the first year after birth (Coyle and Yamamura, 1976). As the cortical cholinergic projections appear to be the last of the developing components of the reticular core, it is thought that this input may play a role in finalizing or cementing synaptogenesis in the cortex.

Cholinergic Receptors

There are both cholinergic muscarinic and nicotinic receptor subtypes. The muscarinic are divided into five subtypes, designated M_1 to M_5, all of which have been cloned. The M_2 receptor is primarily presynaptic. All are linked to G-proteins. There are four subtypes of nicotinic receptors. Neuromuscular blocking agents are specific antagonists.

Functions of the Cholinergic System

The forebrain cholinergic system is implicated in higher cognitive functions, especially memory. The cholinergic system is also involved in the mediation of REM sleep.

Role in Human Psychopathology

Clinical psychopharmacologic and lesion studies in experimental animals have implicated the forebrain cholinergic projections in higher cognitive functions, especially memory. This influence has been strengthened by the demonstration of rather selective and striking impairments in cortical and hippocampal cholinergic integrity in Alzheimer's dementia (Coyle, Price, and DeLong, 1983). Thus, it appears more than coincidental that the postnatal development of cholinergic innervation to the cerebral cortex and hippocampal formation corresponds with the emergence at the end of the first year of life of complex cognitive functions such as speech and memory. Although there is little direct evidence at present to support the hypothesis, one must wonder whether dysfunction of selective aspects of cortical cholinergic projections might not contribute to hereditary and acquired learning disorders. In this regard, evidence has accumulated of rather selective cortical cholinergic deficits in middle-aged individuals with Down syndrome who exhibit the neuropathology of Alzheimer's disease (Price et al., 1982). Although the functional integrity of these cholinergic pathways in younger Down individuals, who do not exhibit the pathology of Alzheimer's disease, remains to be determined, there is pharmacologic evidence of a compromised cholinergic system even in young Down syndrome patients (Harris and Goodman, 1968). Furthermore, in a mouse that suffers from trisomy of the genes coded on chromosome 21 in man, studies on the fetal brain indicate a developmental failure of the cholinergic neurons (Singer et al., 1984).

AMINO ACID NEUROTRANSMITTERS

Amino acids are probably the major neurotransmitters in the central nervous system. However, because they are involved in intermediary metabolism, it has been difficult for them to fully meet the established criteria as designated neurotransmitters. They have been separated into two classes, inhibitory (e.g. GABA) and excitatory (e.g., glutamic acid and aspartate).

GABAergic Neurons

GABA was first synthesized in 1883, but it was not until 1950 that it was identified as an almost exclusive constituent of the normal nervous system in mammals. The GABAergic neurons are local circuit neurons in the cerebral cortex, globus pallidus, substantia nigra, cerebellum, spinal cord, and projecting neurons, so they are not components of the reticular core. In the cerebral cortex, they play an essential role in the local processing of information, and in general, they comprise a major class of local circuit neurons. They utilize γ-aminobutyric acid (GABA) as their neurotransmitter, which is synthesized from the amino acid, L-glutamic acid, by glutamic acid decarboxylase (GAD). GABA is the primary inhibitory neurotransmitter in the brain and may serve as the chemical messenger for up to 30% of brain synapses (Enna and Gallagher, 1983). The GABAergic neurons intrinsic to the cortex are scattered throughout all cortical layers (Ribak, 1978); in particular, they provide important inhibitory input to the pyramidal cells, the primary output system from the cortex. The GABA receptors mediating the effect of this neurotransmitter are linked to receptor sites for the benzodiazepines. A number of anticonvulsants are known to interact directly with the GABA receptor, and the anxiolytic benzodiazepines indirectly enhance the sensitivity of the GABA receptors to their neurotransmitter (Coyle, Price, and DeLong, 1983).

In contrast to the systems described previously, which are components of the reticular core, the cortical GABAergic neurons are local circuit neurons. The progenitors of the cortical GABAergic neurons are found in the subcortical ventricular germinal zone, which produces immature GABAergic neurons throughout the period of cortical formation. Thus, the GABAergic neurons appear much later in brain development than do the reticular core neurons, and GABAergic neuronal maturation coincides with the progressive differentiation of neurons within the cerebral cortex. Synaptic neurochemical studies, however, indicate that the biochemical components involved in the synthesis, release, and inactivation of GABA do not develop in a coordinated fashion as they do in the case of the noradrenergic, serotonergic, and dopaminergic systems (Coyle and Enna, 1976). The levels of GABA in the immature brain are disproportionately high in comparison to the relative activity of its synthetic enzyme, glutamic acid decarboxylase; at early stages of development, the high-affinity uptake–inactivation process for GABA surpasses its activity in adulthood. In contrast, within the cerebral cortex, the postsynaptic GABA receptors and their modulatory benzodiazepine receptors exhibit a much more gradual developmental increase.

GABA Receptors

There are two major types of GABA receptors: $GABA_A$ and $GABA_B$. $GABA_A$ sites have different locations in the central nervous system. Both types have pre- and postsynaptic locations and appear to act independently in synaptic transmission. Unlike $GABA_A$, $GABA_B$ is not linked to a chloride channel. In addition to these receptors, there is a GABA transporter. Moreover, GABA may coexist in the same cell with 5-HT, DA, Ach, and a variety of peptides (e.g., CCK and Substance P).

Functions of the GABA System

The evidence for the role of GABA as a neurotransmitter is less complete than for the neurons of the reticular core. The establishment of neurotransmission is more difficult for amino acids because they may play a dual role both in metabolism and in neurotransmission. However, both neurophysiologic and biochemical studies have demonstrated that most of GABA found in the brain serves a neurotransmitter function (Cooper, Bloom, and Roth, 1991).

Role in Human Psychopathology

GABA involvement has been suggested in anxiety disorders, Huntington's disease, Parkinsonism, seizure disorders, schizophrenia, tardive dyskinesia, dementia, and several behavioral disorders.

Glutamic Acid

Glutamate is another broadly distributed amino acid neurotransmitter. Its stimulatory effects on neuronal activity were first demonstrated through direct topical application to the mammalian brain. Approximately 40% of brain synapses are glutamatergic, yet at one point there were questions about whether or not glutamate was a neurotransmitter. This was finally established by demonstrating that virtually all neurons in the brain that receive glutamate are depolarized and show an increase in firing rate. Depolarization is calcium-dependent and involves glutamate release from defined excitatory pathways. There is also a sodium-dependent, high affinity uptake of glutamate in the defined excitatory pathways and in glia.

Glutamic acid is found in high levels throughout the nervous system and is especially enriched in the hippocampus and neocortex. Regionally, it is found also in large quantities in the spinal cord where it is highest in the dorsal area. Unlike most neurotransmitters, glutamate is involved in intermediary metabolic processes in neural tissue. Therefore, it is difficult to distinguish whether mechanisms for synthesis, transport, and release are for metabolism or for neurotransmission (Headley and Grillner, 1991). In fact, one of the glutamate receptors is referred to as *metabotrophic* because of its involvement in regulating the metabolism of inositol triphosphate. Due to its metabolic and precursor roles, the presence of glutamate is not restricted to a specific type of neuron as are dopamine, acetylcholine, and the other neurotransmitters previously discussed. As a result, the glutamate system is not so accurately mapped by identifying the presence of glutamate or its synthesizing enzymes.

Glutamic acid is released from primary afferent nerve endings. Evidence for neurotransmission is based on meeting four criteria: (1) presynaptic localization, with storage and release from synaptic vesicles; (2) release by a calcium-dependent mechanism by physiologic stimuli, leading to postsynaptic response; (3) an uptake mechanism exists to terminate its action; and (4) it is pharmacologically identical to a naturally occurring substance (Cooper, Bloom, and Roth, 1991). Like GABA, it is released from the cortex of the cat at a rate dependent on the state of CNS activation.

Excitatory Amino Acid Receptors

Study of the excitatory effects of glutamate have been advanced through investigation of analogues of glutamic acid that are specific and potent in depolarizing central neurons. These are kainic acid, iboteric acid, and quisqualic acid. For example, kainic acid is 50 times more potent in its excitatory effects than glutamate. Kainic acid's neurotoxic effects involve an interaction with specific receptors.

A family of kainate, AMPA (quisqualate), and NMDA (N-methyl-D-aspartic acid) receptor channels have been cloned and sequenced. Each receptor subtype has a different regional distribution in the brain (see Fig. 3–6). There are then several glutamate receptors which include kainic acid, AMPA, and NMDA. Each of these substances is mediated by a separate and pharmacologically distinct, ligand-gated ion channel.

Understanding of the amino acid transmission has been enhanced by characterization and isolation of these receptor subtypes. The development of selective agonists and antagonists has led to the recognition of the three subtypes mentioned plus two additional ones. There are five different and distinct types of receptors in the central nervous system: NMDA, kainate, AMPA (an α-aminopropionic acid), AP4, and ACPD. The first three of these are excitatory, AP4 is an inhibitory autoreceptor, and ACPD is a metabotrophic receptor that modifies inositol phosphate (IP) metabolism.

The NMDA receptor is competitively inhibited by AP5. There are also noncompetitive channel blockers, such as phencyclidine and a modulatory glycine site. Both physiologic roles and excitotoxicity have been described for the glutamate system. First, physiologic roles have been described in cognition and sensation. The NMDA receptor mediates long-term potentiation (LTP), a cellular analogue of memory in which marked stimulation of excitatory pathways will produce a permanent enhancement of synaptic efficacy (see Chapter 9). Ethanol, which results in sedation, will interfere with glutamate neurotransmission. Second, excitotoxicity has been described with activation of the glutamate system. For example, systemic treatment of newborn infants with monosodium glutamate causes selective neuronal degeneration in the retina and in the hypothalamus.

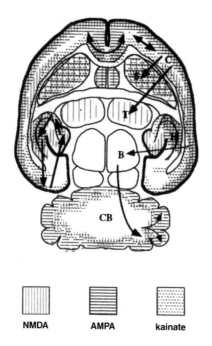

NMDA   AMPA   kainate

Figure 3–6. *Glutamate system.* Major excitatory amino acid transmitter pathways and the distribution of excitatory amino acid receptor subtypes in rodent brain is shown in horizontal section. **C,** cerebral cortex; **S,** striatum; **T,** thalamus; **H,** hippocampus; **B,** brainstem; **CB,** cerebellum (from Young and Fagg, 1991).

Olney (1989) proposed the excitotoxic hypothesis, according to which glutamate depolarizes neurons causing an initial influx of sodium and water through effects on AMPA glutamate channels, which are selectively localized to neuronal dendrites and cell bodies. With this influx, glutamate toxicity is manifested acutely by swelling of neuronal cell bodies, leading to brain edema. Later, delayed toxicity may occur via NMDA receptors by increased and sustained calcium entry. It is thought that glutamate kills by excitation and probably the release of NO (Snyder, 1992). Although there are limitations to the excitotoxic hypothesis, it is one of considerable importance and may be involved as a mechanism in a variety of disorders.

Functions of the Glutamate System

The NMDA type of glutamate receptor, in addition to its role in long-term potentiation, may

be involved in fine control of coordinated movement, memory, and learning, and possibly in epilepsy and neurodegeneration from prolonged depolarization by endogenous and exogenous amino acids (Watkins, 1989).

Role in Human Psychopathology

Selective neuronal vulnerability is noted in several disorders: Huntington's disease, hypoxic/ischemic damage, Alzheimer's disease, and AIDS dementia. In addition, schizophrenia has also been linked to NMDA systems (Freed, 1988). Therapeutic applications for drugs modulating excitatory neurotransmitters have been proposed based on the new understanding of the physiology and pharmacology of the excitatory amino acids. However, a limited number of drugs have reached clinical evaluation. The major therapeutic applications are for anticonvulsive therapy, neuroprotection (e.g., following hypoxic/ischemic damage, from exogenous neurotoxins or endogenous excitotoxins), and for psychiatric disorders.

The anticonvulsant hypotheses are based on the effects of glutamate and aspartate in causing convulsions. The roles in neuroprotection are based on blocking the effects of excitotoxicity previously described. Clinical syndromes with selective premature cell death might involve excessive activation of excitatory amino acid systems, or environmental excitotoxins might be involved. In Huntington's disease, selective degeneration of striatal neurons has been noted with a sparing of dopaminergic terminals. Hence, the pathology of Huntington's disease may be re-created through intrastriatal injections of kainic acid. In Alzheimer's disease, there is a reduction in NMDA receptors in the cortex with aging. Moreover, it has been noted that amyloid sensitizes neurons to glutamate toxicity. In AIDS dementia, quinolinic acid levels are increased in the cerebral spinal fluid, and this acid is thought to act as an endogenous excitotoxin. Quinolinic acid is a metabolite of tryptophan, which acts at the NMDA receptor. Of particular interest is the role of excitotoxicity in hypoxia and ischemia. It is thought that this damage is the result of acute, marked metabolic increase. For example, studies of newborns with hypoxic damage and in older people with strokes have demonstrated excessive release of glutamate. The identification of this mechanism may potentially lead to methods of treatment, because NMDA and KA receptor antagonists do protect against neuronal damage. NO or CO may be of importance in this regard.

A role in psychiatric disturbances has been proposed on theoretical grounds for schizophrenia and anxiety disorders. Freed (1988) has suggested a role for the involvement of excitatory amino acids in schizophrenia, which focuses on the cortico-striatal pathway. He postulates that the antipsychotic effect of dopamine antagonists is due to a secondarily induced, reduced sensitivity of the cortico-striatal excitatory amino acid synapse. Dopamine does inhibit cortically evoked excitatory postsynaptic potentials (EPSPs) in striatal cells consistent with this hypothesis.

There are multiple sites where dysfunction of the glutamate to NMDA receptor neurotransmission may take place. Similarities have been noted between schizophrenia and phencyclidine (PCP) psychosis. The site of action of PCP is at the NMDA channel where it acts as a noncompetitive NMDA atagonist. Consequently, amino acid neurotransmitters might be involved in producing both positive and negative symptoms of schizophrenia. There is currently considerable interest in the developmental issues that relate to excitotoxicity at different phases in the life cycle.

NITRIC OXIDE AND CARBON MONOXIDE AS NEUROTRANSMITTERS

The most recent discoveries in neurotransmission are that nitric oxide (NO), a gas, is involved in sending signals between nerve cells. Because neurotransmitters generally come in chemical classes, following the recognition of the role of NO, efforts were made to look for other gases that might act to signal nerve cells. This led to the recognition that carbon monoxide may also serve as a neurotransmitter. The following section discusses both nitric oxide and carbon monoxide (CO) as neurotransmitters.

The first evidence that nitric oxide is present in the brain came from observations of dissociated cultures of neonatal cerebellar cells, which release a factor whose action on blood vessels is analogous to that of nitric oxide (NO) (Garthwaite, Charles, and Chess-Williams, 1988). The enzyme for synthesis of nitric oxide, NO synthetase (NOS), converts arginine into NO and citrulline. It has been purified and cloned and occurs in discrete neuronal popula-

tions in the brain as well as in the peripheral autonomic nervous system. NO cell processes are widely distributed in the brain. Brain endothelial forms of NOS have multiple regulatory sites, which include phosphorylation by three distinct enzymes and oxidation, which is mediated by multiple cofactors.

Unlike other neurotransmitters, NO is a gas that is not stored in synaptic vesicles or released by exocytosis. It does not act at conventional membrane associated receptors. Yet the biologic roles of NO may be more apparent than more conventional transmitter molecules. The enzyme NOS is regulated by calcium and calmodulin, which accounts for the ability of NO to mediate glutamate stimulation of cyclic GMP by way of NMDA receptors. This rapid activation of NOS by NMDA occurs as a result of the opening of the neuronal membrane calcium channels. There is a rapid influx of calcium, which binds calmodulin to directly activate NOS. It has been suggested (Snyder, 1992) that the cytotoxic effects of glutamate are mediated through the release of nitric oxide into adjacent brain regions.

Purification of the enzyme that synthesizes NO has permitted the production of antibodies and an immunohistochemical location method. Throughout the body NOS immunoreactivity occurs only in neurons and the endothelium of blood vessels. In the brain, NOS neurons display unique localization. NOS is found in the cerebellum, where localization is specific to basket cells and granule cells; it is not found in Purkinje cells. In the cerebral cortex and hippocampus, NOS is found in only 1% to 2% of neurons, yet granule cells of the dentate nucleus in the hippocampus have large amounts of NOS, although pyramidal cells in the hippocampus do not. In the striatum, NOS appears in scattered medium-to-large neurons in both cell bodies and neuropil. Overall, most brain regions contain some NOS cells, but they tend to have discrete localization. These localizations of NOS do not fit that of any known neurotransmitter.

Neurotransmitter-like Functions of NO

Neurotransmitter-like functions of NO have been described. In the brain, NO mediates actions of glutamate that involve the NMDA receptor. Glutamate and NMDA increase cyclic GMP levels about tenfold in cerebellar slices and triple NOS levels.

The criteria for status as a neurotransmitter that are satisfied by NO include the presence of its synthesizing enzyme in relevant neurons, its ability to mimic the effects of physiologic nerve stimulation, and prevention of the effects of nerve stimulation in blocking NO formation (Snyder, 1992). Unlike a conventional neurotransmitter, NO is not stored in synaptic vesicles and released by exocytosis. This suggests that it is a messenger that is synthesized on demand and diffuses out of neurons instead of being released by exocytosis. In summary, NO is an atypical neurotransmitter, which may lead to the revision of classical definitions of neurotransmission or the introduction of a new category of messenger molecule.

Functions of Nitric Oxide

NO is a neurotransmitter candidate that may provide protection from neurotoxicity, yet NO may also induce neurotoxicity, particularly relating to glutamate stimulation of NMDA receptors. It is postulated that NOS neurons release NO to kill adjacent neurons (Dawson et al., 1991). In primary cerebral cortical neuronal cultures, NMDA destroys up to 90% of neurons within 24 hours (Choi and Rothman, 1990). Although NOS occurs in only about 2% of cortical neurons, NOS processes are extensively projected, which accounts for this substantial cell loss. In this system, NOS inhibitors prevent neurotoxicity, as does removal of arginine from the medium.

Possible Role in Human Psychopathology

Because NMDA receptor stimulation is implicated in the neurotoxicity of vascular strokes, NO might play a role. This has been directly tested in mice, where repeated intraperitoneal doses of the NOS inhibitor, nitroarginine, reduce the volume of damaged brain tissue following ligations of the middle cerebral artery (Nowicki et al., 1991). This neuronal protection occurs even when the drug is administered after arterial ligation, suggesting possible therapeutic application in stroke patients. The protection provided by nitroarginine is greater than that of a specific NMDA antagonist, MK-801.

Carbon Monoxide

Another candidate in this novel class of gas neurotransmitter is carbon monoxide (Verma et

al., 1992). It is formed in the brain by the action of the enzyme heme oxygenase-2. A selective inhibitor of heme oxygenase-2 depletes cGMP, suggesting that CO, like NO, may be a physiologic regulator of cGMP. Like NO, CO activates guanylyl cyclase by binding to its heme moiety. This activation is one way that CO may transmit intracellular signals.

The synthesizing enzyme, heme oxygenase-2, shows discrete localization in the brain, in olfactory epithelium and granule cells, in the pyramidal cell layers and dentate gyrus of the hippocampus, in the granule and Purkinje cell layers of the cerebellum, in the pontine nuclei, and in the habenula. Moreover, guanylyl cyclase, the enzyme cells used to make the intracellular messenger cyclic GMP, has been identified in the same brain regions as the synthesizing enzyme nerve cells that make cyclic GMP when stimulated by CO. An inhibitor of CO, zinc protoporphyrin-9, blocks this effect.

Functions of Carbon Monoxide

The activation of soluble guanylyl cyclase by NO allows excitatory amino acids to stimulate cGMP activity in the brain. However, NOS and guanylyl cyclase are not always colocalized, so a considerable proportion of guanylyl cyclase may not act as a target for NO. In regions that lack NOS, heme oxygenase-2 and guanylyl cyclase are colocalized, suggesting that CO may also act as a regulator of guanylyl cyclase and mediate cGMP concentrations. These actions would occur in the cerebellum, hippocampus and olfactory epithelium, accounting for a potential role in smell, probably via nonglutaminergic synapses. Whether a specific neurotransmitter regulates the CO pathway just as glutamate acts on the NO pathway is not known. Additional research is needed on the activity of CO as a neural messenger. However, current evidence indicates that it is a neural messenger involved in the maintenance of endogenous cGMP concentrations in several brain regions.

Possible Role in Human Psychopathology

Perhaps the most intriguing suggestion is that CO may act as the retrograde messenger for long-term potentiation (LTP), the cellular mechanism that may underlie certain forms of learning and memory (Stevens and Wang, 1993). As a gas, CO could easily diffuse backward. Originally, NO was considered as the possible retrograde messenger, but its synthesizing enzyme was not found in some cells such as pyramidal cells. However, CO is abundant in pyramidal cells. An important feature of LTP is that a nerve cell that receives a signal sends a message back to the original cell that signaled it. This message facilitates the release of its neurotransmitter. Stevens and Wang (1993) demonstrated that long-term potentiation was blocked by inhibitors of the enzyme hemeoxygenase-2, which catalyzes the production of carbon monoxide formation. Moreover, when CO was blocked, previous learning was erased.

Future investigations are needed to determine if other gases act as putative neurotransmitters.

NEUROACTIVE PEPTIDES

Neuropeptides affect target cells in both the peripheral and central nervous systems. These targets include neuronal and glial cells as well as blood vessels and glands. These concentrations are lower in the brain, and they are potent at lower concentrations. Specific peptides have not been selectively linked to a given functional system in the brain or correlated with a specific pathological state. Unlike amino acids or monoamine neurotransmitters, which are the end products of enzymatic action, peptides are finally synthesized on ribosomes as prohormones in the perikaryon or dendrites of a neuron. All known peptides arise from these inactive prohormone precursors; the biologically active form is released by proteolytic enzymes. (Transmitter release is calcium-dependent, and some postsynaptic effects are mediated by directly altering ion channel conductance or indirectly regulating ion channels through second messengers, e.g., calcium, cyclic nucleotides or IP_3).

Neuropeptides may coexist with amino acids, monoamine neurotransmitters, and another neuropeptide in both central and peripheral neurons, as shown in Table 3–2. Because of this coexistence, it has been questioned whether there are specific "peptidergic" neurons (Cooper, Bloom, and Roth, 1991). Instead, the co-occurring peptide may enhance or enrich the coexisting compound. How interactions between these substances may occur in the central nervous system is unclear, although

a modulatory role is emerging. For example, dynorphin coexists with glutamate in the mossy fiber pathway in the hippocampus. Synaptic release of dynorphin causes presynaptic inhibition of neighboring mossy fibers. Dynorphin inhibits the induction and expression of mossy fiber long-term potentiation. Consequently, there is a functional basis for the coexistence of a neuropeptide and a neurotransmitter, each playing a different role in this brain region (Weisskopf, Zalutsky, and Nicoll, 1993). Such modulation may also occur without co-occurrence through effects on common target cells. Most often, the peptide enhances the effects of the primary transmitter by prolonging action. Moreover, it may be possible for the peptide to act as a primary neurotransmitter.

The basic families of peptides are oxytocin/vasopressin, the tachykinins (Substance P and neurotensin), glucogon-related peptides, pancreatic polypeptide-related peptides, and opioid peptides. In addition, individual peptides, such as CCK, somatostatin, and CRF, have been studied in psychiatric disorders.

Of these, the vasopressin/oxytocin and opioid families will be discussed here along with the individual peptides mentioned earlier.

Vasopressin/Oxytocin Family

The original mammalian neuropeptides are vasopressin and oxytocin. These two nonapeptides are synthesized in large neurons of the supraoptic and paraventricular nuclei. They are stored in the axons of these neurons in the neurohypophysis and released from there into the blood stream. Each is synthesized from a larger propeptide. In the hypothalamus the neurons of the supraoptic and paraventricular nucleus have axon collaterals that project within the nuclei, between the nuclei, and also to the median eminence. The dynamic regulation of oxytocin and vasopressin involves gonadal steroids, suggesting a gender-specific effect that is activated at puberty.

Functional Effects

Vasopressin analogues have been implicated in learning and memory. Vasopressin has also been implicated in several aspects of social affiliative behavior, including territorial displays and social memory. Winslow et al. (1992) found that vasopressin (AVP) mediates the

Table 3–2. Neuroactive Peptides Coexist with Other Transmitter

Transmitter	Peptide	Location
GABA	Somatostatin	Cortical and hippocampal neurons
	Cholecystokinin	Cortical neurons
Acetylcholine	VIP	Parasympathetic and cortical neurons
	Substance P	Pontine neurons
Norepinephrine	Somatostatin	Sympathetic neurons
	Enkephalin	Sympathetic neurons
	NPY	Medullary and pontine neurons
	Neurotensin	Locus ceoruleus
Dopamine	CCK	Ventrotegmental neurons
	Neutrotensin	Ventrotegmental neurons
Epinephrine	NPY	Reticular neurons
	Neurotensin	Reticular neurons
Serotonin	Substance P	Medullary raphe
	TRH	Medullary raphe
	Enkephalin	Medullary raphe
Vasopressin	CCK, dynorphin	Magnocellular hypo thalamic neurons
Oxytocin	Enkephalin	Magnocellular hypo-thalamic neurons

From Cooper, Bloom, and Roth, 1991.

increase in aggression associated with mating in the vole. Because selective aggression is an aspect of male pair bonding, these results suggest a role for AVP in social attachment in this species.

Oxytocin recently has been linked to attachment behavior (Williams, Carter, and Insel, 1992). Central administration of oxytocin agonists and antagonists linked this peptide to maternal behavior, reproductive behavior, grooming, and quieting of isolated young.

Endogenous Opioid Peptides

From recombinant DNA techniques, multiple endogenous opioid systems belonging to three genetically distinct families have been identified (Akil et al., 1984; Khachaturian et al., 1985; Knigge and Joseph, 1984). These are the (1) opiocortin (β-endorphin and ACTH), (2) enkephalin, and (3) dynorphin groups. Just as differences in function have been demonstrated between the monoamines previously discussed, the catecholaminergic and serotonergic systems, so too the differences among opioid systems are present.

Opiocortin System

Derived from a larger peptide precursor, Proopiomelanocortin or POMC contains one opioid peptide (β-endorphin), ACTH, and potentially three melanocyte stimulating hormonelike (MSH) peptides. These peptides are generated by the enzymatic cleavage of the larger precursor. In the subprimate species studied, peptides from POMC have been found in several major brain sites. The primary site is the corticotrophes of the anterior lobe of the pituitary and all the cells of the pars intermedia. Within the brain, the main cell group is in the region of the arcuate nucleus (Fig. 3–7) of the medial basal hypothalamus; its fibers project widely to areas of the limbic system and brainstem.

There is another concentration of brain POMC found in the nucleus of the solitary tract and in the nucleus commissuralis. The endorphin systems appear to develop contemporaneously in the rat brain (Bayon et al., 1979). A developmental study of this system in the rat brainstem found a 20-fold increase in total content of endorphin in the medulla with minimal alterations in the concentration of β-endorphin (Alessi and Khachaturian, 1985).

Enkephalins

Unlike POMC, the enkephalin precursor, pro-enkephalin produces only active opioid peptides, Met-enkephalin and Leu-enkephalin, seven copies of which are contained in its core. It is found in neuronal systems wholly separate from POMC neurons. Distribution is very widespread, with both endocrine and brain distribution. In the brain, these peptides are located in neuronal systems throughout the neuraxis, including cells of the cerebral cortex down to the spinal cord. Fiber tracts are being mapped that include local circuit and long-tract systems associated with pain, respiration, endocrine actions, motor activity, and limbic system functions. In the periphery, an apparently similar precursor is found both in the adrenal medulla, with catecholamines, and in the gastrointestinal tract. Developmentally, Bayon et al. (1979) indicate that local enkephalin interneurons frequently migrate and differentiate later than do the larger enkephalin neurons; the latter form the neural pathways that project over long distances.

Dynorphin/Neo-endorphin

The dynorphin/neo-endorphin precursor, pro-dynorphin, produces three opioid peptides.

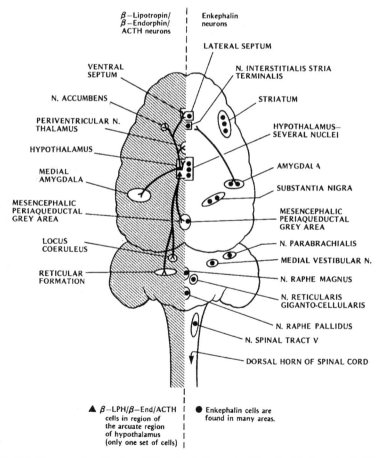

Figure 3–7. *Opioid system.* Localization of the enkephalins and of β-endorphin in rat brain. This horizontal cross section of the brain shows pathways of cells that are immunoreactive to β-LPH, β-endorphin, and ACTH. The right side indicates some locations of cells reacting to antibodies against enkephalin (from Barchas et al., 1978).

These are dynorphin A, dynorphin B, and two neo-endorphins, α and β. They have been found in brain, posterior pituitary, and gastrointestinal tracts. Pro-dynorphin has been noted in several hypothalamic cell groups and is widely scattered in the brain/stem. Pathways identified to date include those from the supraoptic nucleus to the posterior pituitary.

Opioid Receptors

Five receptors have been described to date. These are: mu (μ), delta (δ), kappa (κ), sigma (σ) and epsilon (ε). Mu agonists include morphine, β-endorphin, and enkephalins. Somatostatin is an antagonist. The delta receptor seems specific for enkephalins, and the kappa receptor has dynorphin as a preferential agonist. The sigma receptor is a putative receptor for opiates, because PCP and haldol are also agonists and agonist activity is not blocked by naloxone. Finally, an epsilon receptor for β-endorphin has been described in the vas deferens but not in the brain.

Role in Human Psychopathology

The potential role of brain endogenous opioid systems in human psychopathology remains highly speculative at present, and the development of these systems is not yet adequately characterized. It is therefore not possible to make a meaningful link between disturbances of these systems and the emergence of psychiatric symptoms. Self-injurious behavior is a frequent complication of severe and profound mental retardation. Because of the critical role of the endogenous opioid systems in pain perception and stress-induced analgesia, several authors (Richardson and Zaleski, 1983) have proposed that secondary abnormalities in the endogenous opioid systems might be responsible for the maintenance of certain forms of self-injurious behavior. There are reports of limited behavioral improvement in the autistic form of pervasive developmental disorder and in some cases of self-injurious behavior using naltrexone, an opioid antagonist.

NEURONAL SIGNALING MECHANISMS

Cellular mechanisms for neuronal signaling provide the basis for the study of perception, motor action, and learning. The methods of molecular genetics and molecular physiology are identifying signals, receptors, channels, enzymes, and genes at a rapid rate. Considerable progress has been made with the cloning of channels as well as receptors.

The study of signaling begins at the plasma membrane where the input signals are processed by voltage sensors and by chemical sensors. These are the two major kinds of synaptic transmission, electrical and chemical. In the brain, electrical synapses are less common than chemical synapses, but, where present, electrical synapses are characterized by rapid speed of transmission and stereotypical functioning. Electrical synapses do not easily permit inhibitory actions or long-lasting changes in response to signals.

Neuronal signaling requires the activation of different classes of ion channels, each of which is selective for particular ions. Ion channels represent a class of proteins that traverse or cross the cell membrane. They recognize and select among specific ions, conduct ions, and open and close in response to particular electrical, mechanical, or chemical signals (Kandel and Siegelbaum, 1991). Most ion channels involved in neuronal signaling are gated; like a gate, they open and close in response to these particular stimuli. The gated channels are particularly important for rapid neuronal signaling. These three types of channels are referred to as voltage-gated, transmitter-gated, and mechanically gated. An individual channel ordinarily uses only one type of signal mechanism. Other channels are not gated and are important for the general resting potential.

When a nerve cell is at rest, the membrane potential is determined by ion channels that are selectively permeable to potassium. During the action potential, channels selected for sodium are activated. These ion channels are 10 to 20 times more permeable to sodium than to potassium.

The membrane potential changes quickly during an action potential, up to 500 volts/second. Such rapid changes in potential differences are possible due to the ion channels. Ions are conducted across the cell membrane at rapid rates of up to 100 million ions/second to produce a large flow of ionic current.

Since the cloning of the first voltage-dependent channels, many such channels have been identified, suggesting a "super family" of voltage-dependent cation channels which all have a common basic structure. The study of mutations has allowed key structures that are involved in activation and formation of channel alignment to be identified. Changes of a single amino acid can lead to remarkable changes in the properties of a channel. The study of protein structure and the diversity of proteins involved is an ongoing challenge. With electron microscopy, chemical and electrical synapses have been shown to have different morphologies. In the electrical synapses, ion channels connect the cytoplasm of the pre- and postsynaptic cells whereas in chemical synapses, there is no cytoplasmic continuity between the cells and the neurons are separated by a synaptic cleft.

Chemical Transmission

Neurotransmitters cross the cell membrane by way of a plasma membrane transducing system (Schwartz and Kandel, 1991). This system consists of a cluster of proteins and lipids, which, for chemotransmission, most commonly consist of a neurotransmitter receptor directly bound to an ion channel or linked indirectly through a G-protein to an ion channel, and an enzyme or the ion channel that acts as a catalytic subunit. The receptor is embedded in plasma membrane that consists of a double layer of phospholipids.

Chemical synapses are more flexible than electrical synapses and are capable of maintaining change over time. Their plasticity is essential for memory and other higher brain functions. Chemical synapses can amplify neuronal signals, which allows a small presynaptic nerve terminal to alter the potential of a large postsynaptic cell. In contrast to electrical synapses, where there are gap junctions between two neurons that are bridged by channels, a chemical synapse has pre- and postsynaptic elements that are separated by a synaptic cleft. Two processes are involved in synaptic transmission: the presynaptic release of a chemical messenger and the postsynaptic receptive process, which establishes the binding of the transmitter to a receptor molecule in the postsynaptic cell.

The same chemical messenger may serve several functions. At one site it may act as a conventional neurotransmitter directly affecting neighboring cells, but in another site it may act as a neuromodulator to produce a more diffuse action that fine-tunes a neuron's response. At a third site, it might be released into the bloodstream and then act as a hormone. The molecules previously described — acetylcholine, gamma-aminobutyric acid (GABA), glycine, glutamate, serotonin, dopamine, and norepinepherine — and various peptides act as neurotransmitters. Yet the action of the specific chemical messenger on the postsynaptic cell depends not on the chemical nature of the transmitter but on the property of the receptors which that transmitter will bind. It is the receptor that determines, for example, whether a cholinergic synapse is excitatory or inhibitory and if an ion channel will be activated directly by the transmitter or indirectly through a second messenger mechanism. It is to be noted, however, that in a particular species, a given transmitter substance is associated with specific physiologic function.

All receptors for chemical transmission are membrane-spanning proteins. The part of the protein that is exposed to the external environment of the cell recognizes and binds the transmitter from the presynaptic cell. Then an effector function is carried out within the target cell (e.g., gating an ion channel or initiating a second messenger cascade).

Chemical neurotransmitters fall into two classes, depending on whether their gating of the ion channel is direct or indirect; these two classes are derived from distinct gene families. These two types of receptors show different functions. Receptors that gate ion channels directly produce fast action at the synapse in milliseconds. These systems are important for neural circuits that regulate behavior. Receptors that gate ion channels indirectly show slower synaptic action in seconds or minutes. Such slower actions may modulate behavior by altering the excitability of neurons and the strength of synaptic connections. Such modulatory synaptic systems may be involved in reinforcing stimuli in learning.

On the other hand, electrical transmission that occurs by means of current flow through gap junction channels is the most direct, so electrical transmission is the most rapid form of synaptic communication. Furthermore, groups of cells with electrical synapses may fire together when the collective threshold for that group is attained. Such speed and synchronous firing makes them suitable for fast, stereotypical behaviors (e.g., a defensive response). Still, directly gated chemical transmission is only slightly slower than the electrical form, because the receptors are part of the ion channel molecule. Even though the fastest chemical responses are slower than electrical synaptic responses, the chemical synaptic transmission has a selective advantage, because a single action potential on the cell will release many thousands of neurotransmitter molecules, resulting in an amplification of the synaptic response. In addition, due to the multiple processes involved, chemical transmission is more easily modified pharmacologically than is electrical transmission. This allows synaptic receptors to be selective targets for studying diseases as well as drug treatment.

Direct Gating

Receptors that gate ion channels directly consist of a single macromolecule, which contains several protein subunits that form the recognition element in the ion channel. Because they bind directly to ion channels, these are referred to as *ionophoric receptors*. When attached to a neurotransmitter, these receptors undergo a change in their morphology, which opens the channel.

With direct gating of an ion channel, the mediation occurs by a transmitter receptor that is part of the ion channel, as shown in Figure 3–8A₁. These receptors are multimeric, or multiple, and are made up of four or five subunits. Each subunit contains four or five membrane-spanning α-helical regions, as shown in Figure 3–8A₂. Examples are channels in the central nervous system that are regulated by glutamate, glycine, and GABA. The variation that may occur in subunits is striking. A central problem is to understand which combinations of subunits exist *in situ,* the nature of their functional differences, their localization, and whether it is possible to either discover or construct targeted drugs that would act selectively on one or a few of the existing combinations. This is a complex undertaking because it has been suggested that 4,400 different types of receptors are possible for ionotrophic receptors.

Indirect Gating

Other receptors gate ion channels indirectly (e.g., norepinephrine or serotonin synapses in the cerebral cortex). This involves separate receptors and ion channels that communicate through GTP binding proteins (G-proteins).

The receptor portion of the transduction system is a protein that is made up of seven membrane-spanning regions with inner and outer membrane loops (see Fig. 3–9). Dopaminergic, adrenergic, and serotonergic receptors have this structure. Despite the fact that each receptor consists of a single polypeptide chain, there may be multiple forms — e.g., there are five known dopamine G-protein coupled receptors. Specific receptor agonists bind to the outer membrane extracellular loop and activate the G-protein associated with the receptor. G-proteins may activate or stimulate (Gs) or inhibit enzymes (Gi) or ion channels to which they are coupled. This action leads to an increase or decrease in intracellular second messengers. The biochemical activity of a cell is established by the level of second messengers in the cell membrane or cytoplasm. All norepinephrine, dopamine, serotonin, and muscarinic receptors interact with G-proteins. A regulatory G-protein is associated with the internal leaflet of the plasma membrane and consists of α, β, and γ subunits. The α subunit is loosely associated with the membrane; the β and γ subunits are more tightly bound.

GDP is bound to the G-protein on the α subunit. As shown in the figure, when an agonist binds to the receptor, the GDP (not shown in the figure) is replaced with GTP. The activated α subunit stimulates or inhibits the activity of an ion channel or enzyme which is associated with this specific receptor. By means of these G-proteins, the receptors couple to effector enzymes, which produce intracellular second messengers, such as cAMP. It is the interaction of second messengers in the cytosolic compartment that determines cellular neuronal function.

Second messengers produce the activation or inactivation of intracellular biochemical or physiologic activity as a function of second messenger concentration. Subsequently, the second messenger, e.g., adenosine 3′ or 5′-cyclic phosphate (cAMP), causes the phosphorylation of several proteins, primarily protein kinases, that activate or inactivate other enzymes within a specific cell type (see Fig. 3–10). Depending on the cell type, the kinases vary, thereby providing added specificity for cAMP activity. Moreover, the calcium ion also

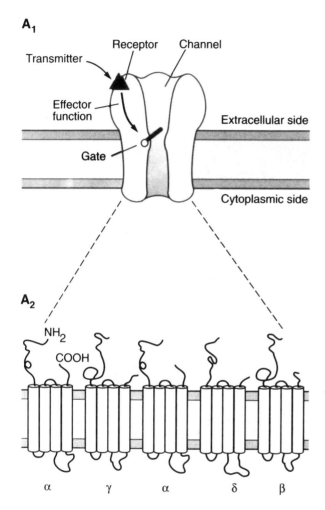

Figure 3–8. *Direct gating.* A₁. Direct gating of an ion channel is mediated by a transmitter receptor that is part of the ion channel. A₂. These receptors are composed of four (or five) subunits, each of which contains four or five membrane-spanning α-helical regions (from Kandel, Schwartz, and Jessell, 1991).

acts as a second messenger through binding to the intercellular protein calmodulin in a 4:1 ratio. The calcium ion/calmodulin complex causes phosphorylation of several enzymes. Once the second messenger, such as cAMP, is released, it may act on the channel directly or, more commonly, activate one of a family of enzymes called protein kinases, which then modulate channels by phosphorylating either the channel protein or a regulatory protein which then has its effect on the channel. Moreover, G-proteins may also interact with ion channels directly independent of second messenger production. In addition to these effects, second messengers also affect the transcription and translation processes.

HUMAN PSYCHOPATHOLOGY AND G-PROTEINS

In psychiatry, the role of the G-protein and the regulation of neuronal function may be important in the pathophysiology of mental disorders. About 80% of all known neurotransmitters, hormones, and neuromodulators (over 100) produce their cellular responses through G-proteins. The G-proteins transmit information to the effector site through coupling mechanisms. The G-proteins couple to effectors in the cytoplasm, such as adenylcyclase, phospholipase C, phospholipase A₂, and several ion channels.

Because G-proteins are involved in the integration, regulation, and amplification of signal transduction pathways, abnormalities in their

Human β₂ adrenergic receptor

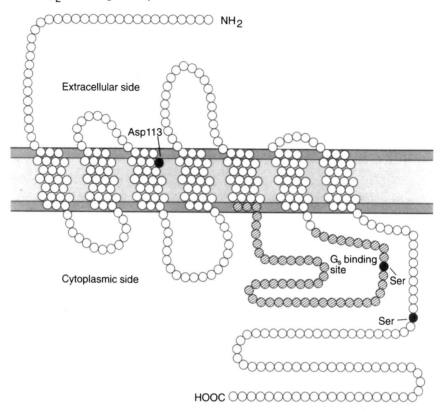

Figure 3–9. *Structure of a G-protein coupled receptor.* The structure of a G-protein coupled receptor contains seven membrane-spanning domains. The structure of the β₂-adrenergic receptor is shown. An important functional feature is that the binding site for the neurotransmitter (in this example norepinephrine) is just within the lipid bilayer on the extracellular surface of the cell (here amino acid residue aspartic acid 113). The part of the receptor indicated by striped circles is the part of the receptor with which G-protein associates. The two serine residues indicated in black are sites for phosphorylation (from Kandel, Schwartz, and Jessell, 1991).

function and/or expression may be involved in a number of pathophysiologic states. This is a consideration because G-proteins provide the first opportunity for signals from different receptors to be integrated. This takes place as interactions link receptors, G-proteins, and their effectors with signals converging to share detectors. For example, G-protein abnormality is a consideration in alcoholism, schizophrenia, and chronic cocaine/opiate ingestion, and in corticosteroid administration following adrenalectomy.

SUMMARY

This chapter reviewed the basic amino acid, monoamine, cholinergic, and peptide neurotransmitters and then discussed neuronal sig-

naling that is pertinent to their actions. Following a description of the localization and function of the various neurotransmitter systems is a brief description of their respective roles in human psychopathology. These findings are only a beginning. With more refined methods, new findings related to the trophic effects of neurotransmitters, the interactions between transmitters and the effects of colocalized neurotransmitters and neuropeptides are becoming increasingly evident. Moreover, novel neurotransmitters continue to be developed. Behavioral research is advancing with the development of new agonists and antagonists, which are tested in more sophisticated behavioral paradigms and to a greater extent in transgenic animals. These developments suggest that the

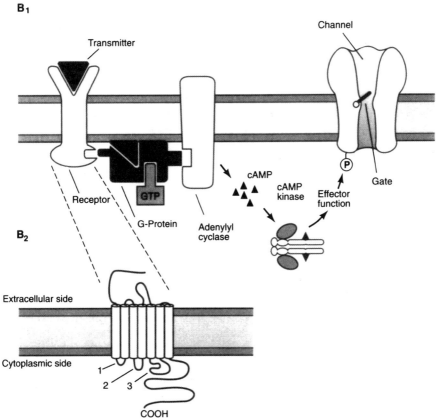

Figure 3–10. *Indirect gating is mediated by a second messenger that couples the receptor to the ion channel.* B_1. The receptor activates a GTP- binding protein (G-protein), which in turn activates a second-messenger cascade that modulates ion channel activity. The channel to be modulated and the receptor are different molecules. In this example, the G-protein stimulates adenylyl cyclase, which converts ATP to cAMP. The cAMP activates the cAMP-dependent protein kinase (cAMP-kinase), which phosphorylates the channel (**P**), leading to a change in function. B_2. The typical receptor of this family of proteins is composed of a single protein with seven membrane-spanning a-helical regions that bind the ligand within the plane of the membrane (from Kandel, Schwartz, and Jessell, 1991).

"Decade of the Brain" will provide exciting new knowledge in the emerging science of molecules and behavior.

REFERENCES

Akil, H., Watson, S.J., Young, E., Lewis, M.E., Khachaturian, H., and Walker, J.M. (1984). Endogenous opioids: Biology and function. *Annual Review of Neuroscience,* 7:223–255.

Alessi, N.E. and Khachaturian H. (1985). Postnatal development of beta-endorphin immunoreactivity in the medulla oblongata of rat. *Neuropeptides,* 5:473–476.

Barchas, J.D., Akil, H., Elliott, G.R., Holman, R.B., and Watson, S.S. (1978). Localization of the enkephalins and β-endorphin. *Science,* 200:964–973.

Bayon, A., Shoemaker, W.J., Bloom, F.E., Mauss, A., and Guillemin, R. (1979). Perinatal development of the endorphin and enkephalin containing system in the rat brain. *Brain Research,* 179:93–101.

Black, I.B. (1982). Stages of neurotransmitter development in autonomic neurons. *Science,* 215:1198–1204.

Choi, D.W. and Rothman, S.M. (1990). The role of glutamate neurotoxicity in hypoxic-ischemic neuronal death. *Annual Review of Neuroscience,* 13:171–182.

Cooper, J., Bloom, F.E., and Roth, R. (1991). *The biochemical basis of neuropharmacology.* Oxford University Press, New York, NY.

Coyle, J.T. (1985). Introduction to the world of neurotransmitters and neuroreceptors. In *Annual Review,* Vol. 4, edited by R.F. Hales and A.J. Frances, pp. 3–97. American Psychiatric Press, Washington, DC.

_____ and Enna, S.J. (1976). Neurochemical aspects of the ontogenesis of GABAergic neurons in the rat brain. *Brain Research,* 111:119–133.

_____ and Harris, J.C. (1987). The development of neurotransmitters and neuropeptides. In J. D. Noshpitz (ed), *Basic handbook of child psychiatry,* Vol. 5, *Advances and new directions,* pp. 14–25. Basic Books, New York.

_____ and Yamamura, H. (1976). Neurochemical aspects of the ontogenesis of cholinergic neurons in the rat brain. *Brain Research,* 118:429–440.

_____ and Molliver, M.E. (1977). Major innervation of newborn rat cortex by monoaminergic neurons. *Science,* 196:444–447.

_____, Price, D., and DeLong, M.R. (1983). Alzheimer's Disease: A disorder of cortical cholinergic innervation. *Science,* 219:1184–1190.

Dawson, V.L., Dawson, T.M., London, E.D., Bredt, D.S., and Snyder, S.H. (1991). Nitric oxide mediates glutamate toxicity in primary cortical culture. *Proceedings of the National Academy of Sciences USA,* 88:6368–6371.

Ehrlich, P. (1900). On immunity with specific reference to cell life. Croonian Lecture. *Proceedings of the Royal Society of London,* 66:424–448.

Enna, S.J. and Gallagher, J.P. (1983). Biochemical and electrophysiologic characteristics of mammalian GABA receptors. *International Review of Neurobiology,* 24:181–212.

Freed, W.J. (1988). The therapeutic latency of neuroleptic drugs and nonspecific postjunctional supersensitivity. *Schizophrenia Bulletin,* 14:269–277.

Furshpan, E.J., MacLeish, P.R., O'Lague, P.H., and Potter, D.D. (1976). Chemical transmission between rat sympathetic neurons and cardiac myocytes developing in microcultures: Evidence for cholinergic, adrenergic, and dual-function neurons. *Proceedings of the National Academy of Sciences USA* 73:4225–4229.

Garthwaite, J., Charles, S.L., and Chess-Williams, R. (1988). Endothelium-derived relaxing factor release on activation of NMDA receptors suggests role as intercellular messenger in the brain. *Nature,* 336:385–388.

Goldman-Rakic, P.S. and Brown, R.M. (1982). Postnatal development of monoamine content and activity in the cerebral cortex of rhesus monkeys. *Developmental Brain Research,* 4:339–349.

Graybiel, A.M., Pickel, V.M., Joh, T.H., Reis, D.J., and Ragsdale, C.W. (1981). Direct demonstration of a correspondence between dopamine islands and acetylcholinesterase patches in the developing striatum. *Proceedings of the National Academy of Sciences USA,* 78:5871–5875.

Harris, W.S. and Goodman, R.M. (1968). Hyperreactivity to atropine in Down's syndrome. *New England Journal of Medicine,* 279:407–410.

Headley, P.M. and Grillner, S. (1991). Excitatory amino acids and synaptic transmission: The evidence for a physiological function. *Trends in Pharmacological Sciences,* Special Report, pp. 30–36.

Hokfelt, T., Johansson, O., Ljungdahl, A., Lundberg, J.M., and Schultzberg, A.M. (1980). Peptidergic neurons. *Nature (London),* 284:515–521.

Hornykiewicz, O. (1966). Dopamine and brain function. *Pharmacological Reviews,* 18:925–964.

Hunt, R.D., Minderaa, R., and Cohen, D.J. (1985). Clonidine benefits children with attention deficit disorder and hyperactivity: Report of a double blind placebo study. *Journal of the American Academy of Child Psychiatry,* 24:617–629.

Hyman, C., Hofer, M., and Barde, Y.A. (1991). BDNF is a neurotrophic factor for dopamine neurons of the substantia nigra. *Nature,* 350:230–232.

Jacobson, M. (1991). *Developmental neurobiology.* Plenum Press, New York.

Kandel, E.R. and Siegelbaum, S.A. (1991). Directly gated transmission at the nerve-muscle synapse. In E. R. Kandel, J. H. Schwartz, and T. M. Jessell (eds) *Principles of neural science,* 3rd ed, pp. 135–152. Elsevier Science Publishing Co., New York.

_____, Siegelbaum, S.A., and Schwartz, J.H. (1991). Synaptic transmission. In E. R. Kandel, J. H. Schwartz, and T. J. Jessell (eds), *Principles of neural science,* 3rd ed, pp. 123–134. Elsevier Science Publishing Co., New York.

Kasamatsu, T. and Pettigrew, J.D. (1976). Depletion of brain catecholamines: Failure of ocular dominance shift after monoculary occlusion in kittens. *Science,* 194:206–209.

Kater, S.B., Mattson, M.P., and Guthrie, P.B. (1989).

Ca++-induced neuronal degeneration: A normal growth cone regulating signal gone awry? *Annals of the New York Academy of Science,* 568:252–261.

Katz, D.M., Markey, K.A., Goldstein, M., and Black, I.B. (1983). Expression of catecholaminergic characteristics by primary sensory neurons in the normal adult rat in vivo. *Proceedings of the National Academy of Sciences USA,* 80:3526–3530.

Khachaturian, H., Lewis, M.E., Schafer, M.K., and Watson, S.J. (1985). Anatomy of the CNS opioid systems. *Trends in Neuroscience,* 8:111–119.

Knigge, K.M. and Joseph, S.A. (1984). Anatomy of the opioid-systems of the brain. *Canadian Journal of Neurological Science,* 11:14–23.

Kovacs, M., Feinberg, T.L., Crouse-Novak, M.A., Paulauskas, S.L., Pollack, M., and Finkelstein, R. (1984). Depressive disorders in childhood: II. A longitudinal study of the risk for a subsequent major depression. *Archives of General Psychiatry,* 41:643–649.

Lankford, K.L., DeMello, F.G., and Klein, W.L. (1988). D-1 type dopamine receptors inhibit growth cone motility in cultured retina neurons: Evidence that neurotransmitters act as morphogenic growth regulators in the developing nervous system. *Proceedings of the National Academy of Sciences USA,* 85:4567–4571.

Lauder, J.M. and Bloom, F.E. (1974). Ontogeny of monoamine neurons in the locus coeruleus, raphe nuclei and substantia nigra of the rat. *Journal of Comparative Neurology,* 155:469–482.

———— and Krebs, H. (1976). Effects of p-chlorophenylalamine on time of neuronal origin during embryogenesis in the rat. *Brain Research,* 107:638–644.

Lidov, H. and Molliver, M.E. (1982). An immunocytochemical study of the development of serotonergic neurons in the rat CNS. *Brain Research Bulletin,* 8:389–430.

Lipton, S.A. and Kater, S.B. (1989). Neurotransmitter regulation of neuronal outgrowth, plasticity, and survival. *Trends in Neuroscience,* 12:265–270.

Moral-Maroger, A. (1977). Effects of levodopa on frontal signs in Parkinsonism. *British Medical Journal,* II:1543.

Murphy, D.L., Campbell, I., and Costa, J.L. (1978). Current status of the indolamine hypothesis of affective disorders. In M.A. Lipton, A. DiMascio and K.F. Killam (eds), *Psychopharmacology: A generation of progress,* pp. 1235–1248. Raven Press, New York.

Nowicki, J.P., Duval, D., Poignet, H. and Scatton, B. (1991). Nitric oxide mediates neuronal death

after focal cerebral ischemia in the mouse. *European Journal of Pharmacology,* 204:339–340.

Olney, J.W. (1989). Excitatory amino acids and neuropsychiatric disorders. *Biological Psychiatry,* 26:505–525.

Patterson, P.H. (1978). Environmental determination of autonomic neurotransmitter functions. *Annual Review of Neurosciences,* 1:1–17.

Price, D.L., Whitehouse, P.J., Struble, R.G., Coyle, J.T., Clark, A.W., DeLong, M.R., Cork, L.C., and Hedreen, J.C. (1982). Alzheimer's disease and Down's syndrome. *Annals of the New York Academy of Science,* 396:145–164.

Puig-Antich J. and Weston B. (1983). The diagnosis and treatment of major depressive disorder in childhood. *Annual Review of Medicine,* 34:231–245.

Ribak, C. (1978). Aspinous and sparsely-spinous stellate neurons in the visual cortex of rats contain glutamic acidic decarboxylase. *Neurocytology,* 7:461–478.

Richardson, J.S. and Zaleski, W.A. (1983). Naloxone and self-mutilation. *Biological Psychiatry,* 18:99–101.

Rogeness, G.A., Javors, M.A., and Pliszka, S.R. (1992). Neurochemistry and child and adolescent psychiatry. *Journal of the American Academy of Child and Adolescent Psychiatry,* 31:765–781.

Schwartz, J.H. and Kandel E.R. (1991). Synaptic transmission mediated by second messengers. In E.R. Kandel, J.H. Schwartz and T.J. Jessell (eds), *Principles of neural science,* 3rd ed, pp. 173–193. Elsevier Science Publishing Co., New York.

Seeman, P., Bzowej, N.H., Guan, H.C., Bergeron, C., Reynolds, G.P., Bird, E.D., Riederer, P., Jellinger, K., Watanabe, S., and Tourtellote, W. (1987). Human brain dopamine receptors in children and aging adults. *Synapse,* 1:399–405.

Seifert, W.E., Fox, J.L., and Butler, I.J. (1980). Age effects on dopamine and serotonin metabolite levels in cerebrospinal fluid. *Annals of Neurology,* 8:38–42.

Shaywitz, B.A., Klopper, J.H., Yager, R.D., and Gordon, J.W. (1976). Paradoxical response to amphetamine in developing rats treated with 6-hydroxydopamine. *Nature,* 261:153–155.

————, Cohen, D.J., Leckman, J.F., Young, J.G., and Bowers, M.B. (1980). Ontogeny of dopamine and serotonin metabolites in the cerebrospinal fluid of children with neurological disorders. *Developmental Medicine and Child Neurology,* 22:748–754.

Singer, H.S., Butler, I.J., Tune, L.E., Seifert, W.E., and Coyle, J.T. (1982). Dopamine dysfunction in Tourette syndrome. *Annals of Neurology,* 12:361–366.

Singer, H.S., Tiemeyer, M., Hedreen, J.C., Gearhart, J., and Coyle, J.T. (1984). Morphologic and neurochemical studies of embryonic brain development in murine Trisomy 16. *Developmental Brain Research*, 15:155–166.

Snyder, S.H. (1992). Nitric oxide and neurons. *Current Opinion in Neurobiology*, 2:323–327.

Stevens, C. F. and Yanyan, W. (1993). Reversal of long-term potentiation by inhibitors of haem oxygenase. *Nature* 364:147–149.

Van Praag, H.M. (1982). Depression, suicide and the metabolism of serotonin in the brain. *Journal of Affective Disorders*, 4:275–290.

Verma, A., Hirsch, D.J., Glatt, C.E., Ronnett, G.V., and Snyder, S.H. (1992). Carbon monoxide: A putative neural messenger. *Science*, 259:381–384.

Watkins, J.C. (1989). The NMDA receptor concept: Origins and development. In J.C. Watkins and G.L. Collingridge (eds), *The NMDA receptor*. Oxford University Press, New York.

Weisskopf, M.G., Zalutsky, R.A., and Nicoll, R.A. (1993). The opioid peptide dynorphin mediates heterosynaptic depression of hippocampal mossy fiber synapses and modulates long-term potentiation. *Nature*, 362:423–428.

Wender, P. (1976). Hypothesis for a possible biochemical basis of minimal brain dysfunction. In R.M. Knights and D.J. Baker (eds), *Neuropsychology of learning disorder*. University Park Press, Baltimore.

Werry, J.S. and Aman, M.G. (1975). Methylphenidate and haloperidol in children: Effects on attention, memory and activity. *Archives of General Psychiatry*, 32:790–796.

Williams, J.R., Carter, C.S., and Insel, T.R. (1992). The neurobiology of social attachment. II: Oxytocin and social bonding. *Abstracts of Panels and Posters. American College of Neuropsychopharmacology, 31st Annual Meeting*, p. 138.

Winslow, J.T., Hastings, N., Carter, C.S., and Insel, T.R. (1992). The neurobiology of social attachment. III: Vasopressin and selective aggression. *Abstracts of Panels and Posters. American College of Neuropsychopharmacology, 31st Annual Meeting*, p. 139.

Wise, R.A. (1982). Neuroleptics and operant behavior: The anhedonia hypothesis. *Behavior and Brain Science*, 5:39–87.

Wong, D.F., Wagner, H.N., Dannals, R.F., Links, J.M., Frost, J.J., Ravert, H.T., Wilson, A.A., Rosenbaum, A.E., Gjedde, A., Douglass, K.H., Petronis, J.D., Folstein, M.F., Tuong, J.K., Burns, H.D., and Kuhar, M.J. (1984). Effects of age on dopamine and serotonin receptors measured by positron tomography in the living human brain. *Science*, 226:1393–1396.

Young, A.B. and Fagg, G.E. (1991). Excitatory amino acid receptors in the brain: Membrane binding and receptor autoradiographic approaches. *Trends in Pharmacological Sciences, A Special Report*, pp. 18–24.

Young, J.G., Kavanaugh, M.E., Anderson, G.M., Shaywitz, B.A., and Cohen, D.J. (1982). Clinical neurochemistry of autism and associated disorders. *Journal of Autism and Developmental Disorders*, 12:147–165.

CHAPTER 4
SLEEP AND CIRCADIAN RHYTHMS

Sleep plays a crucial role in the development of brain and behavior, so disturbances in sleep may affect developmental processes, yet the ancient view was that during sleep all mental functions cease. In fact, Hesiod (Kandel, Schwartz, and Jessell, 1991) suggested that sleep is the brother of death. We now know, however, that during sleep, restoration of function takes place and special forms of mental activity do occur. Rather than a suspension of life, in sleep there is an occasion for physiologic restoration, the integration of experience into memory, and the opportunity to dream.

This chapter offers a definition of sleep, discusses sleep patterns, reviews the neurobiology of sleep, discusses the ontogeny of sleep and circadian cycles, provides background on the development of normal sleep, and discusses the functions of sleep.

DEFINITION OF SLEEP

Both behavioral and electrophysiological criteria are necessary to define sleep. Behaviorally, sleep is characterized by behavioral quiescence, a species-typical stereotypical posture, elevated arousal level, and the reversibility of the sleep state with moderately intense stimulation. The electrophysiological criteria for sleep are based on the two distinct states of nonrapid eye movement (NREM) and rapid eye movement (REM) sleep (see Figure 4–1). A glossary of terms related to the study of sleep is included at the end of the chapter.

In NREM sleep, there are characteristic high-voltage slow waves, spindles, and K complexes, which are recorded from the neocortex. On the other hand, REM sleep is characterized by a low-voltage, fast electroencephalogram (EEG), skeletal muscle atonia, rapid eye movements (REM), and ponto-geniculo-occipital (PGO) spikes from the pons, lateral geniculate body, and occipital cortex. There is a close correlation between these electrophysiological recordings and behavioral changes.

Although there is usually a recumbent sleep posture, under unusual circumstances movement can occur during sleep, as in sleepwalking, night terrors, and other arousal disorders. Furthermore, aspects of sleep may intrude into wakefulness, with dream imagery and muscle weakness occurring in disorders such as narcolepsy (I.C.S.D., 1990)

SLEEP PATTERNS

Determining the amount of time asleep requires considering the two basic sleep patterns, NREM and REM, which alternate about every 100 minutes throughout the night. These two basic kinds of sleep are distinguished by their type, but not by their depth. In both NREM and REM sleep, mental functioning continues, although there is relative quiescence of mental functions in the deepest stage of NREM. Yet, sensory impulses do continue to enter cortical areas during deep sleep. The kind of mental activity depends on which form of sleep is being studied, and it is

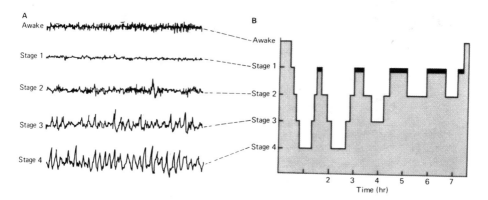

Figure 4–1. *The sleep/wake cycle. A.* The left side of the figure shows electroencephalographic recordings of wakefulness and sleep over a 30-second period. The top recording shows the low-voltage, fast activity during the awake stage and the next four recordings indicate the stages of increasingly deepening slow wave sleep. In stage 2 several 1- to 2-second recordings of sleep spindles, bursts of waxing and waning waves, are apparent. Stage 1 rapid eye movement (REM) sleep can only be distinguished from stage 1 non-REM sleep by using additional criteria from simultaneous electrooculogram and electromyogram recordings.

B. The right side of the figure shows the typical pattern of sleep in a young adult. REM sleep time is indicated by the black bars. The initial REM period is short (5–10 minutes) but lengthens in successive cycles. Stages 3 and 4, which together are commonly referred to as "delta sleep," are predominant in the first third of the night but may be completely absent in the later part of the night and in the early morning (from Kandel, Schwartz, and Jessell, 1991).

gauged by wakings and interview reports. The verbal reports given following awakenings from NREM are most often of thoughts or images, whereas following REM awakenings, reports are of dreams. If deep NREM occurs after a REM sleep episode, REM recall is reduced. In REM and in NREM sleep, if talking occurs, the words uttered and the thoughts dreamed may be correlated. Episodes of sleep talking and sleep-walking occur early in the night and arise from NREM sleep. This is also true of many episodes of bed-wetting. Physical activity or actions taking place in NREM sleep are not remembered. The amount of time spent in REM sleep is greatest in the newborn. In older children, the amount of REM sleep varies in proportion to body weight, and in some mental retardation syndromes may vary with cognitive capacity. The total REM sleep time is reduced with advancing age and following the administration of many drugs. Slow wave sleep declines in puberty and in the middle years of life, and may disappear after age 60. It leads eventually to a biphasic circadian pattern (i.e., an afternoon nap).

Rapid Eye Movement (REM) Sleep

The recognition of rapid eye movement sleep ushered in a new era of sleep research. In the early 1950s Aserinski and Kleitman (1953) measured sleep EEG activity and discovered the rapid eye movements, or REMs, that occurred during sleep. These were associated with more rapid breathing, increased heart rate, and muscular hypotonia. The brain waves recorded were rapid and of low amplitude, similar to those found during waking. It was subsequently demonstrated that these eye movements coincided with dream reports. When adults were awakened during the REM sleep period, over 80% of the time they reported having dreams. Subsequently, Dement and Kleitman (1957) demonstrated that REM sleep occurred in cycles four to five times each night.

Animal models, in cats, subsequently revealed that cerebral cortical activity was present during REM sleep and that the brain was intensely active even though it was not receiving external sensory input. Jouvet (1980) demonstrated that there were regions of the brainstem that functioned like an internal clock. These regions periodically triggered REM sleep and its accompanying brain activity. Brainstem neurons were identified that were involved in REM sleep. When those neurons were destroyed, cats moved during sleep as though they were acting out their dreams by arching their backs and making movements toward invisible mice.

Initially, these brainstem findings were interpreted as random excitation of the cortex and dreams were said to be vivid by-products of purely physiological processes. Hobson suggested that dreams are bizarre because neurons in the brainstem send random signals to the visual cortex (Hobson, 1988; Hobson and McCarley,1977). These signals, PGO spikes, present information that the brain interprets as real visual data. Hobson argues that receiving this information, the brain goes to its memory stores looking for a match and generates dream material. Dreams, then, represent an awareness of this organic brain activity, which may stimulate cerebral motor circuits throughout the night. However, it is not only brainstem signals but also cortical feedback that produces a dream. If the cortex is removed, PGO spikes become simplified, indicating that there is a circuit or flow between cortex and brainstem.

That the cortical areas necessary for attention are involved in REM has received support in a study of the left visual hemi-inattention syndrome that follows right-sided cortical lesions (Dorricchi et al., 1991). The authors found a selective redirection of eye movements during sleep. Involved patients made only rightward eye movements during REM sleep, suggesting a powerful top-down effect on the pontine saccade generator, which occurs in waking and which apparently also takes place in REM (Hobson, 1992).

REM sleep latency (the time interval between the onset of sleep and initiation of the first REM sleep period) varies considerably among individuals and is hypothesized to be an index of the maturation of cerebral function. Rapid eye movements during REM sleep have been intensively studied in regard to intelligence, especially the time intervals between eye movements. Both REM density and the amount of rapid eye movements have been reported to correlate with cognitive ability.

Neurotransmitter Function in Sleep

The acetylcholine system plays an important role in promoting sleep, particularly REM sleep. Cholinergic neurons in the peribrachial region of the pons are involved and project to the paramedian pontine reticular formation and to the thalamus. There they excite other cells that directly mediate signs of REM sleep, including the cortical EEG activation, the ocular saccades (rapid eye movements), and the ponto-geniculo-occipital waves (PGO). Intrinsic cholinergic neurons of the brainstem then directly mediate the PGO waves of each REM period. Datta et al. (1991) have reported evidence that direct triggering of PGO waves by cholinergic chemical stimulation with carbecol is followed by week-long enhancement of REM. Cholinergic neurons may indirectly prime other mediating circuits of the brain to regulate the amount of REM sleep. The cholinergic REM induction and maintenance system is thought to be gated by serotonergic, noradrenergic, and dopamine inputs, which in general are inhibitory. The specificity of this experimental model at both the cellular and molecular levels provides a framework for a molecular biological approach to sleep mechanisms and function (Hobson, 1992).

Early lesion and drug studies had suggested a role of the serotonergic raphe nucleus in the mediation of slow wave sleep. These early studies were refuted by a consistent finding of a selective decrease in raphe firing and 5-hydroxytryptamine (5-HT) release during slow wave sleep. Because the raphe neurons showed an almost complete arrest of firing during REM, it was subsequently proposed that serotonin might actually inhibit the cholinergic/-cholinoceptive REM sleep generator. It is now known that 5-HT is a sedative, but does not enhance serotonergic activity. The 5-HT REM inhibition hypothesis has been confirmed. The most direct evidence for anticholinergic mediation of serotonergic REM suppression comes from intracellular recordings of identified cholinergic neurons. When a 5-HT agonist is applied to cells, they show a hyperpolarization and a decrease in input resistance (Luebke et al., 1992). In behavioral studies, a $5-HT_1$ agonist elicits a dose-dependent REM/PGO suppression in cats, which is followed by rebound. The rebound in PGO waves suggests a potentiation rather than simply a recovery process. Human subjects also show reductions in REM sleep agonists and reuptake blockers.

Noradrenergic neurons are selectively active in waking and inactive in REM sleep. Because this is the case, rather than noradrenaline mediating REM, an inhibitory role is suggested for noradrenaline as well as for serotonin. This is consistent with the evidence that noradrenaline enhances waking brain functions, such as attention, learning, and memory; all of these are deficient during REM. The α_2-adrenergic agonist, clonidine, suppresses REM when injected into the reticular formation in cats, or when given by injection to humans. The failure of enhancement of REM with α_2-adrenergic antagonists in humans may be a function of the route of administration and consequent effects on multiple peripheral physiologic systems (Hobson, 1992).

Other neurotransmitter systems, such as the GABA system, have been studied in sleep. The REM sleep-bursting pattern of cholinergic neuronal discharge is considered to be mediated by local γ-amino-butyric acid (GABAergic) interneurons through membrane hyperpolarization. A GABA agonist has been shown to increase waking and decrease REM sleep and other sleep stages. However, a GABA antagonist produces even greater sleep suppression, leading to lack of clarity about other roles for GABA in sleep.

THE ONTOGENY OF SLEEP

The investigation of the sleep cycle requires consideration of three issues: the time spent asleep, the distribution of sleep during the 24-hour period, and the depth of sleep. The amount, distribution, and depth of sleep varies during the 24-hour cycle and differs among species. The amount of sleep needed for each species is in proportion to the waking metabolic rate, the time needed for restoration, and predator status. When safety is assured, sleep lasts longer. Those who sleep longer have a shorter reaction time and a higher body temperature. The range in the amount of sleep varies with age from infants, who sleep 16 or more hours a day, to adults, who sleep from 3 to 10 hours a day. The distribution of sleep gradually acquires a day/night pattern and becomes entrained to the 24-hour clock from the 25-hour free-running cycle.

The organization of sleep over the 24-hour rest/activity cycle and the duration and structure of sleep show striking changes over the life span (Roffwarg, Muzio, and Dement, 1966). Newborn animals and humans do not immediately express circadian rhythms. Animal studies indicate that the biological clock in the infant is working before birth, keeping the infant and mother in synchrony with one another. The maternal circadian or ultradian rhythms (e.g., daytime increases in blood pressure, pulse rate) and respiratory rate, may influence the periodicity of fetal activity. Ultrasound studies are used to record dynamic phenomena in human fetuses. Fetal biorhythms involving breathing, cardiac, and ocular movements and movements of the whole body can be observed and recorded simultaneously, using real-time echography and Doppler systems.

Studies of the integration of fetal behavioral patterns indicate that movements come under central control early in fetal life. The study of these body movements (gross, eye, and breathing movements) by real-time echography and their computerized analysis may be used for the assessment of the maturation of the behavioral patterns in the human fetus *in utero*.

At about 16 weeks (postmenstrual age), the first slow changes of fetal eye position can be observed with the aid of real-time ultrasonography. At 18 to 20 weeks, rapid eye movements are detectable. These eye movements are organized by episodes of activity, at first unrelated to cyclical change, which become distinct from episodes of quiescence. By 28 weeks of gestation, three patterns can be defined; these are comparable to the sleep stages described in the premature and full-term newborn, i.e., paradoxical, quiet, and transitional sleep. There is a gradual decline in the percentage of time spent in rapid and slow eye movements from 32 to 40 weeks. REM sleep is predominantly present *in utero* and makes up about 80% of total sleep time in premature infants who are born at 30 weeks' gestation (10 weeks before the due date).

The alternation of sleep and waking state is called the circadian rhythm (*circa*, meaning "approximately"; *dies,* meaning "day"). The human newborn infant shows essentially no circadian rest/activity cycle at birth and is as likely to be awake as to be asleep. To adapt, the infant must develop an internal clock for sleep and waking. In preparation for this extrauterine adaptation, the degree of maturation of the CNS is a critical factor. Moreover, the emergence of the sleep/wake rhythm may be delayed in children with mental retardation syndromes and in those with brain impairment.

In newborn infants, the circadian rhythm of sleep and wake develops gradually, with initial alternations of sleep and waking, each of several hours' duration. The 24-hour sleep/wake rhythm is established by 12 to 16 weeks after birth (Kleitman and Engelman, 1953; Meier-Koll et al., 1978) and becomes entrained to the environmental cycle. Even before this age, normal human newborns have already developed a 4-hour sleep/wake cycle (Kleitman and Engelman, 1953), the "ultradian" rhythm. This rhythm occurs in preterm and full-term newborns and is independent of feeding (Emde, Swedberg, and Suzuki, 1975). Both ultradian and circadian rhythms are endogenous and use a system of connected oscillators.

Animal studies have established the brain mechanisms that are involved in the establishment of circadian rhythms and the mechanisms for NREM and REM sleep. Brainstem nuclei, particularly the locus coeruleus and the raphe nucleus, are involved in the generation of the sleep stages. The suprachiasmatic nuclei (SCN) are critical for the circadian rhythms of sleep and wakefulness (Rusak, 1977). There is a hierarchical system of circadian oscillators, which includes at least one dominant and complex pacemaker in the SCN and a set of subordinate oscillators outside the SCN, probably in the hypothalamus. Rest/activity cycles play important roles in generating characteristics of different stages of sleep (Mistlberger and Rusak, 1989).

Free-Running Sleep Cycles

Indicators of environmental time that are essential to establishing the circadian cycle are called *zeitgebers* (*Zeit,* meaning "time"; *geber,* meaning "giver") (Aschoff, 1954, 1965). Those zeitgebers which are the most important are the 24-hour environmental light/dark cycle (Czeisler et al., 1981), the timing of feeding (Goetz, Bishop, and Halberg, 1976), and social contacts with others (Wever, 1979). However, changes of temperature, relative humidity, and other physical influences that occur during the day may also affect the circadian cycle.

Human subjects isolated from environmental cues such as light, darkness, temperature, and humidity, develop patterns of sleep/wake rhythm, body temperature rhythm, and other biological rhythms that differ from the usual 24-hour pattern. This rhythm (called free-running) is close to 25 hours in duration and is considered to be the endogenous rhythm (Aschoff, 1960). Ordinarily, the endogenous free-running rhythm is entrained to the 24-hour rhythm of the environment. The light/dark cycle in the environment is one of the dominant synchronizers of the human circadian system (Czeisler et al., 1981).

Healthy individuals who maintain a normal 24-hour cycle have changes in the sleep/wake rhythm in endocrine rhythms (ACTH and cortisol secretion) and in autonomic rhythms (body temperature, blood pressure, or heart rate). In experimental isolation, sleep/wake rhythm, body temperature, and cortisol secretion follow a 25-hour free-running rhythm. Some subjects developed a longer sleep/wake cycle (30 to 40 hours) but maintained the 25-hour free-running body temperature cycle. This state has been termed "internal desynchronization." These experiments led to the hypothesis that the human circadian system consists of multiple oscillators (clocks) that are usually coupled to each other but may change their phase relation. Internal desynchronization may occur in brain-damaged individuals.

Sleep During Development

The infant's sleep initially does not show the adult stages; both amount and kind of sleep vary with age. Before differentiation into REM/NREM patterns, infant sleep is designated as quiet, active, and indeterminate. From sleep onset REM to undifferentiated NREM, immature patterns become more differentiated. Anders and Keener (1985) studied premature infants, compared them to term infants, and found that sleep/wake maturations of premature and term infants, when matched for concep-tional age, are remarkably comparable. The premature infant had less quiet sleep and more active sleep in the first 2 to 4 weeks than term infants, but these differences are not statisti-cally significant. They found that the amount of time in quiet sleep is easier to measure than that of active sleep, which was more variable, per-haps related to changes in infant care and envi-ronment. The infant sleep cycle differs in terms of REM and NREM patterns, with REM ini-tially preceding NREM. The amount of REM decreases toward the adult level during the first year. The newborn may sleep a total of 16 out of 24 hours, and of this sleep time, 50% is spent in rapid eye movement sleep (REM). In falling asleep, an infant may directly enter REM sleep.

The sleep EEG at birth consists of poorly formed, relatively low-voltage slow waves. An infant's non-REM (NREM) sleep lacks certain EEG characteristics — such as K complexes, sleep spindles, and delta waves — that at a later maturational age define sleep stages 1 to 4. The differentiated patterns, including high-voltage delta waves, sleep spindles, and K complexes, develop rapidly during the first year of life. In subsequent months, NREM matures in the complexity of its EEG patterns, its duration, and its timing, so that increasingly it occurs at the beginning of the nighttime sleep period (Coons and Guilleminault, 1983). Quiet sleep becomes differentiated into the mature states such that by age 2, all EEG characteristics of adult sleep are present. There are then longer periods of wakefulness during daylight hours.

By full term, REM fills half of a normal 16 to 17-hour total daily sleep time as noted ear-lier. REM declines sharply to reach 30 to 35% of the child's sleep time by age 2 years and eventually stabilizes to 22 to 25% by age 10 years. There is little subsequent change until the later years of life, the 70s and 80s. REM declines from approximately 8 hours at birth to 1½ to 1¾ hours at puberty. The nocturnal REM latency, the time from falling asleep and the beginning of the first REM period, gradu-ally increases. REM sleep becomes more prominent at the end rather than at the begin-ning of the night.

Beginning early in life, there is considerable individual difference in sleep duration and sleep traits, which may vary over the year. Genetic factors may play a part, as does temperament (Carey, 1972). "REM storms" (intense rapid eye movements during REMs) at 6 months were significantly negatively correlated with Bayley Scales of Mental Development at age 12 months (Becker and Thoman, 1981). Nighttime waking is common at 9 months after the initial night sleep pattern is established. Psychologi-cally, children adapt to sleep by characteristic behaviors, e.g., bedtime rituals and manipula-tion of bedtimes at age 2, irritability following naps at age 2½, better sleep at ages 6 to 7 and renewed resistance to bedtime at age 8 (Ames, 1964). There are also developmental changes in the occurrence of nightmares, with peaks in the preschool years (Ferber, 1989; Klackenberg, 1987; Terr, 1987).

As children grow older, sleep-related behav-ioral changes are accompanied by significant changes in EEG sleep patterns during middle childhood and puberty. In the preadolescent years, differences in sleep and wakefulness are maximal. During the day, children are very alert and active, and they sleep soundly at night. High-intensity auditory stimuli at 123 dB, which is about 90 dB above the waking threshold, do not arouse children aged 8 to 12 during their first sleep cycle.

Developmentally, sleep pattern differences are related to age, sex, and pubertal states (Coble et al., 1987). Significant differences relate to chronological age. Between the ages of 6 and 11 years, there is a steady decline in nighttime sleep with increasing age, ranging from 9.5 and 9.0 hours (6- to 7-year-olds), to 8 hours (8-year-olds), to 7.5 hours (10- to 11-year-olds), respectively. Measures of sleep con-tinuity remained constant, with high sleep effi-ciency of 94% to 95% in children ages 6 to 11. The NREM sleep measures showed a gradual decline in stage 4 slow wave sleep from 18% in 6- to 7-year-old children to 14% in 10- to 11-year-old children. The reduction is associated with the increase in stage 2 sleep.

The amount of REM sleep remains rela-tively stable at 20% to 22% in the 6- to 11-year- age groups. The onset of REM sleep declines from 140 minutes in 6- to 7-year-olds to about 124 minutes in 10- to 11-year-olds. Although this is not a significant decrease (142 minutes to 124 minutes), these are higher values than those seen in adolescents and adults. With advancing age, the number of REM periods declines (five to four) and measures of REM activity within REM sleep do also (155 to 110 REM units). Moreover, as in adults, REM period lengths tend to increase across the sleep period. In regard to the effect of sex on EEG sleep, boys age 10 years and older showed higher slow wave stage 3 percentages ($p<0.05$), but not higher stage 4 percentages than girls. From ages 6 to 16, values for total sleep and average REM and delta wave counts decrease significantly with increased age.

During the adolescent years, a number of important changes take place in sleep. The duration of sleep, particularly on school nights, decreases during the prepubertal years (Anders, Carskadon, and Dement, 1980). Although it is not clear how much this sleep pattern is influenced by academic and cultural pressures, it does appear that children from ages 8 to 17 average 1½ hours of sleep less than their great-grandparents. This reduction may also be related to an earlier age of onset of adolescence. Moreover, in the middle of the adolescent years, daytime sleepiness, the ability to sleep when offered a chance to nap (Carskadon et al., 1980), becomes apparent. Most commonly, narcolepsy begins during the teenage years. Prepubertal children rarely nap or have irresistible urges to sleep, but these tendencies are present during adolescence. Early sexual maturation in adolescents is accompanied by an increased release of luteinizing hormone (LH) and, in boys, of testosterone during sleep (Boyar et al., 1972).

In adolescence, the changes in the sleep EEG are quantitative, rather than qualitative, but are striking. The time spent in stage 4 sleep declines about 50% and the amplitude of the delta waves declines markedly, so the total effect on biological processes is greater. Peak delta wave changes fall about 75% from 10 to 16 years. Total sleep duration declines by 2 hours. EEG changes are far more significant than those produced during aging in the next four decades.

Feinberg (1974, 1982/83) suggests that the changes in sleep in adolescence may be accompanied by a major reorganization of the brain, reflecting brain plasticity. The amount of deep sleep and rate of brain metabolism drop sharply in adolescence. The capacity of recovery of function after brain injury diminishes, and adult problem-solving ability emerges. A reduction in cortical synaptic density takes place, which might account for these changes. Such synaptic "pruning" may be analogous to the programmed elimination of neural elements in early development. Feinberg suggests that a defect in this process of elimination might underlie the onset of a major disorder, such as schizophrenia, and be a factor related to its age of onset; e.g., a neuronal migration abnormality might become apparent during this proposed phase of synaptic reorganization. Feinberg suggests that one function of sleep is to reverse the effects of waking on brain neurons.

DREAMS: DEVELOPMENTAL ASPECTS

Dreams may be reported as early as age 2 or 3, but these are generally not considered to be true dream reports. The study of the onset of dreaming began with the establishment of EEG sleep laboratories, which studied REM and NREM sleep. Foulkes (1982a) has followed the evolution of dreaming and thinking in children. When children aged 3 to 5 were awakened from REM sleep, dream reports were rare, occurring only 15% of the time. When they did occur, they were typically short, without evidence of plot, movement, feeling, or self-involvement. Animals were frequently mentioned in dreams by preschool children, but human characters were not. At older ages, frequency of dream reports increased to approximately 30% at ages 5 to 7, 43% at ages 7 to 9, and about 80% at ages 9 to 11 (the adult level). In addition, dream content, when reported, matured with age. At ages 5 to 7, children reported several events in series, physical activity, and social interaction. By ages 7 to 9, the child began to describe his own participation in the dream and some feeling states. Foulkes reported that abstract or thoughtlike thinking was not common in NREM sleep until adolescence. He has suggested that the development of dreaming and thinking is in keeping with cognitive stages of development described by Piaget. Based on his research on children's dreams, Foulkes (1982b) proposed that REM is a skilled cognitive act in which memory and knowledge are reprocessed, leading to the generation of consciously recognizable and relatively well-organized dream narratives. He suggests that the imaginable construction in dreams is the result of general symbolic operations, rather than automatic retrieval of concrete visual analogs into consciousness. Imaging is said to be a process that depends upon evocative or symbolic memory, rather than recognition memory.

The relationship of affect and cognition in dream reports has also been investigated by Foulkes (1982c). He makes the following points in his longitudinal sleep laboratory study of children's dreams.

1. Children's earliest reported REM dreams at ages 3 to 5 are unlike those of adults. They do not involve kinematic imagery (i.e., movement and activity). They do not have a well-defined self character, and dream reports of self activity are rare. They lack not only narrative and thematic extension in time, but also consistent presence of human characters or human social interactions. They contain more animal than human characters and more descriptions of body state, such as sleep and hunger, than social interactions. It is particularly rare for 3- to 5-year-olds to have experienced feelings in their REM dreams, and the imagery that they do report does not seem to be the kind that would be appropriate to the experience of feelings. In the sleep laboratory, on most REM awakenings, children reported no dreams at all. These laboratory studies focused on control children and did not focus on children who were abused.

2. The first evidence of feelings accompanying substantial numbers of dreams occurred at ages 7 to 9, when dream affect was in the same 30% to 40% range that is characteristic of children's dream reports from ages 9 to 15. At ages 7 to 9, those who reported happy feelings, which were the most frequently reported individual feelings, were not distinguishable from peers on psychosocial or adjustment dimensions. However, they were consistently more talented intellectually than children with little dream affect. Descriptions of happiness overlapped with those ascribing thought activity to the self. This suggests that dream feelings emerge as part of a more general ten-

dency to take a psychological perspective in dream descriptions.

3. From ages 3 to 5 to 5 to 7, children's dreams begin to lose their non-narrative quality and begin to contain information on physical activity and interpersonal interaction. Overall, it is non-self characters rather than particular self-representations who participate in this more dynamic and socially interactive dream world. Thus, in dreams, movement imagery and narrative structure develop before significant self-representation and the ascribing of feeling states to the self. In children in the transition from ages 5 to 7 to 7 to 9, statistically significant increases in activities and states were noted. From ages 7 to 9, self-participation becomes established in children's dreams. Self-participation was not associated with waking assertiveness, but with improved performance on cognitive tests. This was also true for feeling representation, where children who were ahead of their peers in intellectual development provided the earlier descriptions.

4. In addition, in the transition of ages 5 to 7 to 7 to 9, there was a significant increase, from 31% to 48%, in the frequency with which dreams were reported on REM awakenings in the sleep laboratory. Rather than being related to waking affective behavior, the dreams were positively correlated with individual differences in waking cognitive status, particularly differences between individuals in visuospatial and analytic abilities.

5. At no stage in dream development is dreaming simply a literal re-creation of past waking experiences or an easily understandable portrayal of real-life experiences. Children's earliest reported dreams follow actual real-life experiences or stories that are familiar to them from books and film. Human strangers were almost totally absent in dream reports of 3- to 5-year-olds and in 5- to 7-year-olds. Their presence was predicted by waking cognitive ability, rather than waking affective or psychosocial experiences.

6. Individual children do reliably follow different stages of dream development.

Foulkes (1982c) concludes that children's

dream reports are consistent with a cognitive stage developmental model. Overall, Foulkes suggests that the symbolic generation of affect is a developmentally acquired process and one whose ontogeny lags behind that of other forms of symbolism, such as imagery and speech. Affect generation is a late-appearing, secondary phenomenon in the ontogeny of dreaming and in the reprocessing that occurs during REM sleep. The adult linguistic and imaginable constraints are imposed earlier, and are therefore more basic and general contributors to the final form of dream experience.

In summary, Foulkes (1982a) found a maturational trend in the reporting of affect during dreaming such that by adolescence 60% of girls and 70% of boys report dreams that are accompanied by affect. In preadolescence, he found that reports of feelings lagged behind the reporting of interactional content, so the symbolic elicitation of affect seems to make a late appearance developmentally.

NEUROPSYCHOLOGY OF REM SLEEP

Neuropsychological research has recently focused on similarities and differences between REM sleep with dreaming and the waking state. Following their investigations of the thalamocortical system, Llinas and Pare (1991) suggest that greater weight should be given to external inputs as the critical factor for waking brain function. Because, in waking, relatively little of the neuronal connectivity is actually devoted to a transfer of sensory input, Hobson (1992) suggests that consciousness in both waking and dreaming is a closed-loop process in which intrinsic activity of brain cells is critical. Antrobus (1991) has offered a connectionist model, which postulates the importance of inhibition of external input that thereby allows the output of perception and cognitive modules to serve as the sole inputs.

The role of REM sleep in cortical areas, which are classically needed for attention, has been examined in patients with left visual hemi-inattention syndrome, which follows right-sided cortical lesions (Doricchi et al., 1991), as mentioned earlier. These patients make only rightward eye movements in REM sleep, indicating a powerful top-down effect upon the regions of the pons that generate sac-

cadic eye movements that one would expect to be active in waking. This system, then, is active in REM sleep. The involvement of the frontal eye fields, the midline attentional system, and the parietal lobe visuospatial attention systems in REM sleep has been suggested in studies of brain function in sleeping subjects using PET scanning procedures. The saccadic eye movement system involving the frontal lobe eye fields and dorsolateral prefrontal cortex were demonstrated to be actively scanning targets in the dream scene (Hong et al., 1993). Using ^{18}FDG PET scan methodology, these authors studied nine subjects during REM sleep and six normal control subjects during waking as they periodically moved their eyes. They found that the number of eye movements during REM sleep were positively correlated with local cerebral metabolic rate for glucose metabolism (LCMRglc) in areas corresponding to the saccadic eye movement system (frontal eye field and dorsolateral prefrontal cortex only on the right side), the midline attentional system (cingulate and medial frontal cortex, precuneus), and the parietal visuospatial attentional system (bilateral superior parietal lobules, right inferior parietal lobe), and negatively correlated with LCMRglc in the left inferior parietal lobule. Moreover, positive correlation between waking eye movements and LCMRglc was observed in the same areas other than the inferior parietal lobule.

FUNCTIONS OF SLEEP

Sleep is of most importance to the functioning of the cerebral cortex; this is most clearly shown by the need for recovery sleep following sleep loss or deprivation (Horne, 1988). Although most other parts of the body can relax and recover during wakefulness, the cerebrum cannot do so. Even though the eyes are closed and the mind may be blank, the waking brain remains highly active. Moreover Feinberg (1989) found a high waking metabolic rate in 3- to 8-year-olds, which may suggest the need for greater recovery sleep in children; indeed, children in this age range show substantially greater amounts of stage 3 and stage 4 sleep in the first third of the night than young adults. Maquet et al. (1990) documented reduced cerebral metabolic rate during slow wave sleep and increased activity in REM sleep using PET scanning with the 2-deoxy-D-glucose method. If reduced cerebral metabolic rate during sleep indicates restoration, then slow wave sleep rather than REM sleep is the more important for recovery and restitution of functioning (Horne, 1988, 1992).

Protein synthesis has been found to be enhanced in slow wave sleep, allowing sleep to increase growth and facilitate physiological restoration. The balance shifts from day to night toward greater net protein synthesis and away from degradation due to less cell work during sleep. Ramm and Smith (1990) used L[1–14C] leucine autoradiography to study rates of local cerebral protein synthesis during slow wave sleep, REM sleep, and wakefulness in the rat. Slow wave sleep was found to be associated with higher rates of protein synthesis throughout the brain, but wakefulness and REM were not, suggesting that slow wave sleep favors the restoration of cerebral proteins. These metabolic changes might be facilitated by the production of growth hormone during sleep. Growth hormone release facilitates protein synthesis, in contrast to adrenalin and cortisol production, which, during wakefulness, lead to cell breakdown. Both cortisol and adrenalin release are reduced in sleep.

The developmental importance of REM sleep continues to be debated. Roffwarg, Muzio, and Dement (1966) suggested that *in utero,* where there is little external sensory stimulation, REM provides the internal sensory stimulation necessary for the maturation of the cerebrum. These authors propose that REM leads to activation of neuronal circuits and provides a potent source of internal stimulation that is needed for proper brain growth. Denenberg and Thoman (1981) followed up on this hypothesis and proposed that, if REM played this role, then the more time spent in wakefulness, the less time would be spent in REM sleep. These investigators studied 2- to 5-week-old infants living at home. Wakefulness was divided into "waking active," "quiet alert," and "drowsy" intervals. A high negative correlation (–0.82) between REM sleep and wakefulness was found, which was in support of their hypothesis. The greatest negative correlation was found with the "quiet alert" state. Apparently the primary elements in REM sleep that provide stimulation are the spike discharges from the PGO areas. From his studies of the PGO activity, Morrison (1983) has proposed that REM provides a form of exaggerated awareness that leads to periodic orienting responses due to PGO activity during the night.

This theory of internal stimulation does not seem to account for the continuation of REM after maturation and the lack of clear effects of REM suppression by various drugs. However, Winson (1990; Pavlides and Winson, 1989) proposes that there is an important role for REM after maturation in regard to learning and memory. At about 2 years of age REM sleep is reduced to 3 hours each 24 hour day and the adult pattern is established. Concurrently, the hippocampus, which is still developing, becomes functional, so REM sleep, at this time, might assume a role in learning and memory as the basic infrastructure for memory is laid down in the hippocampus. Winson's findings are described in detail in Chapter 9.

In support of the learning and memory hypothesis, animal studies have shown increases in REM and in the actual number of rapid eye movements after successful learning of an avoidance task. Further evidence to support REM sleep's function to enable learning and memory comes from maze learning trials where rats show a delayed vulnerability to REM sleep loss. It is proposed that there is a vulnerable period of time following successful learning when REM sleep is necessary to consolidate learning. Following acquisition of a variety of tasks, rats showed increased REM sleep at specific post-training times. These increases occur several hours or even several days after the end of training. If following training REM deprivation was applied at the times increased REM was found, learning/memory deficits were observed. These times have been referred to as REM sleep windows (Smith and MacNeil, 1992). Learning deficits occurred only when experienced during the particular time period, this REM sleep window. Moreover, Smith, Tenn, and Annett (1991) have demonstrated that both anisomycin and scopolamine, when given during the REM sleep window, produce similar learning deficits along with decreases in both ACh and ACh esterase/activity.

Smith and Lapp (1991) also have studied the role of REM sleep and the number of REMs and REM density in humans after an intensive learning period. They found significantly increased REM density at the fourth REM sleep period of the night in a group of senior college students following the end of their mid-year examinations. Like the animal studies, these results support the idea of REM sleep or the REMs themselves being involved several days after the end of training in long-term-memory processing. The memory of nonsense words has been found to be greater after an intervening period of sleep. Therefore, memory traces may be potentially strengthened through sleep. Finally, Karni et al. (1994) documented improvement in a visual discrimination task after a normal night's sleep in human volunteers. They provide evidence that a process of human memory consolidation, active during sleep, is dependent of nighttime REM sleep.

The relationship between brain and behavior during sleep has been highlighted in another way by Jouvet (1980) in his proposal that genetic programming of the brain occurs during paradoxical (REM) sleep. He has outlined a theoretical model that periodic programming of the central nervous system occurs to maintain and facilitate the neuronal systems responsible for the "templates" of "innate releasing stimuli" and the fixed motor patterns that are involved in innate behavior. He suggests the relationship of this model to epigenetic events in development and postulates that paradoxical (REM) sleep may be an optimal framework for this programming to occur. Because brain cells do not undergo cell division in mammals, how aspects of heredity (e.g., in homozygous twins raised in different surroundings) persist throughout life is not explained. A genetic program established through neurogenesis is not likely due to the plasticity of the nervous system, so the possibility of iterative (repetitive) genetic programming must be considered.

The internal mechanisms of paradoxical (REM) sleep are well-adapted to such programming. Paradoxical sleep would activate an endogenous system that could stimulate and stabilize receptors genetically programmed by DNA in some neuronal circuits. The excitation of these neurons during paradoxical sleep might lead to behaviors that could be experimentally demonstrated. Among the mechanisms allowing the iterative (repetitive) programming, sleep is particularly important.

Security (i.e., the inhibition of the arousal system) may be a necessary condition for genetic programming to take place. In this way sleep could very well be the guardian of dreaming. On the other hand, sleep seems to be necessary for the accumulation of energetic resources used by the cholinergic mechanisms of paradoxical (REM) sleep. The presence, or absence, of rebound after paradoxical (REM) sleep deprivation may be related to stress during paradoxical sleep suppression. Therefore, one of the functions of paradoxical sleep may be to maintain psychological variability in a given population. Although not proven, Jouvet's hypothesis is an intriguing response to the question of why we sleep. Winson (Pavlides and Winson 1989; Winson, 1990) also suggests a survival role for REM sleep and proposes that with the evolution of REM sleep each species could process the information most important for its survival, such as the location of food or the means of escape from predation. Such information could be reaccessed during REM sleep and integrated with past experience to develop a continuing strategy for adaptive behavior.

The study of sleep in developmentally disabled persons may shed further light on the functions of sleep. For example, Shibagaki, Kiyono, and Watanabe (1982) have found delays in the emergence of sleep spindles in Down syndrome, and other authors have found differences in the amount of REM sleep in low- and high-functioning individuals with Down syndrome. If certain kinds of learning do require REM sleep, including tasks that involve the application of learned rules to solve novel problems (learning of complex tasks), then the study of REM in individuals with mental retardation syndromes and attention deficit disorder might be pursued. The role of the REM sleep window in learning for children with nighttime seizures might also be investigated.

REFERENCES

Ames, L.B. (1964). Sleep and dreams in childhood. In E. Harms (ed), *International series of monographs on child psychiatry.* Macmillan, New York.

Anders, T.F. and Keener, M. (1985). Developmental course of nighttime sleep-wake patterns in full-term and premature infants during the first year of life. *Sleep,* 8:173–192.

Anders, T.F., Carskadon, M.A., and Dement, W.C. (1980). Sleep and sleepiness in children and adolescents. *Pediatric Clinics of North America,* 27:29–43.

Antrobus, J. (1991). Dreaming: Cognitive processes during cortical activation and high afferent thresholds. *Psychological Review,* 98:96–121.

Aschoff, J. (1954). Zeitgeber der tierischen Tagesperiodik. *Naturwissenschaften,* 41:49–56.

———. (1960). Exogenous and endogenous components in circadian rhythms. *Cold Spring Harbor Symposium on Quantitative Biology,* 25:11–28.

———. (1965). Circadian rhythms in man. *Science,* 148:1427–1432.

Aserinski, E. and Kleitman, N. (1953). Regularly occurring periods of eye motility, and concomitant phenomena during sleep. *Science,* 118:273–274.

Becker, P.T. and Thoman, E.B. (1981). Rapid eye movement storms in infants: Rate of occurrence at 6 months predicts mental development at 1 year. *Science,* 212:1415–1416.

Boyar, R., Finkelstein, J., Roffwarg, H., Kapens, S., Weitzman, E., and Hellman, L. (1972). Synchronization of augmented luteinizing hormone with sleep during puberty. *New England Journal of Medicine,* 287:582–586.

Carey, W.B. (1972). Night awakening and temperament in infancy. *Journal of Pediatrics,* 84:756–758.

Carskadon, M.A., Harvey, K., Duke, P., Anders, T.F., Litt, I.F., and Dement, W.C. (1980). Pubertal changes in daytime sleepiness. *Sleep,* 2:453–460.

Coble, P.A., Kupfer, D.J., Reynolds, C.F., and Houck, P. (1987). EEG sleep of healthy children 6 to 12 years of age. In C. Guilleminault (ed), *Sleep and its disorders.* Raven Press, New York.

Coons, S. and Guilleminault, C. (1982). Development of sleep-wake patterns and non-rapid eye movement sleep stages during the first six months of life in normal infants. *Pediatrics,* 69:793–798.

Czeisler, C.A., Richardson, G.S., Zimmerman, J.C., Moore-Ede, M.C., and Weitzman, E.D. (1981). Entrainment of human circadian rhythms by light dark cycles: A reassessment. *Photochemistry and Photobiology,* 34:239–247.

Datta, S., Calvo, J., Quattrochi, J., and Hobson, J.A. (1991). Long-term enhancement of REM sleep following cholinergic stimulation. *NeuroReport,* 2:619–622.

Dement, W. and Kleitman, N. (1957). Cyclic variations in EEG during sleep and their relation to eye movements, body motility, and dreaming. *Electroencephalography and Clinical Neurophysiology,* 9:673–690.

Denenberg, V. and Thoman, E. (1981). Evidence for a functional role for active (REM) sleep in infancy. *Sleep,* 4:185–192.

Doricchi, F., Guariglia, C., Paolucci, S., and Pizzamiglio, I. (1991). Disappearance of leftward rapid eye movements during sleep in left visual hemi-inattention. *NeuroReport,* 2:285–288.

Ellingson, R. J. and Peters, J.F. (1980). Development of EEG and daytime sleep patterns in normal full-term infants during the first 3 months: Longitudinal observations. *Electroencephalography and Clinical Neurophysiology,* 49:112–124.

Emde, R., Swedberg, J., and Suzuki, B. (1975). Human wakefulness and biological rhythms after birth. *Archives of General Psychiatry* 32:780–783.

Feinberg, I. (1974). Changes in sleep cycle patterns with age. *Journal of Psychiatric Research,* 10:283–306.

———. (1982/83). Schizophrenia: Caused by a fault in programmed elimination during adolescence. *Journal of Psychiatric Research,* 17:319–334.

———. (1989). Effects of maturation and aging on slow wave sleep in man: Implications for neurobiology. In A. Wauquier, C. Dugovic, and M. Radulovacki (eds), *Slow wave sleep: physiological, pathophysiological, and functional aspects,* pp. 31–48. Raven Press, New York.

Ferber, R. (1989). Sleeplessness in the child. In M. H. Kryger, T. Roth, and W.C. Dement (eds), *Principles and practice of sleep medicine.* W.B. Saunders Co., Philadelphia.

Foulkes, D. (1982a). *Children's dreams: Longitudinal studies.* John Wiley & Sons, New York.

———. (1982b). A cognitive-psychological model of REM dream production. *Sleep,* 5:169–172.

———. (1982c). REM-dream perspectives on the development of affect and cognition. *Psychiatric Journal of the University of Ottawa,* 7:48–55.

Goetz, F., Bishop, J., and Halberg, F. (1976). Timing of single daily meal influences relations among human circadian rhythms in urinary cyclic AMP and hemic glucagon, insulin and iron. *Experientia,* 32:1081–1084.

Hobson, J.A. (1988). *The dreaming brain.* Basic Books, New York.

———. (1992). Sleep and dreaming: Induction and mediation of REM sleep by cholinergic mechanisms. *Current Opinion in Neurobiology,* 2:759–763.

———, and McCarley, R. (1977). The brain as a dream state generator: An activation synthesis hypothesis of the dream process. *American Journal of Psychiatry,* 134:1335–1348.

Hong, C. C., Gillin, J.C., Dow, B.M., Wu, J., and Buchsbaum, M.S. (1993). Positron emission tomography and eye movements during REM sleep. Neuroscience Abstracts. 19:1493 (Abstract 615.3).

Horne, J.A. (1988). *Why we sleep: The functions of sleep in humans and other mammals.* Oxford University Press, Oxford.

———. (1992). Sleep and its disorders in children. *Journal of Child Psychology and Psychiatry,* 33:473–487.

I.C.S.D. (1990). *International Classification of Sleep Disorders: Diagnostic and Coding Manual.* Diagnostic Classification Steering Committee, M.J. Thorpy (Chairman). American Sleep Disorders Association, Rochester, Minnesota.

Jouvet, M. (1980). Paradoxical sleep and the nature-nurture controversy. *Progress in Brain Research,* 53:331–346.

——— and Delorme, F. (1965). Locus Coerulues et pommeil paradoxal. *C. R. Seances Soc. Biol. Fil. [Paris]* 159: 895–899.

Kandel, E.R., Schwartz, J.H., and Jessell, T.M. (1991). *Principles of neural science,* 3rd ed, p. 794. Elsevier, New York.

Karni, A., Tanne, D., Rubenstein, B.S., Askenasy, J.M., and Sagi, D. (1994). Dependence on REM sleep of overnight improvement of a perceptual skill. *Science,* 265:679–682.

Klackenberg, G. (1987). Incidence of parasomnias in children in a general population. In C. Guilleminault (ed), *Sleep and its disorders in children,* p. 104. Raven Press, New York.

Kleitman, N. and Engelman, T.G. (1953). Sleep characteristics in infants. *Journal of Applied Physiology,* 7:269–282.

Llinas, R.R. and Pare, D. (1991). Of dreaming and wakefulness. *Neuroscience,* 44:521–535.

Luebke, J.L., Greene, R.W., Semba, K., Kamondi, A., McCarley, R.W., and Reiner, P.B. (1992). Serotonin hyperpolarizes cholinergic low-threshold burst neurons in the rat laterodorsal tegmental nucleus in vitro. *Neurobiology,* 89:743–747.

Maquet, P., Dive, D., Salmon, E., Sadzot, B., Franco, G., Poirrier, R., von Frenckell, R., and Franck, G. (1990). Cerebral glucose utilization during the sleep-wake cycle in man determined by positron emission tomography and [18F]2-fluoro-2-deoxy-D-glucose method. *Brain Research,* 513:136–143.

Meier-Koll, A., Hall, U., Hellwing, U., Kott, G., and Meier-Koll, V. (1978). A biological oscillator system and the development of sleep-waking behavior during early infancy. *Chronobiologia,* 5:425–440.

Mistlberger, R., and Rusak, B. (1989). Mechanisms and models of the circadian timekeeping system. In M.H Kryger, T. Roth, and W.C. Dement (eds), *Principles and practice of sleep medicine,* pp. 141–152. W.B. Saunders Co., Philadelphia.

Morrison, A.R. (1983). A window on the sleeping brain. *Scientific American,* 248:86–94.

Pavlides, C. and Winson, J. (1989). Influences of hippocampal place cell firing in the awake state on the activity of these cells during subsequent sleep episodes. *Journal of Neuroscience,* 9:2907–2918.

Ramm, P. and Smith, C. T. (1990). Rates of cerebral protein synthesis are linked to slow wave sleep in the rat. *Physiology and Behavior,* 48:749–753.

Roffwarg, H., Muzio, J., and Dement, W. (1966). Ontogenic development of the human sleep-dream cycle. *Science,* 152:604–619.

Rusak, B. (1977). The role of the suprachiasmatic nuclei in the generation of circadian rhythms in the golden hamster, mesocricetus auratus. *Journal of Comparative Physiology,* 118:145–164.

Shibagaki, M., Kiyono, S., and Watanabe, K. (1982). Spindle evolution in normal and mentally retarded children: A review. *Sleep,* 5:47–57.

Smith, C. and Lapp, L. (1991). Increases in number of REMs and REM density in humans following an intensive learning period. *Sleep,* 14:325–330.

Smith, C. and MacNeil, C. (1992). A paradoxical sleep window for memory 53–56 hours after training. Association of Professional Sleep Societies Annual Meeting Abstracts 6:17 (no. 32).

Smith, C., Tenn, C. and Annett, R. (1991). Some biochemical and behavioral aspects of the paradoxical sleep window. *Canadian Journal of Psychology,* 45:115–124.

Terr, L. (1987). Nightmares in children. In C. Guilleminault (ed), *Sleep and its disorders in children,* pp. 231–242. Raven Press, New York.

Winson, J. (1990). The meaning of dreams. *Scientific American,* November 1990, pp. 86–95.

Wever, R.A. (1979). *The circadian system of man: Results of experiments under temporal isolation.* Springer-Verlag, New York.

GLOSSARY OF TERMS USED IN SLEEP DISORDERS MEDICINE

Active Sleep[1] A term used in the phylogenetic and ontogenetic literature for the stage of sleep that is

[1] The equivalent of REM sleep in newborn infants. In infants younger than 3 months of age, it is difficult to define sleep states and stages using EEG criteria alone. Additional criteria used are respiration, heart rate, body movements, eye movements, and chin EMG. In the full-term infant, most authors use EEG criteria by 3 months of age and switch to REM sleep terminology. Some authors, however, continue to use the term "active sleep" throughout the first 12 months of life.

considered to be equivalent to REM sleep. See *REM sleep*.

Arousal An abrupt change from a "deeper" stage of NREM sleep to a "lighter" stage, or from REM sleep toward wakefulness, with the possibility of awakening as the final outcome. Arousal may be accompanied by increased tonic EMG activity and heart rate as well as body movements.

Circadian rhythm An innate daily fluctuation of physiological or behavioral functions, including sleep/wake states generally tied to the 24-hour daily dark/light cycle. Sometimes occurs at a measurably different periodicity (e.g., 23 or 25 hours) when light/dark and other time cues are removed.

Deep Sleep Common term for combined NREM stages 3 and 4 sleep. In some sleep literature, deep sleep is applied to REM sleep because of its high awakening threshold to nonsignificant stimuli. See *"intermediary" sleep stage; Light sleep*.

Delayed sleep phase A condition that occurs when the clock hour at which sleep normally occurs is moved back in time within a given 24-hour sleep/wake cycle. This results in a temporarily displaced, that is delayed, occurrence of sleep within the 24-hour cycle. The same term denotes a circadian rhythm sleep disturbance, called the *delayed sleep phase syndrome*.

Delta activity EEG activity with a frequency of less than 4 Hz (usually 0.1 to 3.5 Hz). In human sleep scoring, the minimum characteristics for scoring delta waves are conventionally 75-μV (peak-to-peak) amplitude, and 0.5-second duration (2 Hz) or less.

Delta sleep stage Indicative of the stage of sleep in which EEG delta waves are prevalent or predominant (sleep stages 3 and 4, respectively). See *slow wave sleep*.

Electroencephalogram (EEG) A recording of the electrical activity of the brain by means of electrodes placed on the surface of the head. With the EMG and EOG, the EEG is one of the three basic variables used to score sleep stages and waking. Sleep recording in humans utilizes surface electrodes to record potential differences between brain regions and a neutral reference point, or simply between brain regions. Either the C3 or C4 (central region) placement according to the International 10–20 System is referentially (referred to an earlobe) recorded as the standard electrode derivation from which state scoring is done.

Electromyogram (EMG) A recording of electrical activity from the muscular system; in sleep recording, synonymous with resting muscle activity or potential. The chin EMG is one of the three basic variables, along with the EEG and EOG, used to score sleep stages and waking. Sleep recording in humans typically utilizes surface electrodes to measure activity from the submental muscles. These reflect maximally the changes in resting activity of axial body muscles. The submental muscle EMG is tonically inhibited during REM sleep.

Electro-oculogram (EOG) A recording of voltage changes resulting from shifts in position of the ocular globes, as each globe is a positive (anterior) and negative (posterior) dipole; along with the EEG and the EMG, one of the three basic variables used to score sleep stages and waking. Sleep recording in humans utilizes surface electrodes placed near the eyes to record the movement (incidence, direction, and velocity) of the eyeballs. Rapid eye movements in sleep form one part of the characteristics of the REM sleep state.

Fragmentation (pertaining to sleep architecture) The interruption of any stage of sleep due to the appearance of another stage or to wakefulness, leading to disrupted NREM–REM sleep cycles; often used to refer to the interruption of REM sleep by movement arousals or stage 2 activity. Sleep fragmentation connotes repetitive interruptions of sleep by arousals and awakenings.

Hypersomnia (excessive sleepiness) Excessively deep or prolonged major sleep period. May be associated with difficulty in awakening. The term is primarily used as a diagnostic term, e.g., "idiopathic hypersomnia," and the term "excessive sleepiness" is preferred to describe the symptom.

Insomnia Difficulty in initiating and/or maintaining sleep. A term that is employed ubiquitously to indicate any and all gradations and types of sleep loss.

"Intermediary" sleep stage A term sometimes used for NREM stage 2 sleep. See *deep sleep; light sleep*. Often used, especially in the French literature, for stages combining elements of stage 2 and REM sleep.

K Complex A sharp, negative EEG wave followed by a high-voltage slow wave. The complex duration is at least 0.5 seconds, and may be accompanied by a sleep spindle. K complexes occur spontaneously during NREM sleep, and begin and define stage 2 sleep. They are thought to be evoked responses to internal stimuli. They can also be elicited during sleep by external (particularly auditory) stimuli.

Light Sleep A common term for NREM sleep stage 1, and sometimes stage 2.

Microsleep An episode lasting up to 30 seconds during which external stimuli are not perceived. The polysomnogram suddenly shifts from waking characteristics to sleep. Microsleeps are associated with excessive sleepiness and automatic behavior.

Movement arousal A body movement associated with an EEG pattern of arousal or a full awakening; a sleep scoring variable.

Multiple Sleep Latency Test (MSLT) A series of measurements of the interval from "lights out" to sleep onset that is utilized in the assessment of excessive sleepiness. Subjects are allowed a fixed number of opportunities to fall asleep during their customary awake period. Excessive sleepiness is characterized by short latencies. Long latencies are helpful in distinguishing physical tiredness or fatigue from true sleepiness.

Nightmare Used to denote an unpleasant and frightening dream that usually occurs in REM sleep. Occasionally called a dream anxiety attack, not a sleep (night) terror. Nightmare in the past has been used to indicate both sleep terror and anxiety dream attacks.

Non–rapid eye movement (NREM, Non-REM) sleep See *sleep stages.*

NREM sleep intrusion An interposition of NREM sleep, or a component of NREM sleep physiology (e.g., elevated EMG, K complex, sleep spindle, or delta waves), in REM sleep; a portion of NREM sleep not appearing in its usual sleep cycle position.

Phase Advance The shift of an episode of sleep or wake to an earlier position in the 24-hour sleep/wake cycle. A shift of sleep from 11 p.m. to 7 a.m. to 8 p.m. to 4 a.m. represents a 3-hour phase advance. See *Phase Delay.*

Phase delay A shift of an episode of sleep or wake to a later time of the 24-hour sleep/wake cycle. It is the exact opposite of phase advance. These terms differ from common concepts of change in clock time: to effect a phase delay, the clock is moved ahead or advanced. In contrast, to effect a phase advance, the clock moves backward. See *phase advance.*

Phase transition One of the two junctures of the major sleep and wake phases in the 24-hour sleep/wake cycle.

Polysomnogram The continuous and simultaneous recording of multiple physiologic variables during sleep, i.e., EEG, EOG, EMG (these are the three basic stage scoring parameters), EKG, respiratory air flow, respiratory movements, leg movements, and other electrophysiologic variables.

Rapid eye movement sleep (REM sleep) See *sleep stages.*

REM density (REM intensity) A function that expresses the frequency of eye movements per unit time during sleep stage REM.

REM sleep intrusion A brief interval of REM sleep appearing out of its usual position in the NREM–REM sleep cycle; an interposition of REM sleep in NREM sleep; sometimes appearance of a single, dissociated component of REM sleep (e.g., eye movements, "drop out" of muscle tone) rather than all REM sleep parameters.

REM sleep latency The interval from sleep onset to the first appearance of stage REM sleep in the sleep episode.

REM sleep onset The designation for commencement of a REM sleep episode. Sometimes also used as a shorthand term for a sleep-onset REM sleep episode. See *sleep onset; sleep-onset REM period (SOREMP).*

REM sleep percent The proportion of total sleep time constituted by the REM stage of sleep.

REM sleep rebound (recovery) Lengthening and increase in frequency and density of REM sleep episodes, which result in an increase in REM sleep percentage above baseline. REM sleep rebound follows REM sleep deprivation once the depriving influence is removed.

Sleep architecture The NREM–REM sleep stage and cycle infrastructure of sleep understood from the vantage point of the quantitative relationship of these components to each other. Often plotted in the form of a histogram.

Sleep efficiency or **sleep efficiency index** The proportion of sleep in the episode potentially filled by sleep, i.e., the ratio of total sleep time to time in bed.

Sleepiness (somnolence, drowsiness) Difficulty in maintaining alert wakefulness such that the person falls asleep if not actively kept aroused. This is not simply a feeling of physical tiredness or listlessness. When sleepiness occurs in inappropriate circumstances, it is considered excessive sleepiness.

Sleep latency The duration of time from "lights out," or bedtime, to the onset of sleep.

Sleep log (sleep diary) A daily, written record of a person's sleep/wake pattern containing such information as time of retiring and arising, time in bed, estimated total sleep time, number and duration of sleep interruptions, quality of sleep, daytime naps, use of medications or caffeine beverages, nature of waking activities.

Sleep mentation The imagery and thinking experienced during sleep. Sleep mentation usually consists of combinations of images and thoughts during REM sleep. Imagery is vividly expressed in dreams involving all the senses in approximate proportion to their waking representations. Mentation is experienced generally less distinctly in NREM sleep, but it may be quite vivid in stage 2 sleep, especially toward the end of the sleep episode. Mentation at sleep onset (hypnagogic reverie) can be as vivid as in REM sleep.

Sleep onset The transition from awake to sleep, normally to NREM stage 1 sleep, but in certain conditions, such as infancy and narcolepsy, into stage REM sleep. Most polysomnographers accept EEG slowing, reduction, and eventual disappearance of alpha activity, presence of EEG vertex sharp transients, and slow rolling eye movements (the components of NREM stage 1) as sufficient for sleep onset; others require appearance of stage 2 patterns. See *latency; sleep stages.*

Sleep-onset REM period (SOREMP) The beginning of sleep by entrance directly into stage REM sleep. The onset of REM sleep occurs within 10 minutes of sleep onset.

Sleep pattern (24-hour sleep-wake pattern) A person's clock hour schedule of bedtime and arise time as well as nap behavior; may also include time and duration of sleep interruptions. See *sleep-wake cycle; circadian rhythm; sleep log.*

Sleep Spindle Spindle-shaped bursts of 11.5- to 15-Hz waves lasting 0.5 to 1.5 seconds. Generally diffuse, but of highest voltage over the central regions of the head. The amplitude is generally less than 50 μV in the adult. One of the identifying EEG features of NREM stage 2 sleep; may persist into NREM stages 3 and 4; generally not seen in REM sleep.

Sleep stage episode A sleep stage interval that represents the stage in a NREM–REM sleep cycle; easiest to comprehend in relation to REM sleep, which is a homogeneous stage, i.e., the fourth REM sleep episode is in the fourth sleep cycle (unless a prior REM episode was skipped). If one interval of REM sleep is separated from another by more than 20 minutes, they constitute separate REM sleep episodes (and are in separate sleep cycles); a sleep stage episode may be of any duration.

Sleep stage NREM The other major sleep state apart from REM sleep; comprises sleep stages 1 to 4, which constitute levels in the spectrum of NREM sleep "depth" or physiologic intensity.

Sleep stage REM The stage of sleep with highest brain activity, characterized by enhanced brain metabolism and vivid hallucinatory imagery or dreaming. There are spontaneous rapid eye movements, resting muscle activity is suppressed, and awakening threshold to nonsignificant stimuli is high. The EEG is a low-voltage, mixed-frequency, non-alpha record. REM sleep is usually 20% to 25% of total sleep time. It is also called *paradoxical sleep.*

Sleep stages Distinctive stages of sleep, best

demonstrated by polysomnographic recordings of the EEG, EOG, and EMG.

Sleep stage 1 (NREM stage 1) A stage of NREM sleep that occurs at sleep onset or that follows arousal from sleep stages 2, 3, or 4 or REM. It consists of a relatively low-voltage EEG with mixed frequency, mainly theta activity and alpha activity of less than 50% of the scoring epoch. It contains EEG vertex waves and slow rolling eye movements; no sleep spindles, K complexes, or REMs. Stage 1 normally represents 4% to 5% of the major sleep episode.

Sleep stage 2 (NREM stage 2) A stage of NREM sleep characterized by the presence of sleep spindles and K complexes present in a relatively low-voltage, mixed-frequency EEG background; high-voltage delta waves may comprise up to 20% of stage 2 epochs; usually accounts for 45% to 55% of the major sleep episode.

Sleep stage 3 (NREM stage 3) A stage of NREM sleep defined by at least 20% and not more than 50% of the episode consisting of EEG waves less than 2 Hz and more than 75 μV (high-amplitude delta waves); a "delta" sleep stage; with stage 4, it constitutes "deep" NREM sleep, called *slow wave sleep (SWS);* often combined with stage 4 into NREM sleep stage 3/4 because of the lack of documented physiologic differences between the two; appears usually only in the first third of the sleep episode; usually comprises 4% to 6% of total sleep time.

Sleep stage 4 (NREM stage 4) All statements concerning NREM sleep stage 3 apply to stage 4 except that high-voltage, EEG slow waves persist 50% or more of the epoch; NREM sleep stage 4 usually represents 12% to 15% of total sleep time. Sleepwalking, sleep terrors, and confusional arousal episodes generally start in stage 4 or during arousals from this stage. See *sleep stage 3.*

Sleep structure Similar to sleep architecture. However, in addition to encompassing sleep stages and sleep cycle relationships, sleep structure assesses the within-stage qualities of the EEG and other physiologic attributes.

Sleep talking Talking in sleep that usually occurs in the course of transitory arousals from NREM sleep; can occur during stage REM sleep, at which time it represents a motor breakthrough of dream speech. Full consciousness is not achieved, and no memory of the event remains.

Sleep/wake cycle Basically, the clock hour relationships of the major sleep and wake episodes in the 24-hour cycle. See *phase transition; circadian rhythm.*

Slow wave sleep (SWS) Sleep characterized by

EEG waves of duration slower than 4 Hz. Synonymous with sleep stages 3 plus 4 combined. See *delta sleep stage.*

Theta activity EEG activity with a frequency of 4 to 8 Hz, generally maximal over the central and temporal cortex.

Total recording time (TRT) The duration of time from sleep onset to final awakening. In addition to total sleep time, it is comprised of the time taken up by wake periods and movement time until wake-up. See *sleep efficiency.*

Total sleep time (TST) The amount of actual sleep time in a sleep episode; equal to total sleep episode less awake time. Total sleep time is the total of all REM and NREM sleep in a sleep episode.

Wake time The total time scored as wakefulness in a polysomnogram occurring between sleep onset and final wake-up.

I.C.S.D. (1990). *International Classification of Sleep Disorders: Diagnostic and Coding Manual.* Diagnostic Classification Steering Committee, M.J. Thorpy (Chairman). American Sleep Disorders Association, Rochester, Minnesota.

CHAPTER 5

GENETIC ASPECTS OF NEUROPSYCHIATRY

Human genetics has been defined as the "science of variation and heredity in human beings" (Thompson, McInnes, and Willard, 1991) and has taken as its focus the genetic variations involved in medical and behavioral disorders. There are an estimated 100,000 human genes, and an increasing number of these have been identified since the beginning of the Human Genome Project. In a genetic disease, there are variations in the chemical makeup of genes, the units of heredity, which result in the production of abnormal proteins in the form of enzymes, structural proteins, signal receptors, and intercellular signals as described in Chapter 1.

The application of genetic investigation is becoming increasingly important in psychiatry, where advances in psychiatric diagnosis in children and adults, improved research methodology, and new molecular techniques are being implemented (see Chapter 1). In assessment, the interface of psychosocial risk with genetic factors is the most pertinent focus. The study of this interface involves the study of both shared and nonshared environments through the application of genetic research strategies and utilization of advances in molecular biology. Critical to this endeavor is a better definition of neuropsychiatric disorders and the boundaries between the various disorders. This is being approached by using standardized interview and observational instruments, improved sampling of cases, and more appropriate selection of controls in research studies.

An increased focus on the family history includes both genetic and social transmission. Family study is required for children whose parents have major mental disorders just as it has been in mental retardation, where there is considerable knowledge about genetic transmission. The application of genetic approaches is particularly important where there is the co-occurrence of a mental disorder and a mental retardation syndrome.

This chapter provides a definition of patterns of inheritance, discusses genetic strategies used in research, provides a rationale for genetic study, and provides information on genetic findings in developmental neuropsychiatric disorders in children.

THE IMPORTANCE OF GENETIC FACTORS

In the past, psychosocial factors have been emphasized because it was thought that little could be done about heredity. With better understanding of genetics, this is no longer the case. Genetic information may be helpful in the following situations.

1. Identification of treatable conditions

Phenylketonuria (PKU) serves as a model in regard to prevention of neuropsychiatric complications in a genetic metabolic disorder. Untreated PKU leads to severe mental retardation and is associated with autistic disorder and attention deficit disorder. Studies in PKU may lead to a better understanding of the pathways involved in social cognition and executive function. Dietary therapy must be continued beyond childhood to prevent functional deficits related to learning and behavioral problems.

2. Genetic counseling and potential prevention of a genetic disorder

Prevention is based on early recognition of the presence of a genetic disorder and an acknowledgment of individual sensitivity to risk environments. Reduced exposure to risk environments may affect expression of the disorder. For example, there may be a genetic sensitivity in some individuals to alcoholism such that exposure to alcohol results in expression of the disorder. Screening for a genetic disorder *in utero* may lead to early diagnosis and provide the parent with a choice in regard to continuing the pregnancy. Similarly, prenatal diagnosis of Down syndrome may facilitate early adaptation to the disorder by parents, stimulate consideration of adoption plans, or lead to termination of the pregnancy. In addition, early recognition and acknowledgment of a genetic disorder may result in early intervention (e.g., infant stimulation and early communication programs).

3. Definition of the limits of diagnostic groups

In mood disorders, schizophrenia, and developmental neuropsychiatric disorders such as autistic disorder, the presence of hetereogeneity and comorbidity require careful definition of the phenotype. Because there may be a spectrum of presentations of a disorder, defining what is inherited is critical. With a careful genetic family history, early diagnosis may be accomplished through a higher index of suspicion along with the use of standardized methods of assessment.

4. Recognition of differential effects of shared and nonshared environments

The term "shared environment" refers to the exposure of all children in a family to shared risk experiences (such as parental discord) that may increase the risk of disorder. Still, these children may have other nonshared life experiences that are protective. For example, one child may have different experiences in social support from family members, a different quality of peer relationship, and different school experiences. Genetic approaches may help to define the impact of shared and nonshared family, school, and community environments. They help address the issue of individual children in the same family. Are they equally vulnerable to the disorder, and why does one child develop the disorder and a sibling does not? To understand why one family member is affected and another is not, consideration must be given to which aspects of the nonshared environments are protective and which ones increase risk.

5. Discriminating between genetic and psychosocial effects

Children with genetic disorders may initially present with neuropsychiatric symptoms that are attributed to environmental stressors or intrapsychiatric conflicts rather than recognized as early symptoms of a genetic disorder. For example, in the childhood form of adrenoleukodystrophy, learning and behavioral problems are common (Brown et al., 1985). In Huntington's disease, mood disorder in children may be an early manifestation of the disease, whereas conduct disorder may be associated with family discord and disruption (Folstein et al., 1983).

6. Understanding of the natural history of a disorder

By careful study of children at risk, a better understanding may be gained of how genetic factors interact with environmental factors to influence development. To some degree, genetic influences act to shape the environment individuals choose for themselves (Scarr and McCartney, 1983). For example, temperament may shape life experiences by leading to the choice of certain environments, which may place an individual at greater risk for developing a disorder. Careful longitudinal study of cases recognized in childhood also may lead to the recognition of subtypes of mental disorder. In addition, study of the worsening of a condition from one generation to the next (anticipation) has led to the recognition of unstable gene regions, which may balloon in size from one generation to the next, as seen in the Fragile X syndrome (abnormal FMR-1 gene).

7. Better understanding of potential advantages for heterozygotes

In a number of genetic conditions in which the affected person rarely reproduces or does not reproduce at all, study of family members may demonstrate the selective advantage for the heterozygote (Rotter and Diamond, 1987). Selective advantage has been recognized for physical disorders such as sickle cell disease (malaria resistance) and Tay-Sachs disease (tuberculosis protection), but has not been clearly documented for psychiatric conditions and developmental disorders. For example, it was initially believed that autistic disorder was more prevalent in families with higher socioeconomic status, but this has not proven to be the case. Demonstrating the selective advantage for mental traits may come from more detailed family study.

CLASSIFICATION OF GENETIC DISORDERS: CLASSICAL PATTERNS

All clinical conditions are the result of combined activity of the gene and environment, but genetic effects may be variable, small or large. Strongly heritable conditions are not necessarily resistant to environmental influence, and enriched family environment may lead to major developmental gains. To establish the pattern of transmission, the family history is summarized in the form of a pedigree. Standard symbols for the pedigree are shown in Figure 5–1 and a glossary of terms is found at the end of Chapter 1.

There are three main types of genetic disorders:

1. Single-Gene Disorders (abnormal gene and gene product)

These are caused by mutant genes. The mutation may be on one of a pair of chromosomes, matched with a normal allele on the homologous chromosome, or on both of the chromosomes of a pair. In both instances, the result is an error in genetic information. Family studies show abnormal pedigree patterns. These conditions are rare, although for some disorders, their occurrence may be as frequent as 1 in 500 births. Three thousand

of the 4,000 single-gene phenotypes are genetic disorders (McKusick, 1990). In many of these conditions the gene has been isolated and cloned (i.e., segments have been purified so that large amounts of the purified segment can be produced for study). In addition to nuclear genes, mitochondrial genes have been recognized as abnormal. These mitochondrially transmuted genes lead to another type of single-gene disorder.

Single-gene traits are often referred to as *Mendelian* because these traits segregate within families and on average are found in specific and fixed proportions when offspring are studied whose parents have the trait. Many single-gene diseases have been shown to have abnormalities at the protein or DNA levels. The patterns of single-gene transmission depend on the location of the chromosomal locus, either autosomal or X-linked, and whether the phenotype is dominant or recessive. Dominant inheritance is expressed when the variant allele is carried by one chromosome of a pair, and recessive inheritance is expressed when both chromosomes of a pair carry the variant allele. Classically, the following four Mendelian patterns of inheritance have been demonstrated for single-gene disorders: autosomal and X-linked, dominant or recessive.

a. Autosomal Recessive

Autosomal recessive phenotypes account for approximately one third of Mendelian phenotypes. Recessive disorders are only homozygotes, so a mutant allele must have been inherited from both parents. An autosomal recessive phenotype has a recurrence risk of 1 in 4 for each sibling of the proband. Parents may be consanguineous, and for most types males and females are equally affected. When seen in more than one member of a kindred, the disorder is found only in the sibling of the proband and not in the parents, children, or other relatives. An example of an autosomal recessive disorder is phenylketonuria (PKU), which may lead to developmental disability, seizures, behavior disorder, and mental retardation if untreated. The basic defect is a mutation in the gene phenylalanine hydroxylase. Buildup of phenylalanine damages the developing brain. Incidence is 1 in 5,000 to 16,000 in caucasians. Gene location is 12q22–q24. There may be variation in expression.

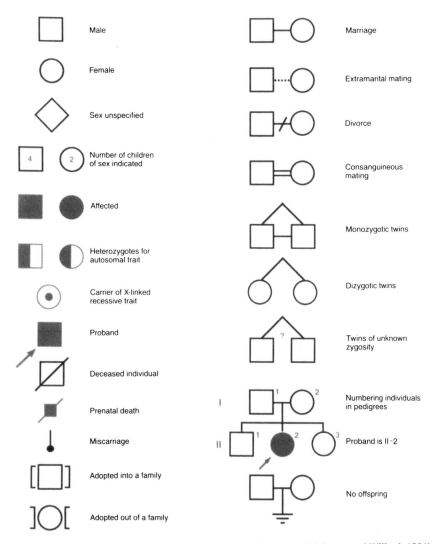

Figure 5–1. Symbols commonly used in pedigree charts (from Thompson, McInnes, and Willard, 1991).

b. Autosomal Dominant

Of 4,500 known Mendelian phenotypes, more than half are autosomal dominant traits (Thompson, McInnes, and Willard, 1991). The phenotype appears in every generation, with each person having an affected parent, (exceptions are fresh mutations and nonpenetrance); children of affected parents are at 50% risk of inheritance. Phenotypically normal individuals do not transmit the condition to their children.

Males and females are equally likely to transmit to male or female offspring. Male-to-male transmission can occur, and males may have unaffected daughters. An example that commonly involves the nervous system is neurofibromatosis (NF1); its occurrence is 1 in 3,000 to 5,000. This is a common autosomal dominant phenotype with full penetrance, but with variation in expression from minimal to severe involvement. Gene location is 17q11.2.

c. X-linked Recessive

The incidence for X-linked recessive disorder is much greater in males than in females. The gene is transmitted from an affected male through all of his daughters. The daughters' sons have a 50% chance of inheriting the disorder. It is never transmitted from father to son, but is transmitted by way of a series of females who are carriers. Ordinarily, heterozygous females are not affected, but in some disorders they may show the condition with varying degrees of severity. An example is Duchenne Muscular Dystrophy (DMD), whose occurrence is 1 in 3,000 to 3,500 male births. The basic defect is an abnormality in the structural gene for the muscle protein, dystropin, which leads to muscle degeneration. Gene location is X_{p21}. This was the first gene to be cloned based on knowledge of its chromosomal location.

d. X-linked Dominant

In this form of inheritance in affected males with normal wives, all of the daughters and none of the sons are affected. Each child, male or female, of an affected family member has a 50% chance of inheriting the phenotype, just as in the autosomal dominant pedigree pattern. Although both sexes are affected, because of the severity of a condition, they may not reproduce. In very rare phenotypes, females are affected about twice as often as males, but often have a milder (although variable) form of the disorder. An example is X-linked hypophosphatemic rickets (vitamin D resistant rickets), which affects the kidney tubules' ability to reabsorb phosphate. Both sexes are affected, but serum phosphate is less depressed and rickets less severe in heterozygous females. Rett's disorder was originally hypothesized to be an X-linked dominant disorder that is lethal in hemizygous males. The disorder occurs exclusively in females, who are almost always single cases in a family and thought to be new mutations. Girls with Rett syndrome are severely handicapped and do not reproduce. In this instance, there is the absence of a family history, but evidence points to this being a genetic disorder. However, X involvement has not been established.

2. Chromosomal Disorders (no abnormal gene or gene product)

Chromosomal abnormalities have been shown in more than 60 identifiable syndromes, represent 0.7% of live births, and account for half of spontaneous first trimester abortions. The major disorders of chromosomes are three autosomal trisomies (13, 18, 21) and the four types of sex chromosomal aneuploidy: Turner's syndrome (ordinarily 45, X); Klinefelter syndrome (47, XXY); 47, XYY syndrome, and 47, XXX syndrome. There is no error in genetic information (i.e., no mutation), but there is an excess or deficiency of genes in the whole chromosome or chromosomal segment. The chromosomal basis of a growing number of significant disorders has been demonstrated. These disorders occur in 7 of 1000 births and are responsible for about 50% of abortions. An example is Down syndrome, in which an extra copy of chromosome 21 results in the most common mental retardation syndrome, although no individual gene on the chromosome is abnormal.

3. Multifactorial Inheritance (no single error in genetic information; a combination of small variations)

The greatest number of genetic phenotypes are those that are found in families in which there is neither a single gene mutation nor a chromosomal disorder; rather, these genetic phenotypes are multifactorial in origin. Multifactorial inheritance is defined as the inheritance of genetic factors and nongenetic factors, each of which is thought to have a small effect. In some instances, the role of environmental factors may be relatively large. In the multifactorial model, the disorder is familial, yet no distinctive pattern of inheritance is demonstrated in a family. Despite this, the recurrence risk is higher when more than one family member is affected, in contrast to single-gene disorders, where the risk is unchanged from one child to the next. The risk is much lower for second-degree relatives than for first-degree relatives, in contrast to autosomal dominant conditions, where the risk drops by half with each step of more distant relationship. In autosomal recessive conditions, it is the siblings who are at risk and not other relatives. In addition, more severely affected patients and their relatives are at greater risk. Finally, the risk to subsequent siblings is increased when the patients are consanguineous. A multifactorial threshold model has been developed that predicts that the risk for first-degree relatives is equal to the square root of the population incidence of a multifactorial trait. Such a relationship is not true for single-gene traits, where the risk for siblings is, for the most part, independent of population frequency.

Multifactorial models have been applied to account for several chronic diseases. Both schizophrenia and manic depressive disease may have multifactorial inheritance. However, there is a continuing effort to look for single-gene defects in these conditions. Overall, these conditions do not show characteristic pedigree patterns as do single genetic traits.

PHENOTYPIC EXPRESSION

Expression of abnormal genotype may be modified by other genetic loci and/or environmental factors. Differences in expression, which are more often found in autosomal dominant conditions, may lead to problems in diagnosis and in the interpretation of pedigrees. This is borne out in clinical experience, where some disorders are not expressed at all in persons who are genetically predisposed. In other instances, there may be variability in clinical severity, age of onset, or both. Some of the most severe neuropsychiatric disorders that may have variable ages of onset include autistic disorder, major depression, and schizophrenia. Finally, pleiotrophy must be considered. Pleiotrophy is a term used to describe multiple phenotypic effects of a single gene or gene pair. Two important concepts in gene expression are penetrance and expressivity.

Penetrance

Penetrance refers to the probability that a gene will have any phenotypic expression. It refers to the percentage of people who are actively affected. The term is used primarily for dominant traits in heterozygous carriers. It denotes the all-or-none expression of mutant genotypes. If less than 100% of the carriers of the responsible allele show the disorder, penetrance is reduced. If 60% of the carriers express it, it is 60% penetrant. Failure of penetrance can lead to apparent skipping of generations in a family tree.

Expressivity

Expressivity indicates the degree or extent of expression of a genetic defect. A defect may show variable expressivity; the trait may vary in its expression from a mild to a severe form. In variable expressivity, the trait is expressed in varying degrees, but it is never not expressed in those who have that particular gene type. Many of the single-gene disorders show multiple characteristic effects. Differences may be seen in the range of abnormalities present and in the severity of the particular manifestation. Examples of gene disorders that show considerable variation in expression include neurofibromatosis and Marfan's syndrome.

NONCLASSICAL PATTERNS OF INHERITANCE

Although uncommon, recent genetic study has resulted in the description of non-Mendelian patterns of inheritance — e.g, genomic imprinting (differential expression of chromosomal material depending on whether the material is inherited from the male or female parent) (Hodgson, 1991); uniparental disomy (the presence of two chromosomes of a pair inherited from one parent with no representation of that chromosome from the other parent); mosaicism (the presence of two or more cell lines having the same origin in the same single zygote but genetically different due to postzygotic mutation or nondysjunction); and mitochondrial inheritance (inheritance of a disorder that is encoded in the mitochondrial genome). Of particular interest is the occurrence of mosaicism and genomic imprinting. Furthermore, studies of the Fragile X syndrome and Huntington's disease have provided insight into "heritable unstable elements" (Richards and Sutherland, 1992). Here, genes are disrupted by inherited unstable DNA elements.

Genomic Imprinting

Genomic imprinting challenges the fundamental assumption of Mendelian genetics that the effect of a gene is fully independent of whether it originally came from the offspring's mother or father. It has now been shown that genes at a chromosomal locus may be differentially inherited from the mother or the father. The parental origin of genetic material can have profound impact on clinical expression of defect. For example, deletion of the 15q11–q13 on one copy of chromosome 15 may be associated with difficulty in behavioral regulation in two different mental retardation syndromes. In one instance, the deletion is in the maternal contribution; in the other, in the paternal contribution. Prader-Willi syndrome (paternal 15q11–13 absent) is characterized by hypogonadism and hyperphagia, leading to massive obesity. Angelman's syndrome (maternal 15q11–13 absent) is characterized by motor clumsiness and problems in affect regulation with periodic bursts of unexpected laughter. Both conditions can be associated with sleep disturbances.

Trinucleotide Repeat Expansion (heritable unstable elements)

A new type of genetic mutation in which genes are unstable and expand or grow larger in subsequent generations, resulting in increasingly more severe forms of disease in their progeny, has been described in myotonic dystrophy, in the Fragile X syndrome (the most common known inherited form of mental retardation) (Hagerman, 1992) and in Huntington's disease (Huntington's Disease Collaborative Research Group, 1993). This phenomenon is now being considered in patients with schizophrenia and bipolar mood disorder.

Prior to identification of heritable unstable DNA elements, the Fragile X syndrome, which occurs in both sexes, was considered to be a dominant X-linked disorder with reduced penetrance in females. Fragile X syndrome has been a puzzle because 80% of males who inherit the mutation have moderate to severe mental impairment, but other males with the mutation have normal intelligence. About 50% of females who inherit the disease from their mothers are cytogenetically positive, but only a third are mentally retarded. To explain these findings, at least two distinct mutation types have been reported in Fragile X syndrome. One, the premutation, consists of a 50 to 600–base pair insertion

or amplification at the Fragile X locus (normal range is 5 to 48; mean 29). Individuals with the premutation do not show the most serious aspects of the clinical syndrome such as severe mental retardation. In the full mutation (i.e., insertion of 600 to 3000 base pairs), both males and females are at greater risk for more severe neuropsychiatric disability related to inactivation of the adjacent candidate FMR-1 gene. This gene is characterized by an unstable CGG repeat sequence that may grow from generation to generation. In males, the degree of clinical involvement appears to correlate with the length of the abnormal CGG repetitive sequence. When the premutation is passed from father to daughter, it remains relatively unchanged in size. However, when it is passed through the mother, it may increase in size and potentially convert to the full mutation in both sons and daughters. Children inheriting an X chromosome with the full mutation from their mother will also have the full mutation, and it often is even further increased in size. Therefore, the premutation increases in size and potentially converts to a full mutation only when it is passed through a female. It has been hypothesized that this conversion occurs during female gametogenesis and that sex-specific imprinting is involved. In addition to the mechanism just described, the Fragile X syndrome phenotype has now also been reported in a patient with a deletion of the FMR-1 gene (Wiegers, 1992).

Fragile X males show a behavioral phenotype of gaze aversion and may present with an autistic-like syndrome whose natural history is distinct from that of classical autistic disorder. In Fragile X females, abnormalities in social interaction, thought process, and affect regulation have been reported (Reiss and Freund, 1990; Reiss et al., 1988).

In the Huntington's disease (HD) gene on chromosome 4, a mutation also affects a triplet of bases, an unstable CAG sequence, and leads to an expansion of tandem repeats similar to the Fragile X syndrome. In the general population, the gene has 11 to 34 triplets, but in Huntington's patients, 35 to 100 or more repeats have been demonstrated. The next step in the study of Huntington's disease is to find how the protein expressed by the Huntington's gene normally functions. HD involves the basal ganglia and is manifested by the progressive onset of chorea, personality changes, memory loss, irritability and dementia. Huntington's disease ordinarily begins in the third to fifth decade but may present in childhood and adolescence. Folstein et al. (1983) studied a sample of 112 offspring of 34 HD patients and found that affective disorder in the offspring was strongly associated with similar symptoms in the parent. They suggested that affective disorder, but not conduct disorder, may be an early manifestation of the HD gene.

METHODOLOGY FOR GENETIC STUDY

Family studies allow analysis of patterns of family aggregation of disease to clarify the mode of genetic transmission. Because of problems in separating genetic and environmental factors, in addition to family studies, twin and adoption studies are important research strategies (Rutter et al., 1990a). The twin and adoption studies allow calculation of the strength of genetic differences (i.e., characteristics or predispositions). Studies of twins and adoptees provide important opportunities for differentiation and genetic and environmental effects. These studies help define the disorder, but neither provides evidence of the mode of genetic transmission. Each of these approaches is now described.

1. Twin Studies

The comparison of monozygotic (MZ) with dizygotic (DZ) twin pairs is recognized as one of the best-established genetic procedures. It is based on the fact that MZ twins share all their genes in common, whereas DZ twins, on average, share half of their genes. Within pairs of twins, correlations allow an estimate of the role of genetic factors in individual variation expressed as a disorder, a manifest trait, or a behavioral characteristic. Twin research designs are strengthened when pairs who are discordant for the trait are studied. The offspring of twins concordant or discordant for the trait may also be investigated. Of particular interest are twins who were separated in infancy and brought up in different environments. Twin studies are also useful when dealing with conditions of variable expressivity and in genetically heterogeneous conditions to investigate the range of the phenotype. For example, twins discordant for autistic disorder were found usually concordant for more broadly defined cognitive and social deficits. Twin studies may be useful to find the effects of shared and nonshared environments. However, there is debate as to whether MZ or DZ twins may differ in comparability of shared environments.

2. Adoption Designs

Investigation of adopted children is an important genetic strategy because it allows for the comparison of biological parents with adoptive parents; this provides a comparison of biological and social parentage (Cadoret, 1986). Furthermore, comparison of rates of disorder in biological and adoptive relatives is feasible. There are a variety of research designs: assessment of the adoptee, cross-fostering, adopted sibling, and parent-offspring adoption. An issue that must be considered is the effect of the type of adoptive home (selective placement), because all homes are not the same. Analysis must consider psychiatric illness in both parents; however, data often is only available from the mother's family. The stress of being an adoptee must also be considered as a diagnostic issue.

In the *adoption paradigm,* the earliest approach was to begin with a biological parent who had a mental disorder and determine the rate of disorder in adopted-away offspring who were separated from the ill parent in early childhood and raised in a different household. In the adoptee family design, a specific disorder in the adoptees leads to a comparison of the rates of that disorder in the biological and adoptive family members, or between the biological relatives of adoptees and those of adoptee control subjects. In the *cross-fostering design,* there is a comparison of children born to normal parents but reared by adoptive parents, one of whom developed the mental disorder that is being studied, and children born to a parent with that disorder but reared by normal foster parents. Another approach is the *adopted sibling design,* which compares the concordance between genetically related pairs of adult adoptees who have been reared separately and genetically unrelated pairs of adoptees who have been reared together. A final design is the *parent-offspring adoption design.* Here, the comparison of parent-offspring associations between adoptive and nonadoptive families provides a tool to investigate genetic effects of environmental correlations between parents and offspring as well as direct environmental effects.

3. Family Genetic Methods

Two basic types of family study have been used to study genetic factors in child psychiatric disorders. The first is the "family aggregation study," which searches for an increased frequency of a disorder among family members who are biologically at risk. The second is adoption or cross-fostering studies, which focus on biologically related individuals who have been reared apart and biologically unrelated individuals who have been reared in similar environments.

Currently these approaches benefit from better-structured interview methods and in careful choice of cases and control groups. Issues that are pertinent in family studies are heterogeneity and comorbidity with other disorders. Estimates have been reported based on the severe presentation of a disorder or on a spectrum of disorders.

As indicated earlier, twin and adoption studies allow evaluation of the extent of genetic influences on some characteristic or predisposition to a disorder, yet neither provides adequate evidence on the mode of genetic transmission (Rutter et al., 1990a). Information on genetic transmission can be provided by family genetic studies. These include case-control studies, high-risk studies, biological trait risk markers, dual mating strategy, sibling comparisons, familial-sporadic distinction, and one- and two-sided familial loading. These approaches are described in detail by Rutter et al. (1990a).

Family genetic studies are particularly important in showing the mode of inheritance for disorders that follow the Mendelian pattern, yet few psychiatric disorders clearly follow this traditional pattern of inheritance. As a result, mathematical modeling may be necessary to test the consistency of first-degree relative or full pedigree information with the different modes of genetic transmission. In addition, genetic linkage analyses use family data to determine if specific disorders in families segregate in the same way as do genetic markers

that are controlled by a single genetic locus for which an approximate chromosomal location is known. In linkage analyses, it is not expected that the markers are either associated with the disorder or related in a causal manner. This approach only establishes that the gene for the disorder and the gene for one of the close neighbors are on the same chromosome. Linkage analyses played an important role in identifying the chromosomal region in the search for the gene for Huntington's disease.

GENETIC CONSIDERATIONS IN THE CHILDHOOD ONSET OF MENTAL DISORDERS

Genetic studies have been carried out to study the concordance of general behavioral deviance in twins. Monozygotic/dizygotic differences in concordance indicate a genetic component, with heredity being over 50% (Graham and Stevenson, 1985). However, for genetic counseling, findings in specific disorders are needed (Rutter, 1966). The child and adolescent psychiatric conditions for which genetic factors have been considered most likely are autistic disorder, schizophrenia, Tourette's disorder, and bipolar mood disorder. Conduct disorder, attention deficit disorder, anxiety disorders, and learning disability also are being actively investigated.

1. Autistic Disorder

Autistic disorder is a rare disorder with a population prevalence of 4 in 10,000 or 0.04% for the classical disorder, but the rate is higher, 12 to 15 in 10,000, for more broadly defined autistic-like conditions. The general population prevalence rate for autistic disorder in siblings and DZ twins is 3%. The risk for a family having a second affected child is 8% to 10% for male children, and overall about 6%. In MZ twins, from data pooled from several twin studies (Folstein and Rutter, 1987; Rutter et al., 1990b), the rate is approximately 50%. Because the base rate is so low for autistic disorder in the general population, Rutter (1991) suggested that autistic disorder may be one of the most strongly genetically influenced child psychiatric conditions. The concordance pattern points to the involvement of several genes, which may act in combination.

Because of the social disability, it is rare that an individual with autistic disorder marries, yet the disorder continues to be expressed. This may relate to there being a spectrum of autistic-like deficits and perhaps an as yet unrecognized advantage for the heterozygote.

2. Schizophrenia

Schizophrenia affects approximately 1% of the population. It has been approached using family studies, twin studies, and adoption studies. Qualitative modeling studies have not supported a specific mode of genetic transmission (Tsuang, Gilbertson, and Faraone, 1990). It is a complex genetic disorder, and most support is for the multifactorial polygenetic model (De Marchi, 1991). However, a mixed genetic model with both a multifactorial component and a single major locus cannot be ruled out. Family studies support family transmission but do not resolve environmental versus genetic mechanisms. Twin and adoption studies provide evidence for a genetic component and suggest that environmental components are much less important. There is little support for the single major locus genetic type of inheritance. Despite this, there continues to be an active search for a single gene etiology. Linkage studies are preliminary and inconsistent. Although localization on chromosome 5 (McGillivray et al., 1990) has been suggested, it has not been verified in follow-up studies. Because it is most likely a heterogeneous condition, the identification of potential subtypes is of importance. Clarifying risk factors that are distinct from genetic history is also essential.

3. Tourette's Disorder Spectrum

There is a pattern of disorders in family pedigrees with Tourette's disorder, which includes tics and obsessive-compulsive disorder (Pauls et al., 1988). Family studies have identified the tics in Tourette's disorder as occurring more often in males, and the obsessive-compulsive disorder more often in females. This Tourette's/tic/obsessive compulsive disorder phenotype is highly penetrant and is most likely inherited as an autosomal dominant condition with differential sexual penetrance. Concordance studies in 30 MZ and 13 DZ twin pairs, identified in a questionnaire study, was 53% and 8% respectively, but concordance for tic plus Tourette's was 77% and 23% from questionnaires; the rate approached 1.0 in MZ twins when cases were directly examined. When the full spectrum of presentation is considered, genetic analyses indicate that Tourette's spectrum may be inherited as a single gene.

4. Major Depression

The risk for mood disorders for relatives of a depressed patient is greater than the risk for the general population. The risk increases with the proportion of genes that are shared with a mood-disordered parent or parents (Beardslee et al., 1983; Weissman et al., 1987). There is some evidence that increased genetic loading leads to earlier expression of depressive disorder in childhood. Conversely, early onset is associated with increased risk in relatives, so it important to ask about the age of onset in family members when a parent reports a family history of depression. The concordance rate among monozygotic twins is three times the rate in dizygotic twins. The MZ twin concordance rate is 0.7 for bipolar disorder and 0.5 for unipolar disorder.

The relatives of bipolar patients have a greater risk for both bipolar disorder and for unipolar disorder; this finding also is shown in twin studies. Therefore, bipolar disorder has a greater familial component than unipolar disorder, but unipolar disorder may have a greater environmental component. Because women are at greater risk and transmission from fathers to sons is less frequent, an X-chromosome locus has been suggested for bipolar disorder. This is being investigated but has not been confirmed by genetic studies, nor have other single genes been conclusively identified. No specific mode of genetic transmission is consistently identified using mathematical modeling. Both multifactorial and mixed single-gene/multifactorial models have been suggested. However, because the condition is probably heterogeneous, analysis is unclear. Linkage studies are inconsistent, and although the X chromosome, chromosome 11, and chromosome 18 have been implicated, independent replication has not confirmed these findings. Biological markers, such as transport of lithium into red cells and cholinergic supersensitivity, have been suggested but not confirmed. Pharmacogenetic study is consistent with similar drug responses in an identified patient when more than one relative is affected. Future investigations must deal with both genotypic and phenotypic heterogeneity. The first suggests that more than one genotype can cause the disorder, and phenotypic heterogeneity indicates that a specific pathological genotype can be expressed in multiple behavioral phenotypes.

5. Attention Deficit/Hyperactivity Disorder

Because of methodological problems, the initial studies suggesting genetic factors in the etiology of attention deficit/hyperactivity disorder (AD/HD) have been supplemented by twin studies that compared MZ and DZ pairs (Goodman and Stevenson, 1989). Concordance for hyperkinesis, when MZ and DZ pairs were pooled, was 50% in a questionnaire-based twin study carried out by Graham and Stevenson (1985) in which one of the twins demonstrated pervasive hyperactivity at home and in school.

The study of the genetics of attention deficit/hyperactivity disorder has been complicated by the frequent co-occurrence of oppositional and antisocial behavior in these children. Children referred to psychiatric clinics often are referred for their behavioral difficulties rather than an attention deficit disorder alone. It has been suggested that there may be different family backgrounds for children with learning disabilities and hyperactivity in contrast to those with hyperactivity and aggressive behavior (August, Stewart, and Tsai, 1981). No firm conclusions can be reached on heritability at this time. Systematic study is needed of children with pervasive hyperactivity/inattention beginning early in life, with careful attention given to oppositional and conduct symptoms and learning disabilities.

Attention deficit disorder may occur in a variety of genetic disorders, such as PKU and neurofibromatosis. In PKU there is a potential link to the proposed catecholamine abnormality in AD/HD because phenylalanine is a precursor to tyrosine, an amino acid essential to catecholamine synthesis. Recently, Hauser et al. (1993) have studied the occurrence of AD/HD in 104 members of 18 families with generalized resistance to thyroid hormone. In this disorder,

there is a genetic defect in assembling thyroid receptors caused by mutations in the thyroid receptor β gene. They found that 70% of children and 50% of adults with the gene for this disorder had AD/HD. In this disorder there may also be a potential link to the catecholamine neurotransmitter system which may be influenced by the thyroid receptor–thyroid hormone complex. Theoretically, mutations of the hTRβ gene could affect behavior through developmental effects during critical periods of brain development. However, this condition is rare, and these findings are controversial (Weiss et al., 1994).

Additional study is needed on the common forms of AD/HD that are not associated with a known syndrome, because there is strong family aggregation of this disorder.

6. Anxiety Disorders

In adults, a familial loading for anxiety disorders has been reported (Last, Phillips, and Statfeld, 1987). Both generalized anxiety disorder and panic disorder with agoraphobia have been considered to have genetic components. Panic disorder with depression has been distinguished from depression alone. Whether these patterns are genetically based or the result of environmental or social transmission in the family is not clear. Twin studies have shown conflicting results; one recent study showed the importance of genetic factors in agoraphobia and panic disorder but not in generalized anxiety disorder.

For children, an increased rate of separation anxiety in parents of children with school refusal (phobia) has been reported (Berg, 1976). Mothers of children with overanxious disorder differ from those with separation anxiety disorder in their histories of past overanxious symptoms. The rate of separation anxiety has been reported to be increased in children whose mothers are agoraphobic. Increased anxiety disorders have been reported in younger children of depressed mothers. Family loading is then present for both children and adults, but additional research is needed to clarify the genetic/environmental interface.

7. Conduct Disorder

In adults, twin and adoptee studies suggest a genetic component in antisocial behavior and in criminality that is greatest for repeated minor crimes rather than for major crimes or violent antisocial behavior (Cloninger and Gottesman, 1987). In twin studies, concordance rates are significant between MZ/DZ twins, with 26% to 51% in MZ twins as contrasted with 13% to 22% for DZ twins (Rowe, 1986). Adoption studies are also consistent in showing a genetic component with associations between personality disorder/criminality in biological parents and similar conditions in their children who were placed in adoptive homes. This genetic risk may depend on exposure to risk environments (e.g., multiple placements, extended institutional care, and lower occupational status). In adolescence, there is an increased risk for delinquent behavior (Rowe 1983, 1986). Because rates are high in both MZ and DZ twins, the family environment is an important factor. Adoption studies suggest a weak genetic component. Although most children with antisocial behavior do not go on to develop adult antisocial disorders, those who do have the onset in childhood or adolescence. Therefore, in the group with persistent antisocial behavior, part of the risk may be due to a genetic component, which is influenced by the psychosocial setting where the child is reared. Furthermore, expression may be different in male and female children in that affected girls may have more somatic and mood complaints and boys more antisocial behavior. The underlying problems may include the child's social deficits. These may result in poor interpersonal relations and problems in social adaptation, which may lead to antisocial behavior in males and somatic and mood symptoms in females. Thus, the phenotype to study is a broad one and complex.

8. Alcohol and Drug Abuse

In adult studies, a significant genetic component in alcoholism has been suggested (Goedde and Agarwal, 1987), but these findings are complicated in that there may be different types of alcoholism with different types of genetic influences. For example, there may be genetic factors in the amount of alcohol consumed once an individual begins to drink. Two paths have been suggested to substance abuse (Cadoret et al., 1986), an indirect and a direct route. The indirect route may progress from alcohol problems in relatives to antisocial behavior to drug abuse. The direct route is from a family history of alcohol use to use and abuse. However, family environmental stresses, such as divorce and psychiatric disorder leading to self-medication, must also be considered. Studies of children of alcoholic parents suggest an increased risk for both alcoholism and individual psychopathology. What might be inherited is an impulsive and sensation-seeking temperament that predisposes to antisocial behavior and alcohol use as well as a specific physiological response to alcohol. However, specific behavioral and physiological markers have not been conclusively established. Alcohol and drug abuse is an area of particular importance in regard to possible prevention; therefore, a careful family history is essential.

MENTAL RETARDATION SYNDROMES

Genetic disorders were initially demonstrated in mentally retarded persons. In mildly retarded persons, genetic influences are thought to be nonspecific and multifactorial. For moderately, severely, and profoundly retarded persons (with IQ of 50 or lower), approximately one fourth have genetic etiologies. Of this group, chromosomal disorders make up the majority of cases, about 75%, followed by those having a single-gene disorder, approximately 20% of this group. Table 5–1 lists the major mental retardation syndromes and their genetic bases.

COUNSELING

When conducting counseling sessions, there is no simple answer to the question of what constitutes a genetic disorder. Not all disorders that involve more than one family member are genetic, and not all genetic disorders involve more than one family member. In making the determination, the diagnosis is of particular importance and often can be made from careful clinical description prior to ordering tests. Genetic counseling must be individualized, taking into account the accuracy of the diagnosis, the type of genetic transmission, and known information about the natural history of the condition. However, families differ in how they will utilize the information provided to them. Working in close collaboration with a geneticist, a

Table 5–1. Mode of Inheritance of
Selected Mental Retardation Syndromes

Syndrome	Mode of Inheritance
Down	
95%	Trisomy 21
1.0%	Mosaic
4.0%	Robertsonian Translocation 21q/21q
Tay Sachs disease	Autosomal Recessive
Hurler	Autosomal Recessive
Hunter	X-Linked Recessive
PKU	Autosomal Recessive
Rett	Unknown
Lesch Nyhan	X-linked Recessive
Prader Willi	Cytogenetic Deletion/genomic imprinting (maternal)
Fragile X	Trinucleotide repeat expansion (heritable unstable DNA sequences)

psychiatrist, psychologist, or social worker can assist the family in understanding the meaning and impact of the psychiatric disorder. The statistics for genetic risk for the same disorder may be interpreted differently from one family to the next, often depending on their life experience with affected family members.

Tsuang and Faraone (1990) suggest several stages for psychiatric genetic counseling. The person counseled may be the identified patient, a relative, an adolescent, or sometimes a younger sibling. The first step is to clarify the accuracy of the diagnosis. The second step is to establish a formulation of the family psychiatric history, which may involve interviews with several family members. The third step is to establish the risks, either empirical or exact. Both are based on psychiatric genetic research, but empirical risks are drawn from epidemiologic studies of morbidity. There is considerable variability between studies, but the range of research findings can be presented. Exact genetic risks can be predicted for several mental retardation syndromes but not for the major psychiatric disorders.

The recognition of genetic disorders associated with conditions that follow Mendelian lines, such as PKU, is well known, as are chromosomal disorders in children with mental retardation syndromes, such as Down syndrome and Fragile X syndrome. Non-Mendelian modes of inheritance are now becoming apparent in some men-

tal retardation syndromes. Recent work on genomic imprinting in Prader-Willi and Angelman's syndromes is of interest. Specific detailed information can be given to families about known transmission of these well-studied conditions. This is best done by an experienced genetic counsellor who appreciates the variable presentations of the particular conditions.

However, for developmental neuropsychiatric disorders such as ADHD, autistic disorder, and mental disorders such as depression and schizophrenia for which physical stigmata are generally not apparent, a specific biochemical marker is not available, and a genetic mechanism is not identified or agreed upon, genetic counseling is more problematic. Each of these conditions may be a final common pathway; multiple subtypes may be present that lead to the similar phenotypes, or the condition may be associated with another known medical disorder. In this sense, there is an analogy to cerebral palsy and mental retardation, which are general terms for conditions that may have multiple etiologies. Because of this genetic heterogeneity, counseling in these conditions must be based on epidemiologic studies of prevalence of the condition. These are often based on family studies, which depend on the accuracy of the diagnosis and the methods used in analysis. Consequently, depending on the criteria used, prevalence rates are ranges of prevalence, lower for the classic, most severe presentation, and higher if the "spectrum disorder" is included in the estimate. At issue is what is inherited: Is it a spectrum of social communication deficits as suggested in autistic disorder or a range of disorders in interpersonal functioning as seen in schizophrenia. One must be prepared to discuss prevalence of both the severe condition and the spectrum disorder while keeping in mind that subtypes may exist. Furthermore, there may be variable expression at different ages. More specifically, the multiple factors that go into multifactorial inheritance need to be reviewed with the family. The nature of the genetic contribution may be a vulnerability to stress, temperamental features that lead to choice of risk environments, or polygenetic risk of a disorder. For these conditions, the gene–environmental interactions are an important part of counseling.

Before the information is communicated to the person being counseled, an understanding of other family members' emotional state, the phase of their acceptance of the disorder, and their intentions regarding the affected child must be considered. In regard to considering having another child, the burden of the illness can be presented, but the benefits of becoming a parent can only be evaluated by the individuals being counseled. Counseling for siblings who have been found to be positive on screening and will develop a disorder at a later age is particularly difficult and requires a careful assessment. It is essential to remember that counseling is an ongoing process and that the counselor must be available for support in follow-up sessions.

REFERENCES

August, G.J., Stewart, M.A., and Tsai, L. (1981). The incidence of cognitive disabilities in the siblings of autistic children. *British Journal of Psychiatry*, 138:416–422.

Beardslee, W.R., Bemporad, J., Keller, M.B., and Klerman, G.L. (1983). Children of parents with major affective disorder: A review. *American Journal of Psychiatry*, 140:825–832.

Berg, I. (1976). School phobia in the children of agoraphobic women. *British Journal of Psychiatry*, 128:86–89.

Brown, F.R. III, Stowens, D.W., Harris, J.C., and Moser, H.G. (1985). Leukodystrophies. In R.T. Johnson (ed), *Current therapy in neurologic disease*, pp. 313–317. B.C. Decker, Inc., Philadelphia.

Cadoret, R.J. (1986). Adoption studies: Historical and methodological critique. *Psychiatric Developments*, 1:45–64.

———, Troughton, E., O'Gorman, T.W., and Heywood, M.A. (1986). An adoption study of genetic and environmental factors in drug abuse. *Archives of General Psychiatry*, 43:1131–1136.

Cloninger, C. R. and Gottesman, I.I. (1987). Genetic and environmental factors in antisocial behavior disorders. In S.A. Mednick, T.E. Moffit, and S.A. Sack (eds), *Causes of crime: New biological approaches*. Cambridge University Press, Cambridge, UK.

De Marchi, N. (1991). The genetics of schizophrenia. *Developmental Medicine and Child Neurology*, 33:452–458.

Folstein, S., and Rutter, M. (1987). Autism: Familial aggregation and genetic implications. *Journal of Autism and Developmental Disorders*, 18:3–30.

———, Franz, M.L., Jensen, B.A., Chase, G.A., and Folstein, M.F. (1983). Conduct disorder and affective disorder among the offspring of patients with Huntington's disease. *Psychological Medicine*, 13:45–52.

Goedde, H.W. and Agarwal, D. P. (eds). (1987). *Genetics and alcoholism*. Alan R. Liss, New York.

Goodman, R., and Stevenson, J. (1989). A twin study of hyperactivity. II. The aetiological role of genes, family relationships and perinatal adversity. *Journal of Child Psychology and Psychiatry*, 30:691–709.

Graham, P. and Stevenson, J. (1985). A twin study of genetic influences on behavioral deviance. *Journal of the American Academy of Child Psychiatry*, 24:33–41.

Hagerman, R. (1992). Fragile X syndrome: Advances and controversy. *Journal of Child Psychology and Psychiatry*, 7:1127–1139.

Hauser, P., Zametkin, A.J., Martinez, P., Vitiello, B., Matochik, J.A., Mixon, J., and Weintraub, B.D. (1993). Attention deficit–hyperactivity disorder in people with generalized resistance to thyroid hormone. *New England Journal of Medicine*, 328:997–1001.

Hodgson, S. (1991). Genomic imprinting. *Developmental Medicine and Child Neurology*, 33:552–556.

Huntington's Disease Collaborative Research Group. (1993). A novel gene containing a trinucleotide repeat that is expanded and unstable on Huntington's disease chromosomes. *Cell*, 72(6):971–983.

Last, C. G., Phillips, J.E., and Statfeld, A. (1987). Childhood anxiety disorders in mothers and their children. *Child Psychiatry and Human Development*, 18:102–109.

McGillivray, B.C., Bassett, A.S., Langlois, S., Pantzar, T., and Wood, S. (1990). Familial 5q11.2–q13.3 segmental duplication cosegregating with multiple anomalies, including schizophrenia. *American Journal of Medical Genetics*, 35:10–13.

McKusick, V.A. (1990). *Mendelian inheritance in man: Catalogs of autosomal dominant, autosomal recessive, and X-linked phenotypes*, 9th ed. Johns Hopkins University Press, Baltimore.

Pauls, D.J., Cohen, D.J., Kidd, K.K., and Leckman, J. (1988). Tourette syndrome and neuropsychiatric disorders: Is there a genetic relationship? *American Journal of Human Genetics*, 43:206–209.

Reiss, A.L. and Freund, L. (1990). Neuropsychiatric aspects of the Fragile-X syndrome. *Brain Dysfunction*, 3:9–22.

———, Hagerman, R.J., Vinogradov, S., Abrams, M., and King, R.J. (1988). Psychiatric disability in female carriers of the fragile X syndrome. *Archives of General Psychiatry*, 45:25–30.

Richards, R.I. and Sutherland, G.R. (1992). Heritable unstable DNA sequences. *Nature Genetics*, 1:7–9.

Rotter, J.I., and Diamond, J.M. (1987). What maintains frequencies of human genetic diseases. *Nature*, 329:289–290.

Rowe, D.C. (1983). Biometric models of self-reported delinquent behavior: A twin study. *Behavior Genetics,* 13:473–489.

_____. (1986). Genetic and environmental components of antisocial pairs: A study of 265 twin pairs. *Criminology,* 24:513–532.

Rutter, M. (1966). *Children of sick parents: An environmental and psychiatric study.* IOP Maudsley Monograph No. 16. Oxford University Press, London.

_____. (1991). Nature, nurture, and psychopathology: A new look at an old topic. *Development and Psychopathology,* 3:125–137.

_____, Bolton, P., Harrington, R., LeCouteur, A., Macdonald, H., and Simonoff, E. (1990a). Genetic factors in child psychiatric disorders. I. A review of research strategies. *Journal of Child Psychology and Psychiatry,* 31:3–39.

_____, Macdonald, H., LeCouteur, A.H., Harrington, R., Bolton, P., and Bailey, A. (1990b). Genetic factors in child psychiatric disorders. II. Empirical findings. *Journal of Child Psychology and Psychiatry,* 31:39–85.

Scarr, S., and McCartney, K. (1983). How people make their own environments: A theory of genotype greater than environmental effects. *Child Development,* 54:424–435.

Thompson, M.W., McInnes, R., and Willard, H.F. (1991). *Genetics in medicine.* W.B. Saunders Company, Philadelphia.

Tsuang, M.T. and Faraone, S.V. (1990). *The genetics of mood disorders.* The Johns Hopkins University Press, Baltimore and London.

_____, Gilbertson, M.W., and Faraone, S.V. (1990). The genetics of schizophrenia: Current knowledge and future directions. *Schizophrenia Research,* 4:157–171.

Weiss, R., Stein, M., Duck, S., Chyna, B., Phillips, W., O'Brien, T., and Gutermuth, L. (1994). Low intelligence but not attention deficit hyperactivity disorder is associated with resistance to thyroid hormone caused by mutation R316H in the thyroid hormone receptor β gene. *Journal of Clinical Endocrinology and Metabolism,* 78:1525–1528.

Weissman, M.M., Gammon, G.D., John, K., Merikangas, K.R., Prusoff, B.A., and Sholomskas, D. (1987). Children of depressed parents: Increased psychopathology and early onset of major depression. *Archives of General Psychiatry,* 44:847–853.

Wiegers, A. (1992). Identical psychological profile and behavior pattern in different types of mutation in the FMR-1 region. Paper presented at the 2nd International Symposium, Society for the Study of Behavioural Phenotypes, *From Genes to Behaviour.* Welshpool, UK. November 19–21, 1992.

PART II
COGNITIVE NEUROSCIENCE

Cognitive neuroscience utilizes an interdisciplinary approach to understand how brain functions result in mental activities, such as perception, attention, memory, emotional experience, language, and the organization of behavior. Three older fields — experimental psychology, neuroscience, and computer science — provide the basis for the methods and theory utilized in cognitive neuroscience, which represents an integration across these fields. This progress has been gradual, beginning in the 1920s and 1930s, and continuing into the 1970s and 1980s with neurobiological analysis of simple behavioral systems and the analysis of elementary forms of learning. The current challenge focuses on the highest cognitive functions. Understanding neural organization of these higher functions may result in an understanding of the principles of mind/brain function that may lead to a better understanding of human behavior.

Kandel and Squire (1992) identify four early influences that precede current achievements in cognitive neuroscience. The first of these is the emergence of cognitive psychology in the 1960s. Prior to that time, behaviorism was the primary focus in psychology. Behaviorism had replaced introspectionism with behavioral analysis that emphasized observable actions. The study of elicited behaviors and the stimuli that generate them had been an essential part of the methodological approach that allowed behavioralism to assume prominence in psychology. The behaviorists rejected the processes the introspectionists emphasized because they were inaccessible to behavioral analysis. As a result, the internal representations that underlie perception, thinking, attention, and strategies for motor activity, as well as conscious (semantic/episodic or declarative) memory were ignored. The behavioral approach has limited experimental psychology, which is based on examining behavior and inferring principles of mental function. The shift to cognitive psychology allowed experimental psychology to again study internal representations of mental events. However, to deal with the challenge that mental processes were largely inaccessible to experimental analysis, new approaches were needed.

Recent progress in brain imaging and in systems neurobiology are approaches that have made it possible to study internal representation directly. Cognitive neuroscience, which merges cognitive psychology and neuroscience, addresses localization within the brain of the cognitive capacities. Consequently, mental functions can be localized to brain regions, whose activity can be monitored using metabolic activation PET studies and functional MRI. Because of these developments in studying brain processes, higher mental functions no longer need to be inferred from behavioral observation, but can be studied directly in both experimental animals and human subjects. These new developments will allow detailed analyses of language and cognitive development in childhood, and the study of methods of problem solving by children.

A second major development in cognitive neuroscience is the expansion of computer sciences to simulate cognitive performance (i.e., the development of artificial intelligence). These advances in the use of computers allow us to think more specifically about how complex information processing takes place. The computer has become a tool for symbol manipulation in the study of mental functioning.

A third element in modern cognitive neuroscience focuses on ethology (see Chapter 12). The ethologists have long emphasized the importance of inherited aspects of behavior and the evolutionary origins of species-typical behavior (MacLean, 1990). Ethologists have pointed out the limitations of operant conditioning, which, in natural settings, occurs primarily during exploratory behavior. They have broadened the definitions of behavior, learning, and attention. Operant methods address a special property of central nervous systems to respond by "feeding back" the consequences of performance to the biological system that initiated the behavior (Lorenz, 1981). If successful, this feedback leads to reinforcement; if not, to extinction of behavior. The ethologists have taught us that the effectiveness of behavioral approaches is not due to their being an "empty organism" but paradoxically to the existence of analogous structures that have convergently evolved in many organisms with a central nervous system which utilizes feedback. What is learned is the circumstances when phylogenetically preadapted motoric patterns of behavior are to be carried out. The ethologists do recognize the importance of learning by reinforcement but are critical of the implication that "there is nothing else in the behavior to investigate." As Lorenz (1981) suggests, what remains to be investigated is what makes "an octopus an octopus, a pigeon a pigeon, a rat a rat, and a man a man . . ." Lorenz also suggests that a more appropriate translation of Pavlov's use of the word *verstarken* is "to encourage or discourage," rather than "to reinforce and to extinguish." This translation is more in keeping with the therapeutic attitude recommended in the "gentle teaching" approach to behavior management.

The approach to cognitive neuroscience addresses certain aspects of ethology such as species-typical behaviors — e.g., attachment, extent of sociability, and (in man) conceptual thought. Ethology focuses on behavior more comprehensively through its study of evolutionary biology and offers biological interpretations for species-typical behavior. The variety of natural behaviors in reptiles, mammals, and higher primates offers a rich mosaic to understand patterns of behavior developmentally.

The fourth and last element that is essential to the development of cognitive neuroscience comes from neuroscience. Cognitive neuroscience encompasses neuropsychology, which merges neurology and psychology. Both fields investigate how the brain produces behavior in mental life. However, cognitive neuroscience, through the study of neuroanatomy, neurophysiology, and "lesion-behavior analysis," offers new experimental paradigms to analyze cognition. Neuroimaging technologies provide an opportunity to study anatomy and brain function directly in living human subjects with brain dysfunction. Moreover, brain-based models of cognitive processes lead to specific brain regions, where processes can be studied more directly, ultimately at the cellular and molecular levels.

New neural network models (Chapter 10) investigate processes, such as memory and visual perception, that are perceived by an individual as continuous by breaking them down into their component functions.

In the following chapters attention, emotion, language, memory, neural networks, and consciousness are considered. For more extensive coverage of these topics and others in the cognitive neurosciences the reader is referred to the comprehensive textbook edited by Gazzaniga.

References

Gazzaniga, M.S. (1995). *The cognitive neurosciences.* The MIT Press, Cambridge, MA.
Kandel, E., and Squire, L. (1992). Cognitive neuroscience: Editorial overview. *Current Opinion in Neurobiology,* 2:143–146.
Lorenz, K. (1981). *The foundations of ethology,* pp. 70–71, 293. Springer-Verlag, New York.
MacLean, P.D. (1990). *The triune brain in evolution: Role in paleocerebral functions.* Plenum Press, New York.

CHAPTER 6

ATTENTION

ATTENTION SYSTEMS

In his *Principles of Psychology,* William James (1890) suggested that attention is at the center of human performance. Now, a century later, developments in cognitive neuroscience allow the physiologic analysis of higher cognitive functions and provide a means to study attention and identify a functional anatomy of the human attentional system. The attention system is basic for the selection of information for conscious processing. Attention is the essential link between mind and brain in connecting the mental level of description (cognitive science) with the anatomic level (neuroscience). Sperry (1988) indicates that attention is an emergent mental property that is new and was previously nonexistent. Mental properties "interact causally at their own higher level" and may exert causal control downward. Attention allows the causal coordination of brain systems by mental states. Its study may allow us to better understand how voluntary control over autonomic systems can be accomplished. Yet it must be kept in mind that attention processes are the activities of people and not of brains.

Multiple experimental methods have converged to allow the study of attention. These include mental chronometry, brain lesions, electrophysiology, and neuroimaging studies.

This chapter will discuss definitions of attention and its characteristics, consider developmental aspects, review anatomic substrates for attention, and introduce psychopathological conditions involving attention.

DEFINITION AND CHARACTERISTICS

Attention (Sims, 1988) is the active or passive focusing of consciousness upon an experience. It is active when externally focused and passive when focusing on the flow of internal events. Attention may be voluntary or involuntary. It is voluntary when effort is focused on an internal or external event by choice or intention and involuntary when an event or object attracts attention without deliberate conscious choice or intentional effort.

Attention is not the same as consciousness although it depends upon it, in that full attention is not possible with reduced consciousness. Yet varying degrees of attention are possible with full consciousness. An object is held in attention voluntarily at a particular focus and becomes the center of attention. Events outside this center, which are peripheral to awareness, may intrude and reduce the clarity of attention.

In regard to thought, active attention focuses and guides its direction. When focused, attention is used to clarify and make thought coherent. Passive attention observes the flow of the thought associations which pass voluntarily into awareness or into consciousness.

Posner and Petersen (1990) suggest that there are subsystems of attention. These include

(1) orientation to sensory events, (2) target detection or selectivity of attention for conscious processing, and (3) maintenance of a sustained state. When attention is used to orient to sensory experience, the term "orientation" is used. Orientation refers to the setting in time and place, and the realities of one's person and situation. As a target detection system, attention selects sensory input from sensory channels and from working memory (see Chapter 9). Attention is closely bound to memory.

ATTENTION AS THE MIND'S EYE

The visual metaphor, the mind's eye, is useful when describing attention. Using this visual metaphor, we see that attention may be focused or peripheral or may come into a central point of clarity. When one is concurrently alert and vigilant, attention may either move easily from one object to another or become absorbed. In absorption, it is narrowed through focus on a particular object so that other awarenesses are not recorded in memory. Attention is normally reduced with fatigue and boredom (reduction of affective interest in an object or person), during sleep, and under hypnosis. In dreams, attention is purely passive except during the uncommon phenomenon of lucid dreaming (LaBerge, 1985). Attention is decreased in states where alertness or consciousness is reduced, as in epilepsy, head injury, drug- and alcohol-induced states, increased intracranial tension, and brainstem lesions involving the reticular formation. But attention may be enhanced by drugs such as stimulants, dissociated in hysterical states, or narrowed in mood disorders, where it may assume the quality of state boundness in depressive illnesses.

ANATOMY OF ATTENTION

Studies in cognitive neuroscience are used to demonstrate the anatomic substrates for attention. To do so, both cognitive operations and neuronal activity must be considered. Although work on attention systems is just beginning, Posner and Petersen (1990) suggest several organizational principles that can be used which allow attention to focus as a unified system to control directed mental processing, channel involuntary memory, and redirect

attention back to its original target when distractions occur.

Attention is conducted through a network of anatomic regions so that there is not a single system in the brain for attention, nor is it an aspect of general brain function. Brain areas involved in attention carry out different functions; for example, orientation, selective detection, and sustained alert vigilance, the subsystems previously described. The attention system is anatomically separate (Posner and Petersen, 1990; Posner and Dehaene, 1994) from interrelated systems that integrate experience (even when attention is directed elsewhere), establishing the identity of separate brain mechanisms for attention.

COGNITIVE NEUROSCIENCE AND ATTENTION

Studies in cognitive neuroscience have focused on the anatomy of attention, cognitive operations that are performed, and how attention relates to other interrelated functions. Such studies focus primarily on the visual system; visual word forms and semantic memory have been most often investigated. For example, for orienting, the visual attention system has been investigated in relation to data processing in the ventral occipital lobe. Moreover, Posner et al. (1989) have suggested a cognitive anatomic approach in considering if word recognition is automatic.

For detecting or selecting, the anterior attention system has been studied in relation to networks that subserve semantic associations (see Fig. 6–1). For alerting or sustaining attention, arousal systems that deal with selective aspects of attention have been investigated. In the sections that follow, orientation, detection, and alerting will be described in more detail.

ORIENTING TO VISUAL LOCATION

To become visually oriented, the stimulus moves into the fovea or center of vision. This improves the efficiency of processing information. Attending to a location, or events at that location, leads to more rapid response and increased brain electrical activity. For example, if people are asked to move their eyes to a target, an improvement in efficiency at the target location (Posner et al., 1984) begins before the

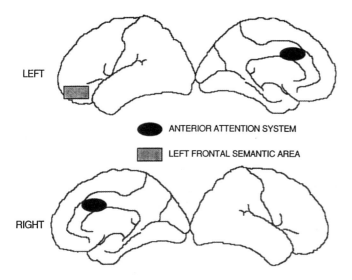

LEFT

ANTERIOR ATTENTION SYSTEM

LEFT FRONTAL SEMANTIC AREA

RIGHT

Figure 6–1. *The anterior attention system.* The *upper two drawings* are the lateral *(left)* and medial *(right)* surface of the left hemisphere. The *lower two drawings* are the medial *(left)* and lateral *(right)* surfaces of the right hemisphere. The semantic association area on the lateral aspect of the left hemisphere is determined by blood flow studies, as is the anterior attention area (from Posner and Petersen, 1990).

eyes begin to move. This covert shifting of attention functions to guide the eye to the appropriate target in the visual field.

The sensory response of brain neurons in several areas has been shown in monkeys to have a greater discharge rate with attention to spatial location. Three of the areas involved with this activity are in the posterior parietal lobe (Mountcastle, 1978), the lateral pulvinar nucleus of the posteriolateral thalamus (Petersen, Robinson, and Morris, 1987), and the superior colliculus. Similar changes in the parietal cortex have been shown in normal humans with positron emission tomography (Petersen et al., 1988). Brain injuries to these three regions lead to a reduction in the ability to shift attention covertly (prior to the attentional act). Yet different regions produce different kinds of defects. For example, more posterior damage in the parietal lobe leads to difficulty in disengaging an attentional focus from a target located in the side opposite the lesion. On the other hand, deterioration of the superior colliculus leads to a deficit in the ability to shift attention. The shifting of attention is slowed whether or not attention is being initiated elsewhere. This suggests that the processes involved in moving attention to a target are impaired. These deficits may be linked to saccadic eye movements. Lesions in the lateral pulvinar also demonstrate difficulties in covert ori-

entation. Unilateral thalamic lesions produce problems in engaging the target area even though there is time to orient to that location.

These investigations into orientation confirm that anatomic areas carry out specific cognitive operations and suggest the hypothesis that, first, the parietal lobe disengages its attention from its present focus, then the midbrain superior colliculus moves attention to the area of the target, and, finally, the pulvinar is involved in reading out information from indexed or identified locations. Additional studies are needed to confirm these hypotheses.

We may orient attention to locations in visual space, then concentrate attention on a narrow area or distribute it over a wider area. Patient studies (Robertson and Delis, 1986; Sergent, 1982) indicate that the right hemisphere may be biased toward global processing and the left to local processing, suggesting a form of hemispheric specialization in the overall structure of the attention system. Left and right hemispheres carry out operations needed to shift attention in the opposite or contralateral direction, but they also may have more specialized functions in regard to the level of detail of attention. These specializations may show a time course during development and may not be innate, although exactly how they develop is not currently known. It has been suggested that the development of literacy or reading may be a factor in establishing these hemispheric differences.

The attention system that is described here involving the posterior parietal lobe is referred to as the posterior attention system. It involves dorsal visual pathways that focus on area VI in the cortex and extend to the parietal lobe (see Fig. 6–2). PET studies (Petersen et al., 1988) indicate that the parietal region is activated during visual orienting and that blood flow also changes in visual word processing areas so that an area in the left ventral occipital lobe is active when visual words are processed, but is not active for letterlike forms (Snyder et al., 1989). This posterior system is thought to affect ventral pathways during tasks which require detailed processing, as in visual search tasks.

The interface between the attention and cognitive systems involving visual pattern recognition has also been described. This may occur at various levels from the initial recognition of a pattern to the storage of new visual patterns. The dorsal system is involved in visual orienting, and a ventral system is involved in pattern recognition. These systems can be coordinated through the pulvinar (Petersen, Robinson, and Morris, 1987) or through other pathways. The attention system modulates the selection of information that may be important at a specific moment.

AUTOMATIC ATTENTION PROCESSING

Automatic processing can occur without attention. Automatic processing involves the ventral visual pathway during the recognition of visual objects. Cognitive studies (LaBerge and Brown, 1989) indicate that cuing people to locations influences aspects of visual perception. Therefore, attention not only provides high priority to the features attended to but it does so in order that the physical distance between objects may be over-ridden.

Snyder et al.'s (1989) reporting an area in the left ventral occipital lobe that is unique to strings of letters which are either words or orthographically regular nonwords denotes a visual word form area (see Fig. 6–2) that appears to operate without attention. This confirms the suggestion that word recognition can be automated and not require spatial attention. However, the related tasks of searching for a single letter, forming a conjunction, or reporting letters seen in a random string do appear to require attention.

EXPERIMENTAL STUDY IN MONKEYS

Furthermore, recordings from individual cells in alert monkeys confirm that attention can play a role in ventral pattern recognition (Wise and Desimone, 1988). The pathway involving

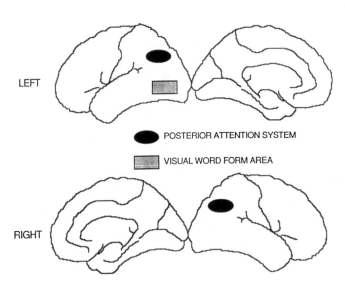

LEFT

POSTERIOR ATTENTION SYSTEM

VISUAL WORD FORM AREA

RIGHT

Figure 6–2. *The posterior attention system.* The *upper two drawings* are the lateral *(left)* and medial *(right)* surfaces of the left hemisphere. The *lower two drawings* are the medial *(left)* and lateral *(right)* surfaces of the right hemisphre. The location of the posterior visual spatial attention system is shown on the lateral surface of each hemisphere as determined by blood flow studies. The location of the visual word form area on the lateral surface of the left hemisphere is also depicted (from Posner and Petersen, 1990).

the posterior attention system and pattern recognition is thought to be through the thalamus. Models of the nature of the interaction between attention and pattern recognition have been reported by LaBerge and Brown (1989). Crick (1984) had previously suggested the role of the thalamic reticular complex as the searchlight attention hypothesis.

IMAGERY

In addition to pattern recognition which occurs as a result of sensory events, it is also possible to construct visual representations or images by asking individuals to imagine scenes from long-term memory (Kosslyn, 1988). There is now evidence that some of the same anatomic mechanisms used in imagery are involved in some aspects of pattern recognition. Patients with right parietal lobe lesions fail to report contralesional side visual images; when asked to imagine a familiar scene, they report on the right side but not the left side. The abnormality is thought to arise at the time of scanning the image. Furthermore, when normal adult subjects imagine themselves walking on a familiar route, activation of the superior parietal lobe on both sides is noted (Roland, 1985). These studies suggest that activation of the superior parietal lobe may be unique to imagery. Further, the parietal lobe seems central to spatial attention to external locations. Therefore, the brain systems used in attending to an external location seem to be related to those used when the subject scans a visual image.

DETECTION OF TARGETS

The posterior attention system may be linked via connections between the posterior parietal lobe and areas of the lateral and medial frontal cortex (Goldman-Rakic, 1988). These anatomic connections may be responsible for linking involuntary orienting and the posterior attention system to conscious attention.

GENERAL ALERTNESS AND FOCUSED ATTENTION

There are distinct general alert states and states in which attention is clearly oriented and focused. In the alert but disengaged state, tar-

gets of sufficient intensity summon selective attention. Once focal attention is elicited, there is widespread interference with most other cognitive operations (Posner, 1978). This indicates that there are generally alert states, disengaged states, and attention states of active engagement in information processing. In the alert state, any target may reach detection, whereas the range of target detection is narrowed during focused attention.

BRAIN AND WORD PROCESSING

Midline frontal areas, including the anterior cingulate gyrus and supplementary motor area, are active during semantic processing of words (Petersen et al., 1988). The degree of blood flow in the anterior cingulate increases as the number of selective targets to be recognized or detected increases. Therefore, the anterior cingulate seems to be sensitive to operations that involve selective attention to targets. Anatomic studies link the anterior cingulate to the posterior attention system as well as to language tasks. Language tasks have effects that are different from engaging attention at a visual location. Effects are bilateral for language rather than being mainly on the side opposite the lesion as in visual orienting. The language task involves some but not all of the same mechanisms used in visual orienting. This suggests that visual orienting involves systems separate from but interconnected with those used for language processing. These investigations suggest a hierarchy may be present in attention systems whereby the anterior system can pass its control to the posterior system when it is not occupied with information processing. Treisman and Gormican (1988) suggest the use of a spotlight as an analogy to attention that focuses, disengages, moves, and is then re-engaged.

SUSTAINED ALERTNESS

The attention function that prepares and sustains alertness has been investigated using letter and word matching tasks (Posner, 1978). Here, the relationship between the alert state and other aspects of information processing are studied. A highly alert state produces more rapid responding but also is accompanied by a greater error rate. Alertness (Posner, 1978) does not affect the buildup of information in memory and sensory processing, but apparently does affect the rate of attentional response. The ability to develop and maintain the alert state depends on the integrity of the right cerebral hemisphere (Heilman, Watson, and Valenstein, 1985). The isolated right hemisphere apparently has the mechanisms required to maintain an alert state, and when lesioned, reduces general performance by the whole individual. Blood flow and metabolic studies suggest a link of the right cerebral hemisphere with alerting.

The maintenance of an alert state is linked to the right hemisphere and is linked to attention. Since the norepinephrine system is involved with alerting, these findings are consistent with a norepinephrine hypothesis of attention and alertness. The norephinephrine system has its origin in the locus coeruleus, which may be important in the alert state. Animal studies are consistent with norepinephrine's role in arousal or vigilance. Lesion studies in rats, involving lesions of the right hemisphere but not the left, result in depletion of norepinephrine on both sides (Robinson, 1985). The effects are greater with more frontal lesions. Studies in monkeys indicate that the norepinephrine innervation is most strongly present in the posterior parietal lobe, pulvinar, and superior colliculus. These are the areas related to the posterior attention system. All of these findings converge to suggest that norepinephrine pathways provide the mechanism to maintain alertness and are most specifically involved in the posterior attention systems of the right cerebral hemisphere. Clark, Geffen, and Geffen (1989) have shown that the use of drugs to manipulate norepinephrine levels affects the shifting of attention.

ALERTNESS AS A SUBSYSTEM

Posner and Petersen (1990) suggest that alertness involves a subsystem of attention which acts on the posterior attention system. This system supports visual orienting and may also influence other attention subsystems. This system is physiologically dependent on norepinephrine pathways that arise in the locus coeruleus and are lateralized to the right hemisphere. Activation of the norepinephrine system

then, through this posterior system of attention, would increase the rate of selection of priority visual information for processing. This more rapid selection of information may be at the expense of lower quality information and may result in an increased number of errors.

In summary, the study of attention in the past has often been neglected. Recently, we have come to recognize attention as the operation of separate sets of neural areas which interact with domain-specific brain systems; for example, semantic word form or semantic association. Knowledge of the anatomic aspects of attention allows closer coordination of brain imaging in humans with individual cell recording studies in animals. Coordinated studies of PET and event-related potentials (ERPs) imaging may provide additional information about posterior visual word form systems and anterior semantics (Posner and Petersen, 1990). Attention is involved in this kind of information transfer between such systems. Current ERP methods do not allow precise localization of cortical areas; however, combined recordings allow description of both the cortical anatomy and time course of attention selection processes. Thus, combining PET and ERP data offers a powerful high resolution approach to defining the spatial-temporal properties of brain activity. Heinze et al. (1994) have used this approach to image brain activity during visual selective attention.

There is a continuing effort to understand automatic priming of semantic systems. An area of recent investigation relates to how attention relates to semantic activation in sleep. Hobson (1988) suggests that during sleep ongoing neural activity may be interpreted semantically by neural networks that have been primed by daily activity. In addition, split brain studies suggest an interpreter system in the left hemisphere that imposes reasons for our behavior. These investigations, and those of memory, are of particular interest. Lesion studies of the hippocampus demonstrated the inability to consciously retrieve memories. Yet lesioned patients may demonstrate memory storage by their task performance, despite lack of retrieval. This suggests a distinction between automatic and conscious processing in memory (Squire, 1986), and suggests that they involve different neural mechanisms.

PSYCHOPATHOLOGICAL CONDITIONS

Disorders of higher cognition may be related to attentional deficits. These include attention deficit/hyperactivity disorder, schizophrenia, traumatic brain injury, and neglect syndromes (Mesulam, 1981; Prigatano and Schacter, 1991), as well as other syndromes. Studies of the attention systems of the brain in these conditions are of particular interest. For example, it has been suggested that the core deficit in schizophrenia may be a failure of the anterior system of the left hemisphere to control the normal inhibitory pattern of the left lateralized semantic network (Early et al., 1989). Ideas such as these focus on integration at the levels of neurotransmission, neuroanatomy, and cognition (Posner and Peterson, 1990). Furthermore, attention deficit disorder might be linked to the right hemispheric mechanisms that control sustained attention. Consequently, combined cognitive and anatomical approaches may assume new importance in the study of the integration of physiological and psychosocial influences in psychopathological disorders rather than being considered separately as they have been in the past.

REFERENCES

Clark, C.R., Geffen, G.M., and Geffen, L.B. (1989). Catecholamines and the covert orienting of attention. *Neuropsychology*, 27:131–140.

Crick, F. (1984). Function of the thalamic reticular complex: The searchlight hypothesis. *Proceedings of the National Academy of Science*, 81:4586–4590.

Early, T.S., Posner, M.I, Reiman, E.M. and Raichle, M.E. (1989). Left striato-pallidal hyperactivity in schizophrenia. Part II. Phenomenology and thought order. *Psychiatric Developments*, 2:109–121.

Goldman-Rakic, P.S. (1988). Topography of cognition: Parallel distributed networks in primate association cortex. *Annual Review of Neuroscience*, 11:137–156.

Heilman, K.M., Watson, R.T., and Valenstein, E. (1985). Neglect and related disorders. In K.M. Heilman and E. Valenstein (eds), *Clinical neuropsychology*, pp. 243–293. Oxford University Press, New York,

Heinze, H.J., Mangun, G.R., Burchert, W., Hinrichs, H., Scholz, M., Munte, T.F., Gos, A., Scherg, M., Johannes, S., Hundershagen, H., Gazzaniga,

M.S., and Hillyard, S.A. (1994). Combined spatial and temporal imaging of brain activity during visual selective attention in humans. *Nature*, 372:543–546.

Hobson, J.A. (1988). *The dreaming brain.* Basic Books, New York.

James, W. (1890). *Principles of psychology*, Vol. 1. Holt, New York.

Kosslyn, S.M. (1988). Aspects of a cognitive neuroscience of mental imagery. *Science*, 240:1621–1626.

LaBerge, S. (1985). *Lucid dreaming.* J. P. Tarcher, New York.

_____ and Brown, V. (1989). Theory of attentional operations in shape identification. *Psychology Review*, 96:101–124.

Mesulam, M.M. (1981). A cortical network for directed attention and unilateral neglect. *Annals of Neurology*, 10:309–325.

Mountcastle, V.B. (1978). Brain mechanisms of directed attention. *Journal of the Royal Society of Medicine*, 71:14–27.

Petersen, S.E., Robinson, D.L., and Morris, J.D. (1987). Contributions of the pulvinar to visual spatial attention. *Neuropsychology*, 25:97–105.

_____, Fox, P.T., Posner, M.I., Mintun, M. and Raichle, M.E. (1988). Positron emission tomographic studies of the cortical anatomy of single word processing. *Nature*, 331:585–589.

Posner, M.I. (1978). *Chronometric explorations of mind.* Earlbaum, Englewood Heights, NJ.

_____ and Petersen S.E. (1990). The attention system of the human brain. *Annual Review of Neuroscience*, 13:25–42.

_____, Walker, J.A., Friedrich, F.J., and Rafal, R.D. (1984). effects of parietal lobe injury on covert orienting of visual attention. *Journal of Neuroscience*, 4:1863–1874.

_____, Sandson, J., Dhawan, M., and Shulman, G.L. (1989). Is word recognition automatic? A cognitive-anatomical approach. *Journal of Cognitive Neuroscience*, 1:50–60.

Posner, M.I., and Dehaene, S. (1994). Attentional networks. *Trends in Neurosciences*, 17:75–79.

Prigatano, G.P. and Schacter, D.L. (eds). (1991). *Awareness of deficit after brain injury: Clinical and theoretical Issues.* Oxford University Press, New York.

Robertson, L. and Delis, D.C. (1986). Part-whole processing in unilateral brain damaged patients: Dysfunction of hierarchical organization. *Neuropsychology*, 24:363–370.

Robinson, R.G. (1985). Lateralized behavioral and neurochemical consequences of unilateral brain injury in rats. In S.G. Glich (ed), *Cerebral lateralization in non-human species.* Academic Press, Orlando.

Roland, P.E. (1985). Cortical organization of voluntary behavior in man. *Human Neurobiology,* 4:155–167.

Sims, A. (1988). *Symptoms in the mind: An introduction to descriptive psychopathology.* Bailliere-Tindall, W. B. Saunders, Philadelphia.

Sergent, J. (1982). The cerebral balance of power: Confrontation or cooperation? *Journal of Experimental Psychology and Human Perceptual Performance,* 8:253–272.

Snyder, A.Z., Petersen, S., Fox, P., and Raichle, M.E. (1989). PET studies of visual word recognition. *Journal of Cerebral Blood Flow and Metabolism,* 9:Supplement 1-S576. (Abstr.).

Sperry, R.L. (1988). Psychology's mentalist paradigm and the religion/science tension. *American Psychology,* 43:607–613.

Squire, L.R. (1986). Mechanisms of memory. *Science,* 232:612–619.

Treisman, A.M. and Gormican, S. (1988). Feature analyses in early vision: Evidence for search asymmetrics. *Psychological Review,* 95:15–48.

Wise, S.P. and Desimone, R. (1988). Behavioral neurophysiology: Insights into seeing and grasping. *Science,* 242:736–741.

CHAPTER 7
EMOTION

Although attention is at the center of human performance, it is emotion that motivates action. This chapter reviews definitions of emotion and related terms, historical issues in the study of emotion, the development of the primary emotions, the emergence of self-conscious emotions, the relationship of emotion and cognition, and the neurobiology of emotional learning and memory.

DEFINITIONS

Emotion has been categorized according to type, duration, and intensity. Seven main groups of emotions are generally described (Izard, 1991): joy, surprise, fear, sadness, anger, disgust/contempt, and interest. These emotions may be communicated by bodily postures and through facial expression, gesture, tone of voice, and general appearance. Emotion is assessed empathetically, so if someone is friendly and cheerful on greeting, then the feeling of cheerfulness may be initially experienced by the recipient. One literally puts one self in the place of another through empathy.

Emotion is generally used to describe physiological and psychosomatic concomitants of mood (Sims, 1988). Emotion should not be confused with feeling and affect—each word has a specific meaning. Emotion refers to a state of the self, whereas the word "feeling" may be used to describe both emotions and sensations. Jaspers (1959) wrote about the psychological feeling of emotions such as sadness and joy, and the more global, vital feelings in which an emotion is described subjectively as completely encompassing the whole organism. Emotion may also be designated according to its biological purpose, and in this context would be described as an instinct.

A mood is a pervasive and sustained emotion that, when intense, colors a person's perception of the world (DSM-IV) (APA, 1994). A mood is a prolonged state and shows considerable variation. Mood is used to describe one's psychological state in relation to the environment.

Feeling is the term used to describe a positive or negative reaction to an experience. Feeling refers to both the active experience of sensation, (e.g., touch) and the subjective experience of emotion. Affect indicates differentiated specific feelings that are directed towards people and objects. Whereas feeling is an individual emotional response, affect describes complex emotional arousal. Affect describes a pattern of observable behaviors that express subjectively experienced feeling states based on emotion. Affect is variable over time in response to changes in emotional state, in contrast to mood, which is pervasive and sustained. Therefore, there is a range of affect that may be described as broad, constricted, blunted, or flat (DSM-IV). Normal affective expression is indicated through the variability in facial expression, voice tone, and expressive hand and body movements.

In *General Psychopathology,* Jaspers (1959) concentrated on three aspects of mood and affect: the involvement of the self, the contrast of opposites, and the object toward which the response was directed. In regard to the self, feelings are experienced by the self, but empathy may be attributed to others. The judgment that another person is sad or happy because of a facial expression or that a picture looks sad results from the response it evokes in the observer. On the other hand, affect is experienced in polar contrasts and may be described in opposites. Visual analogue scales of mood confirm this in their request for self-report rating of changes in mood. Furthermore, feelings may be directed toward an object, (e.g., fear of a dog) or may have no object, as in the case of anxiety.

HISTORY

The major contribution to the study of emotions in the last century was Charles Darwin's *The Expression of the Emotions in Man and Animals,* published in 1872 (Darwin, 1965). He emphasized that there are specific fundamental emotions, which are expressed in overt behavior. Subsequently, in 1884, William James suggested that the outward signs of emotions, such as facial expressions or bodily responses, are not the result of prior emotional signals, but rather "our feeling of the bodily changes as they occur is the emotion." A similar point was made by C. G. Lange in 1885, so this position is known as the James/Lange theory of emotion (i.e., an external event perceived by an individual produces a bodily response, and it is the perception of these events that constitutes the emotional experience). The implication is that a specific emotional experience is produced by a specific and unique set of bodily and visceral responses. In the 1920s, W. B. Cannon (1927, 1929) published a critique of the James/Lange theory. He suggested that emotional behavior was still present when internal organs were surgically or accidentally disconnected from the central nervous system, so emotions did not differ in important ways in the associated visceral response. He noted that autonomic responses are slow and emotional experience occurs quickly. The two theorists leave us with this

question, Is emotion experienced because we perceive our bodies in a particular way, or are there specific emotional neural systems in the brain that respond to environmental events? As Gregory (1987) asks, Do we grieve because we cry, or do we cry because we grieve?

Historically, this debate on the emotions went into decline when behavioralism was the primary paradigm in psychology. With the behavioral focus on objective and observable data, less emphasis was placed on the study of emotion. With the resurgence of cognitive psychology, cognitive aspects of emotion have again been addressed. The cognitive view is that novelty, discrepancy, and interruption of our perceived cognitive sets lead to visceral responses, which cognitively are interpreted and experienced as sadness, fear, joy, etc. Richard Lazarus (1991) has taken up this theme in his book, *Emotion and Adaptation.* With the establishment of a cognitive approach to emotion, cognitive neuroscience is free to study the brain mechanisms of emotion and emotional learning.

EMOTION AND MEMORY

The relationship between emotion and memory is particularly important. Emotional arousal may facilitate the remembrance of events that occurred during a similarly aroused state. Events occurring during intense emotional arousal seem to be preserved in memory with special accuracy and clarity. The memory of intense experiences has been referred to as the "flash bulb" memory hypothesis (Christianson, 1989). Yet the effect of emotion on memory may be more general than this because, in classical learning theory, memories are established when behaviors are followed by biologically reinforcing stimuli (Skinner, 1938). Those stimuli that have reinforcing properties have emotional properties as well, so learning theorists have assumed that the capacity of the stimulus to act as a reinforcer may be directly related to its emotional properties. In this way, those memories that depend on reinforcement mechanisms may also depend on the degree of emotional arousal. In this case, the relationship between emotion and memory is as a facilitator for the establishment of memory.

On the other hand, emotion has been proposed to suppress memory. In the psychodynamic concept of repression (Freud, 1917), the recall of events that are associated with the arousal of emotion may produce anxiety. To defend against anxiety, the memory of events is prevented from reaching conscious awareness. Repression has been studied in the experimental literature in the context of perceptual defenses and subliminal processing of experiences (Erdelyi, 1985).

In addition to facilitating and inhibiting the memory of events, emotion itself may be directly remembered (i.e., emotional experiences may be directly experienced without conscious recall). This was demonstrated in a classic case by Claparede (1951). He was evaluating a brain damaged patient with a profound memory disturbance who lacked conscious recall of experiences that had occurred only moments before. The examiner, on one occasion, stuck the patient with a pin during the interview. She asked what had just happened to her, but had no conscious memory of the event; however, in the future, she refused to shake the hand of the examiner. This suggests that the emotional memory of the unpleasant experience (painful pinprick) permitted the patient to respond appropriately by storing information that allowed her to avoid future hand contact with the examiner. Stored memory was apparently undisturbed despite the brain damage, which impaired her ability to recall the details of experience. This early experiment is significant in suggesting that brain circuits used for implicit memories may differ from those used for conscious explicit memories. Memories may represent the storage of emotionally significant experiences in the nervous system, which may influence future information processing even though these event memories are out of awareness. In this context, emotion is treated as a memory process in itself rather than one that influences memory through inhibition and facilitation.

THEORIES OF EMOTION PROCESSING

Conscious emotional experiences depend on emotional processing mechanisms that take place out of awareness. Four theories have been proposed to account for emotional processing: the central theory, the cognitive arousal theory, the facial feedback theory, and the perceptual-motor theory.

The *central theories* were proposed by Cannon (1927) and Papez (1937) who suggested that emotional experiences are the result of neural activity in brain circuits. Consequently, sensory stimuli are transmitted through the brain to the thalamus. They are then conveyed to the cortex and elaborated into perceptions and thoughts. These thalamic-sensory inputs may also be conveyed to the hypothalamus, where their emotional significance is established. The hypothalamus receives input from the cortex, which allows it to evaluate the significance of perceptions and thoughts in addition to more primitive sensory information. The central theories suggest that emotional experiences are initiated through ascending connections from the hypothalamus to the cerebral cortex. The information transmitted to the cortex from the hypothalamus, after its significance is evaluated, determines the quality of emotional experience. The central theories have been updated recently since it has become apparent that the critical subcortical area which is involved in receiving sensory input is the amygdala, which projects to structures in the hypothalamus and brainstem that regulate the autonomic expression of fear. In line with the older theories, it is now suggested that transmission from the amygdala to the brainstem and cortex underlies emotional experiences (LeDoux, 1987, 1992b; LeDoux, Xagoraris, and Romanski, 1989).

The next approach is the *cognitive arousal theory* (Schachter and Singer, 1962), which proposes that emotional experiences occur when the brain becomes aware that the body is in the state of physiologic arousal. Here, stimuli from the environment are conveyed to the brain, where they initiate emotionally ambiguous and peripheral emotional responses, especially in the autonomic and hormonal systems. The nonspecific arousal is transmitted to the brain, which elicits an evaluation process. The brain interprets emotionally ambiguous states from situational cues from both the physical and social environment. This approach was introduced to answer a problem in William James's theory of emotion. James proposed that the physiologic feedback from the periphery determines the nature of emotional experience.

Cannon had successfully argued that peripheral autonomic feedback was not sufficiently specific to determine the nature of experience. The cognitive arousal theory solution was to add cognition in the chain between nonspecific arousal and experience.

The inability to detect differences in patterns of autonomic effects for the different emotions and the existence of evidence for differentiation of emotions at a subjective level has created major difficulties for emotion theory. Because we feel distinct emotions in the absence of objective evidence for autonomic differentiation, emotions must involve the integration of separate response components. Among these are autonomic activity and the cognition of external events plus pattern feedback from motor systems, such as the face. The cognitive arousal hypothesis was proposed to deal with these complications and states that emotional experience is generated through the integration of a generalized state of autonomic arousal with cognitions that are specific for each of the emotions. An undifferentiated autonomic arousal is necessary to create the subjective experience of emotion, but the specific situation is necessary to generate the qualitative aspect, such as fear, anger or sadness. Cognition is not a stimulus to emotional reactions, but it is the mental event that is the equivalent to the quality of the emotion. Subjective feelings, then, are critical markers for emotion, but expressive behaviors are used as the indicators. This approach has allowed the exploration of social and cognitive factors that are responsible for emotional experiences. Using this framework, the social context for the resolution of ambiguous emotional states is considered. Still, this model has difficulty in at least four areas. Leventhal (1991) suggests that autonomic participation may not be necessary for emotional experience and behavior. Second, this model indicates that socialization history may be essential to create the cognitions that are essential for emotional feelings. However, the similarity of emotional expressions and judgments across widely separate cultures is inconsistent with the socialization hypothesis based on a history of certain experiences. There is little reason to identify the quality of emotion with cognition, because the two seem different and the organization of the nervous system suggests

that these two sets of events are the product of separable processing mechanisms. Third, this model fails to account for the role of the social environment in shaping individual emotional experience. Fourth, it fails to address the internal organizing functions of emotion.

On the other hand, James suggested that both autonomic feedback and feedback that occurred during the behavior itself which involved the somatic muscles contribute to emotional experience. James's focus on somatic experience is considered somewhat differently in the third approach, the *facial feedback theory*. In facial feedback theory, emotional feelings result when the state of the facial muscles during emotional experiences is communicated to the brain (Izard, 1977). This approach contrasts with the cognitive arousal theory, in which the brain interprets nonspecific peripheral feedback on the basis of external events in the environment; that is, the interpretation of feedback to the brain from the face, which is specific to the emotion expressed. It is the condition that determines the emotion that can be experienced.

Each of these first three theories requires that some form of emotional coding take place before emotional experience is generated. In the central theories, subcortical brain areas must identify the exact emotional implications of the stimulus. The cortex then produces an emotional experience appropriate to that stimulus. In the cognitive arousal theory, the brain must distinguish between emotional and nonemotional situations and generate responses. In facial feedback theory, the brain determines the emotional significance of the stimulus so that the facial muscles can be appropriately contracted and provide emotionally specific feedback. Each of these approaches is considered to be a competing theory. On the other hand, even though they are considered to be separate theories, it may be that each approach is useful in explaining various types of emotional experiences. All three of these approaches agree on one thing, that emotional processing precedes conscious emotional experience. Emotional processing occurs out of awareness and is not conscious. The results of nonconscious processing may be experienced as conscious content, but the processes themselves remain inaccessible (Jackendoff, 1987). Zajonc (1980) showed that affective reactions (preference formation) may take place prior to, and independent of, conscious recognition of an environmental stimulus. The computation of the affective experience stimuli is not consciously processed in his experiments. This indicates that the brain can compute the emotional signifi-cance of the stimulus independent of the mecha-nism for recognizing what that stimulus is. As a result of these experiments demonstrating non-conscious computation of behavioral and auto-nomic expression of emotion, the role of con-sciousness in the initial generation of emotion is no longer an essential element. In summary, we no longer need to depend on consciousness to explain emotional behavior and memory.

The fourth approach to understanding emotion is referred to as the *perceptual-motor model.* This model focuses on understanding how emotions are constructed and the changes in emotional con-structive processes over the life span. The percep-tual-motor model suggests that there is a core set of emotional reactions that are present at birth and that these core reactions are elaborated during development. This model differs from the other models presented in that increased emphasis is given to the components or modules of cognitive and expressive motor processes that generate emotions. By looking at the components of emo-tional reactions, we recognize that the terms "emotion" and "cognition" both stand for com-plex sets of partially independent processes that are integrated in the generation of emotional or cognitive reactions. In addition, emotion is a process that organizes those components that are involved in affecting behavior.

The major challenge to emotion processing theory is to specify the factors responsible for the organization of emotion. There are three components for emotional processing that must be considered. These are cognitive-expressive modules, action systems, and somatic receptor systems. The cognitive-expressive modules are sensitive to interper-sonal expressive cues (for example, facial or vocal cues), and generate parallel reactions in response to these cues. Leventhal (1991) sug-gests that some expressive modules are closed units like phonetic modules, which are used for the perception and production of phonetic units in speech. Although these modules may be unique to emotional reactions, others may be also components of the cognitive system.

Action systems organize general approach and avoidance behavior, and therefore function at a higher level than the expressive modules and may include more than one expressive module. These action systems may respond to a wide array of stimuli and produce a broad range of behaviors. Various memory structures may be assessed by each action system as it guides approach or avoidance.

Somatic receptor systems may integrate both expressive modules and action systems with the organism's physiologic systems. These systems are integrated through hormones that are manu-factured in various parts of the body, and they communicate and integrate specific functions by acting upon receptor sites or target cells. These systems integrate the brain, that is, cogni-tive-expressive modules and action systems, with widely separate physiologic processes.

COGNITION AND EMOTION

An analysis of the components of emotion may lead to a better understanding of the relation-ship between emotion and cognition. It is not that either emotion or cognition is primary, but rather that there is a continuing interaction between cognitive and emotional processing. Each serves as goals for and drives the other, so cognitions create emotions and emotions gener-ate cognitive reorganization. Leventhal (1991) points out that it is correct that situational per-ceptions and/or cognitions stimulate and shape emotional reactions. On the other hand, it is also correct that emotional actions may precede and shape cognition.

In addition, there is an ongoing interaction between psychological and biological processes that are involved in constructing both cognitive and emotional reactions. To consider the interac-tion of emotion and cognition, it is critical to take into account what level of cognitive and emotional activity is involved in the interaction. For example, to evaluate the impact of emo-tional states and cognitive activity, it is important to clarify whether the focus is on preattentive cognitive processes, attentional processes, or consciously generated cognitive activity along with the module and level of emotional process-ing that may be involved (Leventhal, 1991). In regard to emotion and memory, memory can alter attention, thus affecting what is learned and thereby alter retrieval.

Emotions, such as joy, fear, and sadness, may have an impact on initial learning. For example, a frightened person might be more attentive to and better retain frightening memory content. Yet even though the mood may affect learning, it would not necessarily be more accessible if the individual's emotional state at the time of retrieval matched that at the time of learning.

A network formulation of emotion must take into account active search processes that are associated with schemata for specific action systems. Those action systems, to approach or to avoid, direct attention for information. The interaction of emotion and memory, then, is not fully described by a network model in which moods and emotions are nodes linked to nodes for cognitive content. Emotions may alter search strategies, so information does not flow passively along networks, but requires active engagement.

NEUROSCIENCE AND EMOTION

The physiology of emotion has been linked to the amygdala, and extensive studies have been conducted regarding its role in emotion, particularly regarding the physiology of fear. During the past forty years, the amygdala, a small region in the temporal lobe, has been identified as the source of the brain's emotional network. Following the original studies of Kluver and Bucy (1937), which showed that damage to the temporal lobes in monkeys leads to emotional disturbance, it was demonstrated that damage to the amygdala alone will produce the same behavior. In the Kluver/Bucy studies, lesioned monkeys lost fear of previously frightening stimuli, attempted to copulate with members of the same sex, and tried to eat inappropriate objects. Much of this syndrome can be understood as a disconnection of the sensory and the affective or motivational properties of incoming stimuli. Although visual stimuli are perceived as visual objects, the response to them is no longer socially appropriate. The amygdala has been shown to be an essential component of the brain's emotional system and is consistently implicated in emotional processing.

The amygdala's role in emotional processing is the consequence of its anatomic connectivity. It receives input from sensory processing areas in the neocortex and thalamus. It projects to brainstem regions that control autonomic responses, hormonal responses, and behavior. Because of this extensive connectivity, the amygdala can transform sensory stimuli into emotional signals. Through the amygdala, sensory processing becomes emotional processing. It can both initiate and control emotional responses. With better understanding of the functional organization of the amygdala, its role in emotion is becoming increasingly clarified (LeDoux, 1992b). There are ten or more subareas of the amygdala; each has its own unique set of afferent and efferent connections (Amaral, 1987). The role of the amygdala in fear and anxiety has recently been summarized by Davis (1992) (see Fig. 7–1).

AMYGDALA AND CONDITIONED FEAR

The amygdala has a crucial role in the expression of conditioned fear. Conditioned fear occurs when an initially neutral environmental stimulus is repeatedly paired with an aversive stimulus. Davis describes the amygdala and its efferent projections as presenting a central fear system that is involved in the expression and acquisition of conditioned fear.

As shown in Figure 7–1, there are direct connections between the central nucleus of the amygdala and hypothalamic and brainstem target areas that may be involved in the elicitation of fear and anxiety. Davis demonstrates that stimulation of efferent fibers from the amygdala to various anatomic targets leads to sympathetic activation, parasympathetic activation, increased respiration, activation of catecholamines, increased reflexes, cessation of behavior, open-mouth movements, and ACTH release. The behaviors associated with amygdaloid stimulation include the various symptoms of fear and anxiety, such as tachycardia, respiratory distress, increased startle, facial expressions of fear, and the stress response. Various sensory projections terminate in the lateral amygdaloid nucleus to produce these effects. These projections originate in the areas of the cortex and thalamus that process sensory input. Although the connections between the cortex and amygdala have been studied extensively, less is known about the connections between the thalamus and the amygdala.

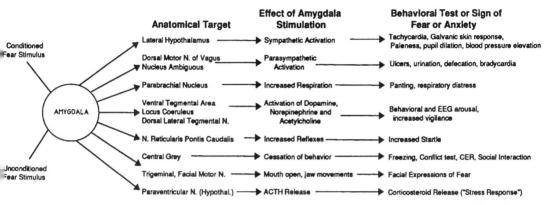

Figure 7–1. Schematic diagram showing direct connections between the central nucleus of the amygdala and a variety of hypothalamic and brainstem target areas that may be involved in different animal tests of fear and anxiety (from Davis, 1992).

LeDoux and others (LeDoux 1991, 1992a; LeDoux, Farb, and Romanski, 1991) have carefully studied the auditory projections to the lateral amygdala from the thalamus. The thalamic cell group receives auditory input directly from the inferior colliculus, which is associated with the medial geniculate body. About half of the projections between the thalamus and amygdala use the excitatory neurotransmitter, glutamate. In addition to auditory input, the amygdala receives input from the thalamus for the other sensory modalities (Turner and Herkenham, 1991).

Fear conditioning is thought to occur via emotional learning processes involving these thalamic-amygdala projections. Through this subcortical pathway, inputs from the thalamus to the amygdala lead to activation either before or simultaneously with the arrival of input at the cortical level. This subcortical system may play an important role in preconscious and precognitive emotional processing. Because these connections are direct, they may allow primitive sensory representations to activate quickly in emotional situations. These direct connections are reminiscent of the classic theories of Cannon (1929) and of Papez (1937). Both authors emphasized the importance of subcortical sensory transmission in the experience and expression of emotion.

Recent anatomic studies, using new axonal transport neuronal tract tracing methods, allow more specific study and identification of cells involved in uptake and transport. New insights into the organization of the amygdala have come from these new transport tracing agents, which allow visualization of axonal arborizations and identification of synaptic boutons at the light microscopic level. Direct connections between the lateral nucleus and the basolateral nucleus of the amygdala that project to the cortical association areas have been documented (Pitkanen and Amaral, 1991). This means that sensory information that reaches the lateral nucleus from either the cortex or the thalamus can influence ongoing cortical processing. Furthermore, the basolateral nucleus projects to the central nucleus, providing a link to sensory inputs that can activate emotional behaviors and autonomic responses to influence cortical arousal.

In summary, these anatomic studies document the role of the amygdala in emotion. Understanding the organization of the amygdala and how sensory information reaches it and is then distributed is critical to establishing an anatomic understanding of the input and output relationships that underlie information processing. Projections to the amygdala from areas of sensory input from the thalamus are more extensive than previously understood and may be important in emotional learning. These connections may contribute to cortical arousal and neuronal plasticity in emotional situations. Cellular mechanisms for emotional learning and for long-term potentiation have been suggested in the amygdala (Brown et al., 1988; Chapman et al., 1990; Miserendino et al., 1990). It is still not clear whether or not NMDA receptors are primarily involved. Some studies with blocking agents have not affected responses (Chapman and Bellavance, 1992).

AMYGDALA AND SOCIAL COGNITION

Animal studies have demonstrated that the amygdala contains neurons that respond to faces and is involved in emotion and social behavior. However, determination of the amygdala's functions in humans has been limited because selective lesions of the amygdala are uncommon. Adolphs et al. (1994) studied a patient, S.M., with a rare disorder, Urbach-Wiethe disease, in which the amygdala in both cerebral hemispheres are nearly completely destroyed by calcium depositions, although the hippocampus and neocortex are unaffected. This patient does not experience fear in herself nor can she produce a facial expression of fear when asked to do so. She is unable to recognize fear in other's facial expressions and does not recognize multiple emotions in a single facial expression. Yet she has no difficulty in recognizing the faces of familiar people from their photographs. Such findings further specify the effects of damage to the amygdala and highlight its role in the recognition of facial expressions of emotion. They indicate that the amygdala does participate in the perception of social signals and offer an additional link of brain systems involving the amygdala to social cognition.

Allman and Brothers (1994) suggest that the role of the amygdala in detecting both direction of gaze and facial expressions of emotion indicates a role for the amygdala in those brain mechanisms that represent the intentions and dispositions of others. They suggest additional studies of the role of the amygdala in the interpretation of social touch and voice intonation. Since brain systems linking the orbital frontal cortex and amygdala have been proposed to participate in social decision-making by correlating somatic states with behavioral situations (Damasio, 1994), additional studies of deficits in patients with damage to the amygdala are needed to evaluate its role in fear conditioning

and interpersonal decision making (Allman and Brothers, 1994).

The important point is that those brain structures which have a role in learning and memory can now be studied. Anatomic studies in the amygdala demonstrate that the substrate of emotional organization can now be investigated. Emotion has become a legitimate area of focus in the neurosciences. Future studies in normal subjects might address the interaction of mental images and the neural systems that underlie the emotions (Kosslyn, 1994)

The next step is to move beyond animal studies to investigate the development of emotion in infants and children. The psychological aspects of emotional development are described in Chapter 14. The study of emotional development in children with specific handicaps (e.g., Down syndrome and autistic disorders), may contribute to our understanding of brain systems involved in emotional development.

DEVELOPMENT OF EMOTIONS

During development, changes in emotion involve both the addition of new components and changes in the organization and interaction among components. Fear, anger, and happiness in an infant might differ from the emotions that use the same labels in adulthood. Furthermore, some emotions are not experienced until new cognitive components are available for their emotional processing. Lewis et al. (1989) found that the sense of self may emerge as a result of the infant and toddler's intentional actions and through social exchange with caregivers. The establishment of a sense of self is essential for the appearance of the self-conscious emotions, such as shame, pride, and guilt. These new emotions are developmentally complex and generally require maturation, yet components of emotion may maintain their original integrity, even though they may be incorporated into new organizational structures. The type of interpersonal experience may lead to variation in the organization of emotions. Leventhal (1991) gives the example of parents who toss their 2-year-old in the air when the child is joyful and may link intense physiologic activation with the joy of the experience. On the other hand, those parents who interact quietly with their infant during joyful exchanges could generate a different link between the expression of joy and the motor and somatic systems. Cultural influences may be important, then, in the expression and channeling of emotions. Although expressive modules are thought to be innate, the emotions system may be reorganized still retaining the basic biologic substrate. Consequently, if emotional experience is inhibited in early life, then new conditions may need to be simulated in therapy situations for the full expression of that neglected emotion.

During development, emotions show multiple component constructions at various levels, which may have a degree of functional independence. Socialization of the child may link components in typical or unexpected ways, so the expected organization may not always occur. Cognitive components, especially those associated with the sense of self, are important in the expression of emotion and its elaboration. The components represented in emotion are active processing units that use emotional schemata that may be based on modules for emotional processing. Additional research is needed to clarify components of emotional experience, such as perceptual memory for faces, things, and places, and the differentiation between volitional and spontaneous emotional-motor behavior.

In summary, emotional reactions may reflect the operation of modular components along with reciprocal interaction between emotion and cognition. These processes have evolved throughout evolution and have underlying endocrine and somatic receptor systems. Both evolutionary development and individual development have resulted in perceptual-cognitive and motor systems that may more effectively carry out the execution of adapted genetic plans. In this sense, through the study of emotion, we come to understand the unity of "the mind in the body" and "the body in the mind."

REFERENCES

Adolphs, R., Tranel, D., Damasio, H., and Damasio, A. (1994). Impaired recognition of emotion in facial expressions following bilateral damage to the human amygdala. *Nature,* 372:669–672.

Allman, J. and Brothers, L. (1994). Faces, fear, and the amygdala. *Nature,* 372:613–614.

Amaral, D.G. (1987). Memory: Anatomical organi-

zation of candidate brain regions. In F. Plum (ed), *Handbook of physiology:* Sec. 1, *The nervous system,* Vol. 5, *Higher functions of the brain,* pp. 211–294. American Physiological Society, Bethesda, MD.

American Psychiatric Association, Committee on Nomenclature and Statistics. (1994). *Diagnostic and Statistical Manual of Mental Disorders,* 4th ed. Author, Washington, DC.

Brown, T.H., Chapman, P.F., Kairiss, E.W., and Keenan, C.L. (1988). Long-term synaptic potentiation. *Science,* 242:724–728.

Cannon, W.B. (1927). The James-Lange theory of emotions: A critical examination and an alternative theory. *American Journal of Psychology,* 39:106–124.

_____. (1929). *Bodily changes in pain, hunger, fear and rage.* Appleton, New York.

Chapman, P.F. and Bellavance, L.L. (1992). Induction of long-term potentiation in the basolateral amygdala does not depend on NMDA receptor activation. *Synapse,* 11:310–318.

_____, Kairiss, E.W., Kennan, C.L., and Brown, T.H. (1990). Long-term synaptic potentiation in the amygdala. *Synapse,* 6:271–278.

Christianson, S.A. (1989). Flash bulb memories: Special, but not so special. *Memory and Cognition,* 17:435–443.

Claparede, E. (1951). Recognition and "me'ness." In D. Rapaport (ed), *Organization and pathology of thought,* pp. 58–75. Columbia University Press, New York. (Reprinted from Archives de Psychologies, 1911, 79–90).

Damasio, A. (1994). *Descartes error.* Putnam, New York.

Darwin, C. (1965). *The expression of the emotions in man and animals.* University of Chicago Press, Chicago.

Davis, M. (1992). The role of the amygdala in fear and anxiety. *Annual Review of Neuroscience,* 15:353–375.

Erdelyi, M.H. (1985). *Psychoanalysis: Freud's cognitive psychology.* W. H. Freeman, New York.

Freud, S. (1917). In J. Strachey (ed), *The standard edition of the complete psychological works of Sigmund Freud.* Hogarth, London.

Gregory, R.L. (1987). *The Oxford companion to the mind.* Oxford University Press, New York.

Izard, C.E. (1977). *Human emotions.* Plenum Press, New York.

_____. (1991). *The psychology of emotions.* Plenum Press, New York.

Jackendoff, R. (1987). *Consciousness and the computational mind.* MIT Press, Cambridge.

Jaspers, K. (1959). *General psychopathology* (transl. J. Hoenig and M.W. Hamilton, (1963). Manchester University Press, Manchester.

Kluver, H. and Bucy, P. (1937). Psychic blindness

and other symptoms following bilateral temporal lobectomy in rhesus monkeys. *American Journal of Psychology,* 119:352–353.

Kosslyn S.M. (1994). On cognitive neuroscience. *Journal of Cognitive Neuroscience,* 6:297–303.

Lazarus, R.S. (1991). *Emotion and adaptation.* Oxford University Press, New York.

LeDoux, J.E. (1987). Emotion. In F. Plum (ed), *Handbook of physiology:* Sec. 1, *The nervous system,* Vol. 5, *Higher functions of the brain,* pp. 419–459. American Physiological Society, Bethesda, MD.

_____. (1991). Emotion and the limbic system concept. *Concepts in Neuroscience,* 2:169–199.

_____. (1992a). Emotion and the amygdala. In J. Aggleton (ed), *The amygdala: Neurobiological aspects of emotion, memory, and mental dysfunction.* Wiley-Liss, New York.

_____. (1992b). Emotion as memory: Anatomical systems underlying indelible neural traces. In S. Christianson (ed), *The handbook of emotion and memory: Research and theory.* Lawrence Erlbaum, Hillsdale, NJ.

_____, Farb, C.R., and Romanski, L. (1991). Overlapping projections to the amygdala and striatum from auditory processing areas of the thalamus and cortex. *Neuroscience Letter,* 134:139–144.

_____, Xagoraris, A., and Romanski, L.M. (1989). Indelibility of subcortical emotional memories. *Journal of Cognitive Neuroscience,* 1:238–243.

Leventhal, H. (1991). Emotion: Prospects for conceptual and empirical development. In R.G. Lister and H. J. Weingartner (eds), *Perspectives on cognitive neuroscience.* Oxford University Press, New York.

Lewis, M., Sullivan, M.W., Stranger, C., and Weiss, M. (1989). Self- development and self-conscious emotions. *Child Development,* 60:146–156.

Miserendino, M.J.D., Sananes, C.B., Melia, K.R., and Davis, M. (1990). Blocking of acquisition but not expression of conditioned fear-potentiated startle by NMDA antagonists in the amygdala. *Nature,* 345:716–718.

Papez, J.W. (1937). A proposed mechanism of emotion. *Archives of Neurology and Psychiatry,* 79:217–224.

Pitkanen, A. and Amaral, D.G. (1991). Demonstration of projections from the lateral nucleus to the basal nucleus of the amygdala: A PHA-L study in the monkey. *Experimental Brain Research,* 83:465–470.

Schachter, S. and Singer, J.E. (1962). Cognitive, social, and physiological determinants of emotional state. *Psychological Review,* 69:379–399.

Sims, A. (1988). *Symptoms in the mind: An introduction to descriptive psychopathology.* Bailliere-Tindall, W.B. Saunders, Philadelphia.

Skinner, B.F. (1938). *The behavior of organisms: An experimental analysis.* Appleton-Century-Crofts, New York.

Turner, B.H. and Herkenham, M. (1991). Thalamoamygdaloid projections in the rat: A test of the amygdala's role in sensory processing. *Journal of Comparative Neurology,* 313:295–325.

Zajonc, R. (1980). Feeling and thinking: Preferences need no inferences. *American Psychology,* 35:151–175.

Zola-Morgan, S., Squire, L.R., Alvarez-Royo, P., and Clower, R.P. (1991). Independence of memory functions and emotional behavior: Separate contributions of the hippocampal formation and the amygdala. *Hippocampus,* 1:207–220.

CHAPTER 8

LANGUAGE

Nevertheless, the difference in mind between man and the higher animals, great as it is, is certainly one of degree and not of kind. If it be maintained that certain powers, such as self, consciousness, abstraction, etc., are peculiar to man, it may well be that these are the incidental results of other highly advanced intellectual faculties; and these again are mainly the result of the continued use of a highly developed language.

Charles Darwin, *The Descent of Man*, 1871

The emergence of language in human evolution is an issue of continuing interest to cognitive neuroscientists. The establishment of language is crucial in distinguishing humans from other species. But is its structure different in kind, resulting from genetic changes that produce unique neural circuits specific to humans, or is it different in degree, evolving from phylogenetically older structures, as Darwin might suggest? To address these questions, this chapter focuses on cognitive neuroscience, whereas Chapter 16 discusses the evolutionary origins of language and how language functions as a representational system (Bickerton, 1990).

The innateness of language development has been investigated throughout recorded history. New research methods now ask not only about language innateness, but also about the domain specificity of language (Bates, Thal, and Marchman, 1991). Domain specificity is contrasted with the view that language is an innate system, but one that involves the reconfiguration of mental and neural systems that are present in other species and continue to serve a nonlinguistic function in our own species.

This chapter reviews current issues in language development regarding innateness, discuss simulated language learning in neural networks, considers event-related potential studies that relate to language development, and, finally, emphasizes special issues in language development. These relate to children with focal brain injury, specific language impairments, and deafness; children from families with genetic disorders involving language; and children who are linguistically deprived.

HISTORY

Without special training or carefully sequenced linguistic training, children normally acquire natural language. The extent of language development is related to overall cognitive ability, but children who are mentally retarded acquire language without special training just as normal children do. Language is innate but it is not necessarily domain-specific (Bates, 1992).

The earliest known language experiment took place in the late 7th century B.C. (Rymer, 1993) when Psamtik I, the first of the Saitic kings of Egypt asked, "What might be the original language of the world?" Living in a country with multiple cultures produced through immigration, he decided to explore which language a child would speak spontaneously if deprived of early language experience. According to the Greek story as given in Herodotus, two infants were taken from their mothers at Psamtik I's request. They were placed in isolation in a shepherd's hut, and the shepherd was told not to speak with them. They were thus reared in silence on a diet of goat's milk. Two years later, when the shepherd returned to the hut, the children went to him and spoke their first utterance. The word they spoke, *bekos*, was the word for bread in the language of the Phrygians. The ruler then stated that this was the protolanguage and established himself as perhaps the first linguistic researcher. Psamtik I is remembered now for his scientific errors; it is unclear, for example, whether the children simply preferred the bread of this particular Phrygian culture and had not had a natural grasp of other words. However, the question that he raised in regard to spontaneous innate language production persists, and understanding language development continues to be a challenge for developmentalists.

Although children are not denied experience for the sake of science, our understanding about the acquisition of language does come from children. The most extreme examples are children who have been raised in the wild, called *feral* children, such as the *Wild Boy of Aveyron* (Lane, 1977) and, more recently, the case of *Genie* (Curtiss, 1977). In other instances, children who have been abused or neglected and whose family histories replicate the isolation prescribed by the ancient Egyptian ruler are studied.

Following Psamtik, a Greek philosopher, Epicurus, felt that language was a product of nature — a biological function like vision or digestion — and not the product of intellect or a specially created ability. However, later philosophers, such as Leibnitz in the 17th century, suggested that language ability was a special gift and that its form of expression was determined by natural instinct.

It was not until the 1950s when Noam Chomsky published *Syntactic Structures* (1957) that the study of language acquisition assumed scientific prominence. Previously, the research focus had been on vocabulary, until Chomsky changed the focus to syntax. The syntactic argument was that grammars of different languages used the same principles. Because of this striking uniformity between languages in different cultures, Chomsky had suggested that language was specific to the human species and that the rules of language are ingrained on a level "more basic than thought." This view, that of the nativist or innatist school, suggests that language would develop spontaneously. However, this approach was questioned by environmentalists or empiricists, who indicated that children learned language through interaction, primarily from interactions with their parents, and particularly from their parents' speech.

The extent to which language is innate has been the subject of debate following Chomsky's focus on there being a special and separate mental organ that is responsible for language. If he is correct, this would suggest that mental structures that support language are modular and discontinuous from other perceptual and cognitive systems. Furthermore, it suggests that the brain of a newborn child contains neuronal structures that are destined to mediate language and only language. This view is contrasted with an approach in which language is viewed as innate but requires the reconfiguration of mental and neuronal systems that persist from other species to develop, much as Darwin might have suggested. These systems then would continue to serve some nonlinguistic functions as well.

Current studies support the view that language development does appear to occur as a result of a mix of neuronal systems that also serve other cognitive and perceptual functions. Linguistic theory has focused on understanding this acquisitional process. The knowledge the child brings to the language learning task is often referred to as the *language acquisition device* (LAD). The input from parents and others is referred to as *primary linguistic data* (PLD).

EVENT-RELATED POTENTIALS AND LANGUAGE DEVELOPMENT

Electrophysiologic studies of event-related brain potentials (ERPs) have recently been reported in regard to language development in children. Molfese (1990) reported electrophysiologic correlates of words that 1-year-old children do and do not know. Other investigators — Mills, Coffey, and Neville (1992, 1993) — have demonstrated changes in event-related potentials to familiar and unfamiliar words at different stages in early language development. These authors studied children who were the same chronological age but had attained different language milestones. Distinct components of event-related potentials that are related to familiar words were associated with independently assessed levels of comprehension ability. For example, they found that 10-month-olds who had begun to understand words differed from 10-month-olds who were still unable to comprehend speech. Furthermore, components of event-related potentials associated with comprehension of familiar words between 13-month-olds who could and could not produce these words were identified. At 20 months distinct lateral and anterior-posterior brain specializations were apparent in discriminating comprehended words. Increasing cerebral specialization for language processing was linked to the temporal and parietal regions of the left hemisphere. Besides being related to changes in chronological age, those neuronal systems that mediate language then appear to change over time as a function of language learning.

LANGUAGE ACQUISITION/ NEURAL NETWORKS

The most recent developments in language acquisition involve research in what is called *learnability theory*. In this approach, formal analyses are used to determine the conditions under which different kinds of grammar can be learned. This research had been based on the assumption that language learning in humans is similar to digital computer models. Learnability theory appears to require that children have extensive stores of innate and domain-specific grammatical knowledge. This theory has been challenged recently by breakthroughs in the application of different computer architecture. In these studies, using neural networks, connectionism, and parallel distributed processing procedures have been of particular interest. The findings of Rumelhart and McClelland (1986) on learning the English past tense suggest that connectionist networks go through stages that are similar to those shown by children who are acquiring language. For example, a child may produce the word "wented," then, aware of the error, spontaneously correct the word to "went." The procedure is that of producing and then recovering from rulelike overgeneralizations. Marchman (1992) "lesioned" neural networks at various points in a test of learning of the past tense. These simulations captured some classic critical period effects in language learning. The authors found that smaller and earlier lesions in the neural network led to better outcomes and later, larger lesions led to persistent problems in grammar. This demonstrates that these effects can occur in the absence of specific maturational constraints. These damaged networks found it more difficult to acquire regular verbs than irregular verbs. This result is consistent with the pattern of deficits described by Gopnik and Crago (1991) in a family they studied. Their findings can result from nonspecific forms of "brain damage" in a general-purpose learning device.

Research on language learning in neural networks is early in its development. It promises to be an important tool to determine how much innate knowledge has to be in place for certain kinds of learning to take place.

SPECIAL ISSUES IN LANGUAGE LEARNING

Language acquisition in the absence of experience has been approached in a variety of ways. One approach has been to study children who were deliberately or accidentally denied language experience. In some instances, the focus has been on the deaf child who is reared with deaf parents; in others, on children who have been emotionally deprived and denied language experience, but also in instances where language exposure has been minimized.

It should be noted here that children who are blind, children who are deaf, and children who are deprived of sensory input do develop language syntax in unique ways; it is the structure that allows this to occur that Chomsky (1988) suggests is innate. The child brings the syntax with him and the words are gradually fit into that syntax.

Pettito and Marentette (1991) investigated deaf infants exposed to sign language and found that they babbled with their hands and produced meaningless but systematic actions that are not observed in children who hear. This form of manual babbling occurs at 8 to 10 months of age, the same age when vocal babbling appears in the hearing child. These authors concluded that language learning involved innate abilities that are independent of the input modality, whether it is manual or vocal. They also suggested that their results provide support for the innateness of language and of language as a mental organ. Still, the social aspect must also be taken into account in the deaf children; normal children imitate novel actions at 8 to 10 months. The more involved the adult is, the more systematic the child's imitation will become. Babbling in the visual modality could conceivably be an example of this remarkable imitation ability. The question about imitation versus an innate language organ in the deaf indicates that these findings are not conclusive in regard to innateness. However, Pettito and Marentette claim that language learning is based on innate systems that are free of the modality in which the language is expressed.

Yet another argument for innateness is presented by Gopnik and Crago (1991), citing a family in which there are difficulties with particular aspects of grammar such that regular verb inflections such as the "ed" ending are difficult for them, whereas irregular verbs, such as "came" are not. It has been suggested that regular and irregular verbal forms are handled by separate mental and perhaps also separate neural mechanisms. Although Fletcher (1990) has questioned Gopnik and Crago's findings, this issue needs to be pursued because of the findings using the neural network model.

LANGUAGE REHABILITATION

Children with focal brain injury (Marchman, Miller, and Bates, 1991) have been reported to show better recovery than adults. Retrospective studies report that many children following brain injury may show complete recovery in language, whereas others show more subtle deficits. Prospective studies of infants with brain injury in the first stages of language learning show language delays when either left or right hemisphere is damaged (Vargha-Khadem et al., 1991). However, as is often the case, abnormalities in infants are not analogous to changes in adults. Comprehension deficits occur more often with right hemisphere injury. With left hemisphere injury comprehension deficits may be less severe. Left posterior lesions may be associated with greater delays in expressive language but not necessarily in lexical comprehension (Thal et al., 1991). In child language development, there is also not a clear-cut relationship to the size of the lesion, and there is reason to believe that large lesions could lead to an early compensatory switch to an undamaged hemisphere and result in better short-term outcome. Results in child language studies suggest that there is remarkable plastic-

ity in brain regions that can support language (Mills, Coffey, and Neville, 1992). However, recovery occurs after an initial delay and the regions responsible for language learning are not necessarily the same regions that mediate language use and that maintain language in adults.

LANGUAGE IMPAIRMENT WITHOUT KNOWN NEUROLOGICAL IMPAIRMENT

Specific language impairment in receptive and/or expressive language development may occur without specific known neurological or cognitive impairment. Consequently, the definition of specific language impairment may need revision because there may be impairments in some aspects of cognition and perception that are not specific to language in these children. Tallal, Stark, and Mellits (1985; Tallal et al., 1991) have found that many children with specific language impairments have difficulty in processing rapid transitions in acoustic information. This includes both linguistic and nonlinguistic stimuli. Furthermore, when comparing language learning in English, Italian, and Hebrew, the specific areas of grammar that are most delayed vary from one language to another. The most vulnerable elements within a language seem to be those that are low in salience (phonological substance). Subtle deficits associated with specific language impairment may affect certain kinds of manual gestures as well as acoustic language. The brain bases for specific language impairment are unknown. MRI studies have shown specific lesions and subtle differences in brain symmetry (Jernigan et al., 1991), which require further study. Investigations of specific language impairment suggest that it may not be a purely linguistic or acoustic issue. Neither is it a congenital variant of the aphasias observed in adults with focal brain injury.

LANGUAGE INNATENESS AND SPECIFIC SYNDROMES

Another approach to language innateness involves the study of specific syndromes. In some instances, language may appear to be spared in congenital syndromes despite limitations in other cognitive abilities. Children with spinal bifida, hydrocephalus, and Williams syndrome have been described who have such disassociations. Language disassociations in Williams syndrome indicate that language can decouple from mental age at some point in development. In Williams syndrome, linguistic function is selectively preserved despite severe general cognitive deficits (Bellugi et al., 1992). However, recent studies in Williams syndrome do not suggest that language is a separate mental system from the beginning of life. Moreover, language development is delayed in infants and preschool children with Williams syndrome, although they may demonstrate hyperlalia. These findings suggest that cognitive prerequisites are necessary before language can be acquired. Older children with Williams syndrome maintain isolated sparing of some nonlinguistic areas, such as face recognition. Bates (1992) suggests that their spared language may be the result of abnormalities in the form of information processing, which operates in areas beyond language proper. Still, one must take into account the relationship or lack of relationship between face recognition studies and studies of language. Skelly, Wilson, and Goldman-Rakic (1992) have reported a link between the right inferior temporal cortex, where feature detection is thought to occur, and the right prefrontal cortex in monkeys, which may be essential for working memory involved in face recognition. Further study is needed to establish whether specific developmental disorders may show disconnection between brain regions involved with detection from those involved in recognition.

When children with Williams syndrome are compared with children with Down syndrome and matched for mental age, each group has a specific and complementary profile of impairments in cognition. These changes are in some ways analogous to differences between adult patients with damage to either the left or the right hemisphere of the brain. However, MRI studies in these syndromes do not show left/right differences, although there are group differences in brain morphology in regard to anterior/posterior axis and cerebellar/cerebral ratios when they are compared (Jernigan and Bellugi, 1990). There are also differences in proportionate size of neocerebellar versus paleocerebellar structures. Studies in these specific syndromes challenge theoretic ideas about neuronal structures that mediate language and cognitive structures that relate to language.

IMPACT OF EARLY EXPERIENCE ON LANGUAGE

Language develops in a social context. There are rare examples of children being raised without language exposure from adults. These are ordinarily abusive situations, and it has been difficult to separate out evidence of abuse and mental retardation from language findings when interpreting the findings. One case of a girl (Genie) who is thought to have functioned in the normal range of intelligence and was initially considered to have had no lasting emotional damage from being socially isolated was described by Susan Curtiss (1977). This was a young woman who was first examined as an adolescent and had been kept alone in a bedroom from approximately 18 months until her early teens, without exposure to language during those years.

Intensive speech and language therapy was initiated, but she did not fully acquire language. After initially demonstrating the pre-2-year-old stages of language, she did not move beyond what is referred to as *protolanguage* (described below). Her language basically consisted of two or three content words loosely linked by meaning but without grammatical items. Her lack of response to language training is not consistent with language being a unitary system. If language acquisition requires exposure to some form of linguistic input within a critical period, then Genie, who was not speaking previously, would not have acquired any language. However, if there is not a critical period for acquisition, she should have acquired language fully. Her response raises questions about why she acquired any language and why her language acquisition stopped at a particular point. Furthermore, why language stopped when it did rather than at an earlier or later stage must be considered.

One explanation is that there may be an early stage of language development called *protolanguage* that is part of our biological endowment but lacks most of the distinguishing formal properties of language. If this is assumed, then Genie acquired protolanguage, which is more robust than formal language. It does not have a critical period, although some lexical input is necessary for it to develop. The explanation for her language development ceasing might be that protolanguage and formal language are separate or disjointed, so the acquisition of one does not involve the acquisition of the other. Her language, then, would have ceased when it did because she had moved as far as she could in the development of protolanguage alone. In addition to protolanguage, she developed some rote learned phrases but did not develop formal language that one would have expected. She represents a case of an individual who, even though mature, still employed a variety of language that, despite its content, is formally no more developed than that of children under two. Similar findings are seen with adults who have formal language but are forced to utilize protolanguage by social circumstances in new language environments. However, it must be kept in mind that Genie was abused for many years and experienced both social and sensory isolation, which have been associated with brain dysfunction.

SUMMARY

In summary, neural network simulations of language learning have recently demonstrated that language can be acquired by general-purpose learning devices. Furthermore, electrophysiologic studies have demonstrated that neural systems subserving language level change with development, as distinct from chronological age. Studies of language acquisition in children with focal brain damage show substantial plasticity of brain regions that subserve language learning. Studies of specific language delay suggest that specific language impairment may not be as specific as previously thought. Finally, studies of mentally retarded children challenge simple views of the relationship between language and cognition. Studies of syndromes, such as Williams syndrome, raise new questions about neuronal substrates for both linguistic and cognitive profiles. Advances in the biological foundations of language development and evidence for innateness of language are substantial. However, evidence for a specific mental organ is difficult to demonstrate. Language learning appears to be based

on the brain plasticity of neuronal systems that may also serve other functions.

REFERENCES

Bates, E. (1992). Language development. *Current Opinion in Neurobiology,* 2:180–185.

_____, Thal, D., and Marchman, V. (1991). Symbols and syntax: A Darwinian approach to language development. In N. Kasnegor, D. Rumbaugh, E. Schiefelbusch, and M. Studdert-Kennedy (eds), *Biological and behavioral determinants of language development,* pp. 29–65. Erlbaum, Hillsdale, NJ.

Bellugi, U., Bihrle, A., Neville, H., Doherty, S., and Jernigan, T. (1992). Language, cognition and brain organization in a neurodevelopmental disorder. In W. Gunnar and C. Nelson (eds), *Developmental behavioral neuroscience.* Erlbaum, Hillsdale, NJ.

Bickerton, D. (1990). *Language and species.* University of Chicago Press, Chicago.

Chomsky, N. (1957). *Syntactic structures.* Mouton, The Hague, Holland.

_____. (1988). *Language and problems of knowledge.* MIT Press, Cambridge, MA.

Curtiss, S. (1977). *Genie: A linguistic study of a modern day "wild" child.* Academic Press, New York.

Darwin, C. (1871). *The descent of man, and selections in relation to sex,* 2 vol. John Murray, London.

Fletcher, P. (1990). Speech and language defects. *Nature,* 346:226.

Gopnik, M. and Crago M. (1991). Familial aggregation of a developmental language disorder. *Cognition,* 39:1–50.

Jernigan, T. and Bellugi, U. (1990). Anomalous brain morphology on magnetic resonance images in Williams Syndrome and Down Syndrome. *Archives of Neurology,* 47:529–553.

_____, Hesselink, M.D., Sowell, E., and Tallal, P. (1991). Cerebral structure on magnetic resonance imaging in language and learning-impaired children. *Archives of Neurology,* 48:539–545.

Lane, H. (1977). *The wild boy of Aveyron.* Harvard University Press, Cambridge, MA.

Marchman, V. (1992). *Constraints on plasticity in a connectionist model of the acquisition of the English past tense* (technical report). University of California, San Diego, Center for Research in Language, 9201, La Jolla, CA.

_____, Miller, R., and Bates, E. (1991). Babble and first words in children with focal brain injury. *Applied Psycholinguistics,* 12:1–22.

Mills, D., Coffey, S., and Neville, H. (1992). Changes

in cerebral organization in infancy during primary language acquisition. In G. Dawson and K. Fischer (eds), *Human behavior and the developing brain.* Guilford Publications, New York.

_____, _____, and _____. (1993). Language acquisition and cerebral specialization in 20-month-old children. *Journal of Cognition Neuroscience* 5:317–334.

Molfese, D. (1990). Auditory evoked responses recorded from 16-month-old human infants to words they did and did not know. *Brain and Language,* 38:345–363.

Pettito, L. and Marentette, P.F. (1991). Babbling in the manual mode: Evidence for the ontogeny of language. *Science,* 251:1493–1499.

Rumelhart, D.E. and McClelland, J.L. (1986). *Parallel distributed processing,* Vol. 1 and 2. MIT Press, Cambridge.

Rymer, R. (1993) *Genie: An abused child's flight from silence.* Harper Collins Publishers, New York.

Skelly, J.P., Wilson, F.A.W., and Goldman-Rakic, P.S. (1992). Neurons in the prefrontal cortex of the Macaque selective for faces. *Society for Neuroscience Abstracts,* 297.3.

Tallal, P., Townsend, J., Curtiss, S., and Wulfeck, B. (1991). Phenotypic profiles of language-impaired children based on genetic/family history. *Brain and Language,* 41:81–95.

_____, Stark, R., and Mellits, D. (1985). Identification of language impaired children on the basis of rapid perception and production skills. *Brain and Language,* 25:314–322.

Thal, D.J., Marchman, V., Stiles, J., Aram, D., Trauner, D., Nass, R., and Bates, E. (1991). Early lexical development in children with focal brain injury. *Brain and Language,* 40:491–527.

Vargha-Khadem, F., Isaacs, E., Papaleloudi, H., Polkey, C., and Wilson, J. (1991). Development of language in six hemispherectomized patients. *Brain,* 114:473–495.

CHAPTER 9

MEMORY

Our modern word for memory comes from the Latin *memoria,* which means "recollection and retrieval from a store," yet in its original Greek origins, memory was bestowed by Mnemosyne, the goddess who, as mother of the Muses, was the source of inspiration and of creative invention. Barth writes that "if Zeus in this allegorizing myth, represents fertilizing power, life force, creative energy, it is Memory—fertilized, energized, and no mean creator herself, who gestates, shapes and delivers . . ." (Barth, 1992).

The original Greek meaning then implied something more, namely, that the retrieval of narrative information, the "spinning" of a tale, is a creation from universal stores of plots, rather than a rote reproduction from memorized facts. Such is the source of the inspiration that may be linked to various regions of the brain. Perhaps narrative memory links affect, image, movement, and consciousness, whereas the mnemonic is limited only to factual stores from semantic sources, rather than the broader-ranging, multiply placed episodic events.

It is only recently that we have come to understand that memory is, indeed, created; that it resides in a brain system that may be disrupted; and that there is a developmental sequence in its production. Memory includes both storage and retrieval of information and experience. Retrieval of memories may occur in several ways. Facts may be reproduced as rotely learned, but experiences (episodes) are

apparently reconstructed paralleling the two modes of thinking—the analytical and the narrative—necessary for their meaningful presentation. Cognitive processes and linked cognitive/affective processes must be considered in the study of memory.

Motor patterning or habit training is the basis of another form of learning, operant conditioning, and is referred to as "habit formation" by Mishkin, Malamut, and Bachevalier (1984) to distinguish it from memory that involves conscious cognition or knowing. Habit learning has been studied in sea snails (aplysia) (Kandel, Schwartz, and Jessell, 1991), in the octopus (which responds differently depending on the sense approached, e.g., touch or sight), and in other species (Lorenz, 1981). Studies in these simple species have contributed to an understanding of the basic mechanisms of sensitization.

This chapter discusses these various aspects of memory. It provides a definition and classification of memory, reviews its neuroanatomy and synaptic basis, discusses animal models, highlights the relationship of REM sleep and memory, discusses emotional memory, and considers how disturbance of memory may be pertinent to developmental disorders.

DEFINITION AND CLASSIFICATION

A memory system can be defined as an organized relationship among brain structures and includes those processes that make possible the acquisition, retention, and utilization of knowledge (Schacter and Moscovitch, 1984).

Memory has been applied in a general way to describe the ability to conserve and later utilize experiences. Piaget and Inhelder (1973) wrote of memory in this wider sense, which includes the acquisition of skills, vocabulary, and adaptive responses. In the stricter sense, memory describes the ability to consciously reflect on past incidents. An infant's performance on tasks such as habituation, object search, novelty preference, and conditioning are accounted for by the wider concept of memory. Memory in this wider sense precedes the reflective form of memory.

Historically, William James (1890) had proposed that there were two kinds of memory, primary and secondary. Primary memory referred to keeping information in mind, and secondary memory referred to stored information that has dropped from mind but remains available for retrieval. Using the current terminology, primary memory is short-term and secondary memory is long-term. Memory may be categorized in several ways (Maurer, 1992). General classifications include (1) by the subprocesses used in storage (i.e., ultrashort-term, short-term, and long-term); (2) by the process used in retrieving memories (through thought, through action, or through perception); and (3) by the modality of cognitive memory that is lost in amnesia (i.e., global, partial, or specific). These approaches are summarized in Table 9–1.

However, for our purposes, a more detailed classification of multiple memory systems will be used as shown in Figure 9–1 (Squire and Zola-Morgan, 1991) and in Table 9–2 (Tulving, 1992).

This classification of memory generally follows a developmental sequence in that new forms transcend earlier ones to allow for increasing reflection on choices and actions. These multiple forms of memory involve different brain systems and have different characteristics (Squire, 1992). Procedural memory systems are the first to appear, and episodic memory systems are the last to develop. Many of the higher and later developing memory functions depend on, and are supported by, the operations of the lower and earlier developing ones. Still, the lower systems can essentially operate independently.

Table 9–1. Dimensions Used in Classifying Memory

By the Process Used in Retrieval of the Memory

Retrieval through thought
Cognitive memory
"Conscious" or "psychological" memory
"Unorganic" ("unorganized" and semi-organized") memory
Declarative memory
Representational memory
Explicit memory
Anterograde and retrograde memory (taken together)

Retrieval through action or through perception
Habit formation (through action) and priming (through perception)
"Unconscious" memory
"Organic" ("organized") memory
Procedural memory (through action)
Nonrepresentational memory
Implicit memory

By the Modality of Cognitive Memory Lost in Amnesia

All modalities
Global amnesia
"General" amnesia

Some modalities
Partial amnesia
Domain-specific memory
Material-specific memory

Specific "metamodalities"

MEMORIES LOCALIZED IN TIME
Episodic memory
"Unorganized" memory

MEMORIES NOT LOCALIZED IN TIME
Semantic memory
"Semiorganized" memory

By the Subprocess of Cognitive Memory Used in Storage of the Memory

Ultrashort-term storage
Ultrashort-term memory
Sensory memory

Short-term storage
Short-term memory
Primary memory
Working memory
Attentional memory
Immediate memory

Long-term storage
Long-term memory
Secondary memory
Recent memory (anterograde, sometimes called "short-term") and remote memory (retrograde, sometimes called "long-term")
Reference memory

From Maurer, 1992.

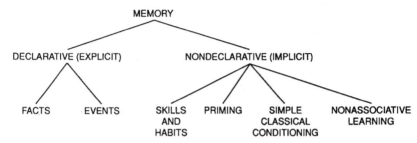

Figure 9–1. *Classification of memory.* Declarative (explicit) memory refers to conscious recollections of facts and events and depends on the integrity of the medial temporal lobe. Nondeclarative (implicit) memory refers to a collection of abilities and is independent of the medial temporal lobe. Nonassociative learning includes habituation and sensitization. In the case of nondeclarative memory, experience alters behavior nonconsciously without providing access to any memory content (from Squire and Zola-Morgan, 1991).

Procedural memory, the first to develop, includes skill learning and simple conditioning. It is followed by the establishment of a perceptual representation system (PRS), which is involved in perceptual priming and in the identification of objects. Next is semantic memory, which refers to general knowledge of the world, and then episodic memory, the last to appear, which includes the conscious recollection of personal past experiences. Semantic and episodic memory have been categorized together as declarative or propositional memory because they share common features.

Memory may also be distinguished as *implicit* (nondeclarative) or *explicit* (declarative), the terms used in this chapter. Implicit memory refers to information acquired without personal awareness of its acquisition. In implicit memory, the individual expresses what he knows but does not necessarily remember how, when, or where the knowledge was acquired. On the other hand, explicit memory addresses the conscious expression of both short-term, or working memory (highly accessible information of recent origin and input), and episodic memory. Explicit memory is the expression of what a person consciously remembers as a personal experience. Procedural memory, perceptual representation systems (PRS), and semantic memory are classified as implicit.

From a developmental perspective, episodic memory is best described as embedded in semantic memory. Meaningful episodes are first described as entering consciousness as scripts (Nelson, 1986) and later may contribute to autobiographical memory. Around age 4, children demonstrate autobiographical memory in describing their daily experiences. Self-recollection is a developmental landmark for this age 4 transition.

Table 9–2. Major Memory Systems

1. Procedural memory:
   Skills, simple conditioning
2. Perceptual representational system**:
   Perceptual priming of identification of objects
3. Short-term memory*:
   Highly accessible information from recent cognitive inputs.

Declarative memory includes:

4. Semantic memory**:
   General knowledge of the world
5. Episodic memory*
   Conscious recollection of the personal past

*Explicit memory
**Implicit memory
From Tulving, 1992.

DESCRIPTION OF SPECIFIC MEMORY SYSTEMS

The procedural system is an action system, and its operations are expressed in behavior that is independent of cognition. Simple stimulus-response connections are examples of tasks requiring procedural memory that are expressed in behavior. Performance of perceptual-motor tasks and simple stimulus-response are characteristic behaviors. Behavioral approaches to the treatment of developmentally disabled children and adolescents emphasize this form of memory. Reinforcement by conditioning relies on a basic property of nervous systems (Lorenz, 1981) to respond to reinforcement. This kind of learning is preserved after hippocampectomy because procedural retrieval apparently is not based on the context of the experience. Contextual retrieval requires representational storage and the integrity of the hippocampal system.

Perceptual priming refers to a special form of learning, which is expressed in enhanced identification of objects as "structured entities" (Tulving and Schachter, 1990). Perception at time one primes the perception of the same or a similar object at time two. Consequently, subsequent identifications require less information and less time when priming has occurred.

Short-term memory, also referred to as *primary memory* or *working memory,* provides the means to register and retain information in a highly accessible form but for only a short time period.

Semantic memory makes possible acquisition and retention of factual information and makes general knowledge of the world available to thought. It includes the classification of events, situations, objects, or symbolic descriptions of them, and knowledge of the location of objects in nonperceived space.

Finally, episodic memory makes possible the remembrance of personal past experiences. Consequently, events can be recalled as occurring in subjective time. Episodic memory depends on semantic memory but goes beyond it. The unique awareness and recollection of personal past experiences is different from those kinds of awareness that follow perceptual input, imagining, problem solving, dreaming, and the retrieval of semantic facts. This form of memory is associated with consciousness of an enduring self experience over time.

GENERAL EVENT REPRESENTATION AND AUTOBIOGRAPHICAL MEMORY

Autobiographical memory is generally categorized as a form of episodic memory. Episodic memory is generally considered to be stored, then retrieved using temporal and spatial cues. Semantic (or conceptual) knowledge, of which general event representation is a part, is thought to be stored and retrieved by other processes. (In the child development literature, the term "general event representation" (GER) is used to describe the acquisition of facts and events into memory. GER represents information, including lists of people or objects that can fill slots, alternative approaches, and optional pathways. A single event that already has adequate representation in GER would not be stored separately.)

On the other hand, autobiographical memory that deals with the specific representation of experience may be thought of as embedded in general event representation, because it requires the structural background of general event representation. Hudson (1986) has suggested that specific events are recalled, not by time and space cues, but in terms of a link with general event representation. Subsequently, routine events are not attended to but are forgotten or are absorbed into general event representational memory. However, novel experiences are better remembered. They may be linked to general representations and indexed by their distinctive features so that the context is established in a more general way.

Repeated novel experiences, as they are attended to over time, may be incorporated into GER. Attention to detail and memory for details results in the formation of new pathways. Linton (1975, 1982) describes this as a transition from episodic to semantic memory; here the episodic memory is less intense as the more typical features are abstracted from experience.

Therefore, an autobiographical memory may include both discrete details and information from general event knowledge. However, reconstruction from GER may be faulty or confused as to "what must have happened." The general representation may become confused regarding the specific details. In this way, what happened may be confused with what must or could have happened.

NEUROANATOMY AND SYNAPTIC BASIS

To accomplish localization of memory in the mammalian brain, it is necessary to establish what neuronal circuitry is necessary for a particular type of memory, its formation, storage, and retrieval. Neuronal circuits involved in certain forms of learning have been identified. There is some early evidence for localization of memory traces. Fear conditioning, classical conditioning of discrete responses, instrumental learning, explicit memory, short-term (working) memory, experience-dependent reorganization of memory, and the invertebrate models have been and continue to be studied. Of particular interest is the role of glutamate receptors and long-term potentiation in the formation of memory. Changes in gene expression and protein synthesis that relate to memory are being evaluated and may be essential in long-term sensitization in invertebrates (Kandel, Schwartz, and Jessell, 1991).

The various forms of memory are mediated by separate brain systems. Conscious memory for facts and events (declarative or explicit memory) and nonconscious memory (acquisition of skills, habits, and other procedures, i.e., nondeclarative or implicit memory) use different systems. The hippocampus and its related structures are essential for declarative or explicit memory, but other structures are necessary for nondeclarative or implicit memory. Even though the hippocampus and related structures are needed for the establishment of enduring memory, eventual long-term memory storage is believed to involve the neocortex. Thompson (1992) has pointed out that nondeclarative memory appears to be stored in specific sensory and motor pathways. Moreover, the cerebellum is an important site for classical conditioning of skeletal musculature.

New models to study memory investigate processes such as memory and visual perception. Visual input is ordinarily perceived as continuous but is studied by breaking it down into component functions. The next step is to study the components in particular brain regions. There is limited understanding of how these components are localized or distributed; however, they are being investigated through study of neural networks (Hinton, McClelland, and Rumelhart, 1986; Hinton and Shallice, 1991).

Computationally oriented cognitive neuroscience emphasizes neural network computer models (Chapter 10). These approaches attempt to formulate detailed models of actual neural circuits. For example, there are neural network models that address how an individual per-

forms specific tasks; networks are constructed and trained to interpret worklike inputs. This model is then damaged, and error patterns are examined. In some respects, these model circuits mirror brain damage, so the modeling potentially accounts for difficulties in brain-damage models that allow new hypotheses to be evaluated. Other neural networks have modeled the olfactory cortex to establish how new associations to scents are developed. The use of neural networks may have more general application in understanding the process of memory storage (Thompson, 1992).

ANIMAL MODELS OF MEMORY FUNCTION

Animal models of human amnesia are available in the nonhuman primate. It is now possible to investigate systematically which anatomical structures are important for memory through utilizing these animal models. In these models, monkeys are prepared with bilateral lesions limited to a particular structure or combination of structures. The effects of the surgical removal on memory is then determined by evaluating the monkey's performance on tasks that are either identical to, or analogous to, tasks of memory impairment in humans. To establish if the impairment in monkeys is long-lasting, as it is in humans who have had damage to the medial temporal lobe, these monkeys can be tested again several years subsequent to their surgery. Because there are multiple memory systems, specific systems can be tested in animals whose performance corresponds to humans with amnesia.

The development of one animal model in the monkey involves large bilateral lesions of the medial temporal lobe, which approximate damage in known amnesic human patients. The damaged area includes the hippocampal formation, the amygdala, and the surrounding perirhinal and perihippocampal cortices. Following the lesions, the monkeys were impaired on a number of explicit memory tasks, like human patients, but were entirely normal on implicit memory tasks of acquiring and retaining skills. The best test to demonstrate impaired memories in monkeys is the delayed nonmatching to sample task. This is a task of recognition memory in which a single object is presented, and then after a delay, two objects are presented, the original object and a new or novel one. The animal must choose the new or novel object to obtain a food reward. The testing is done in multiple trials, and unique pairs of objects are used for each trial. The results in this animal model have demonstrated that structures of the medial temporal lobe rather than adjacent areas are critical for recognition memory (Squire and Zola-Morgan, 1991).

Moreover, the main components of medial temporal lobe memory have been identified. The memory system consists of the hippocampal formation, which includes the entorhinal cortex along with adjacent anatomically related regions. The amygdaloid complex is not a component of the medial temporal lobe memory system. It does not contribute to explicit memory, which depends on this system. As noted in the chapter on emotion, the amygdala is important for conditioned fear and attachment of affect to neutral stimuli. It may also have a role in establishing links between stimuli and in making associations between various sensory modalities as well as in the recognition of emotion in facial expressions. In the same monkey model, damage to the amygdaloid complex caused alterations in emotional behavior, in that the monkeys were less fearful than normal and willing to touch and interact with novel stimuli.

In summary, the medial temporal lobe cortex participates in memory functions through its extensive reciprocal connections with memory storage sites in the neocortex. Systematic research with monkeys and related research in humans has identified the connections and components of the medial temporal lobe memory system. This system is fast, has limited capacity, and performs crucial functions during the time of learning to establish long-term explicit memory. Moreover, its role continues following learning during a lengthy period of reorganization and consolidation during which memories are stored in the neocortex and eventually become independent of the medial temporal lobe memory system. Because long-term (permanent) memory storage is gradually assumed by the neocortex, the medial temporal lobe memory system is always available for the acquisition of new information. Because the anatomy and function of the system and how it relates to the neocortex is now better under-

stood, studies using neural networks for computational modeling may now be undertaken.

LONG-TERM POTENTIATION

Memories are stored or encoded in neural networks in the brain. It is thought that new or novel experiences lead to neuronal firing in these networks. Subsequently, an attempt to recall an experience, or an experience that reminds one of the past, may trigger the same firing pattern that represents the memory.

This memory system in the brain has the capacity to store and retrieve massive amounts of information. New information is encoded in seconds, and the encoded information is stored and remains persistently encoded. A time period of several minutes is needed to stabilize or consolidate newly acquired experience or information. This encoding process is stimulated by patterns of electrophysiologic activity in the brain that is acquired during the learning process (Lynch and Granger, 1992) and is accompanied by actual morphological change. All of these aspects of memory are consistent with the long-term potentiation (LTP) effect suggested by Hebb (1949).

Long-term potentiation refers to how the production of changes in synaptic efficiency occurs. LTP was discovered in 1972, when it was shown that rapid neuronal firing in the hippocampus of the brain on one occasion established a pattern in which neurons fired more readily with subsequent stimulation. When neurons were activated, synaptic connections were strengthened by this process. In long-term potentiation, a new cell that is signaled over and over again remembers the signal, laying down a memory.

Molecular changes also take place within the neurons and their synaptic junctions during LTP. As a result of strengthening of these synapses, some neuronal groups respond better to specific stimuli because they have been selected and their connections strengthened.

Lynch and Granger (1992) point out five characteristics of LTP that make it the major candidate for being the substrate of forms of memory. First, LTP is synaptically specific, so induction in one group of contacts on a cell does not affect other contacts. This property allows for substantial memory capacity. Second, LTP begins to develop within 10 seconds and is established by 20 to 30 seconds. Third, LTP can persist for weeks, allowing long-term storage. Fourth, there is a consolidation phase, also referred to as a vulnerable phase, lasting several minutes. Finally, brain activity patterns that emerge during learning are directly related to those cellular events that initiate LTP.

Long-term potentiation has been demonstrated in many brain regions but has been studied most extensively in the hippocampus. The early work of Bliss and Lomo (1973) showed an increase in the size of excitatory postsynaptic potentials (EPSPs) after a brief period of high-frequency (tetanic) electrical stimulation of the perforant path of the hippocampus. The primary form of LTP involves activation of the N-methyl-D-asparate (NMDA) subtype of glutamate.

This process is shown in Figure 9–2. It leads to a subsequent influx of Ca^{2+} into the postsynaptic cells via the NMDA receptor channels. The induction of this LTP requires concurrent pre- and postsynaptic receptor activation and may be prevented by postsynaptic cell manipulation. Therefore, the induction of LTP is postsynaptic; however, the mechanism of maintenance of LTP is still under investigation. LTP occurs in several brain regions and does not always involve NMDA receptor activation. However, the NMDA receptor is involved in the hippocampus and is linked to memory.

The link of LTP to learning and memory has been studied extensively. NMDA receptor antagonists have been shown to prevent various forms of learning in awake animals. NMDA receptor blockade does not prevent learning all tasks because there are different forms of LTP in different brain regions. Because the induction of LTP occurs postsynaptically, a signal must be sent from the site of LTP maintenance to activate the increase in transmitter release. In other words, the nerve cell that receives the signal sends a message back to the cell that first signaled it. That message makes the first cell more effective in releasing its neurotransmitter. Several candidates for this signal, the retrograde message, have been proposed. Initial study focused on arichidonic acid and then on nitric oxide. Nitric oxide is a newly described neurotransmitter that, as a gas, can easily diffuse back-

ward. It is synthesized in the postsynaptic cell and might act as an intercellular messenger. However, its synthesizing enzyme is not present in the pyramidal cells of the hippocampus described earlier, which are thought to be involved in the production of memory.

Recently another gas, carbon monoxide, which is found in the hippocampus among other brain regions, has been reported to be a neurotransmitter (Verma et al., 1993). The enzyme that synthesizes it is localized in the hippocampal region involved in LTP mediated learning. Stevens and Wang (1993) have found that an inhibitor of carbon monoxide prevents long-term potentiation in this hippocampal region. Furthermore, using carbon monoxide as a blocking agent resulted in previous learning being erased. Further confirmation is needed on the role of carbon monoxide in LTP. Clinical findings from carbon monoxide poisoning suggest the importance of continued study of carbon monoxide as a neurotransmitter.

REM AND MEMORY STORAGE

The role of sleep in memory is receiving new emphasis as the sleep cycle is better understood neurobiologically. Dreaming (REM sleep) may reflect a biological process in which new information is incorporated into existing memory. Evidence for this hypothesis has been presented by Winson (1990; Pavlides and Winson, 1989) who has demonstrated that information from an animal's waking hours is reprocessed by the dreaming brain. During the dream, new experiences may be integrated with old ones in an adaptive strategy to prepare for the next day. Dreams in early life may help build a plan for behavior that influences subsequent adaptation in later life. This neurobiological understanding of dreams contrasts with the classical psychoanalytic view which provided a psychological explanation that the function of dreams is to protect the ego against unacceptable wishes.

REM sleep may have evolved as an efficient means to store information in the brain. REM sleep first occurs in mammals, and with the exception of the Echidna (spiny ant eater), has been demonstrated in all mammals tested. Winson (1985) has suggested that the prefrontal cortex is large in the Echidna relative to the rest of the brain and proportionately larger than in

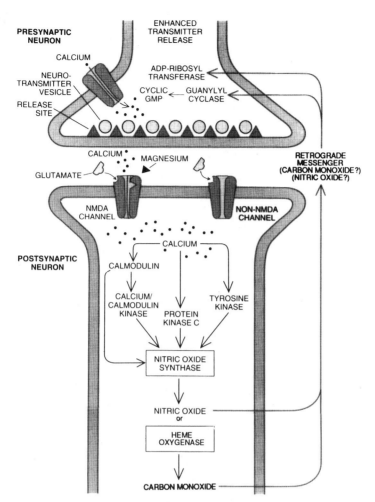

Figure 9–2. *The NMDA receptor and long-term potentiation.* In long-term potentiation, the postsynaptic membrane is depolarized by the actions of the non-NMDA receptor channels. The depolarization relieves the magnesium blockade of the NMDA channel, allowing calcium to flow through the channel. The calcium triggers calcium-dependent kinases that lead to the induction of LTP. The postsynaptic cell is thought to release a retrograde messenger, possibly nitric oxide or carbon monoxide, capable of penetrating the membrane of the presynaptic cell. This messenger is believed to act in the presynaptic terminal to enhance transmitter (glutamate) release, perhaps by activating guanylyl cyclase or ADP-ribosyl transferase (adapted from Kandel and Hawkins, 1992).

humans. He has suggested that the Echidna must respond to environmental challenges based on previous experience, which is updated through the large prefrontal areas. Because the prefrontal cortex is involved in planning and in adaptive behavior, without memory, an enormous amount of information would need to be stored in the brain for successful adaptive behavior. To deal with the environment, higher mammals had to use brain areas more efficiently because of limitations in prefrontal cor-

tical development. Consequently, Winson has suggested that REM sleep allows the brain to reprocess information taken in during the day so that the brain can function in a more efficient manner. In computer terms, this "off line" processing may be important in memory consolidation. In hypothesizing that REM sleep triggers reprocessing and consolidation of daytime information into memory, Winson suggests that the hippocampus is the brain region crucial for memory and dreaming. The hippocampus produces a distinct rhythm, the theta rhythm, which shows alternate spikes and waves at a six per second rate. The theta rhythm occurs during REM sleep. Moreover, stimulating the hippocampus at the peak of the theta rhythm induces LTP.

The theta rhythm is then synchronized with exploratory behavior. A variety of mammals show this theta rhythm when they are exploring a strange place. For example, cats demonstrate it when stalking prey, and rabbits demonstrate it when startled by a predator. The olfactory bulb is linked with this pattern of behavior as the rat sniffs and moves its whiskers to explore the environment. As a rat explores its surroundings, theta waves in the hippocampus are synchronized with sensory signals from the whiskers and nose. A memory trace is the apparent result of this activity. Subsequently, in REM sleep, these neuronal circuits may be reactivated, potentially resulting in integration of the day's experience with memories of previous experiences.

Pavlides and Winson (1989) tested the REM hypothesis by studying spatial activity in the rat. In an open maze, rats oriented to landmarks in the room, such as a window or a clock. This orientation is related to place neurons in a hippocampal brain map. By recording from a place neuron, the investigators could clarify whether or not the neuron fired. They hypothesized that the same neuronal area would later fire for the reactivation process during REM.

The procedure was to identify place neurons for a specific spot in a maze. Subsequently, access to that spot was prevented, to clarify that signaling only occurred when that particular region was reached. During sleep, a second neuronal probe was used to demonstrate that theta waves emerged as the animal entered REM sleep. Recordings from the place neurons repeatedly were found to be activated during REM sleep. When the rat moved to the rest of the maze, the neuronal firing subsided. During REM sleep, the place neuron became activated again at a rate that is effective for inducing LTP. In another experiment, the neurons that paced the auscultations of the theta rhythm were destroyed and it was found that rats who had learned spatial cues to find a particular area in a maze could no longer do so. Spatial memory, then, was obliterated without the theta rhythm. Subsequently, Winson went on to con-

duct other experiments to demonstrate that particular spatial memories were related to the theta rhythm. Other researchers have shown that theta waves are also generated in the entorhinal cortex, the area that prepares information for entry into the hippocampus.

This experiment provides direct evidence that the brain is reprocessing daytime information while an animal sleeps. Wilson and McNaughton (1994) offer additional confirmatory data in rats that information acquired during active behavior is re-expressed in hippocampal circuits during sleep as postulated in theories of nighttime memory consolidation. These experiments highlight the adaptive function of REM sleep and its purposefulness. Human studies have demonstrated a relationship between REM and learning; for example, Smith and Lapp (1991) have reported increases in the number of REMs and REM density in humans following an intensive learning period. Karni et al. (1994) have demonstrated improvement in performance of a basic visual discrimination task after a normal night's sleep. These authors conclude that a process of human memory consolidation that is active during sleep is largely dependent on REM sleep. Consequently, dreams may have significance in social adaptation. Winson's findings are congruent with Jung's view of the adaptive nature of dreaming (1974).

IMPLICIT MEMORY AND EMOTION

The investigation of memory has largely emphasized the study of explicit memory. However, there are multiple memory systems. Memory systems encode a structural description of perceptual input and represent the event itself as an episode in context. It is possible that emotional memories are supported by a different memory mechanism than that used for explicit memory and that this memory mechanism primarily represents emotional experiences. If this is the case, then multiple memory systems are necessary — one to support explicit memory and another to support implicit emotional memories.

As previously stated, initial research on memory focused on declarative or explicit memory, referring to an individual's conscious intentional recollection of previous events. Assessment of explicit memory has been most commonly carried out using standard tests of recognition and recall. It has been found that accessibility of memories is affected by the congruence of the individual's mood state at the time of encoding and at the time of retrieval of memory. In addition, the retrieval of emotional memories can affect the individual's mood state, yet what the individual brings to awareness in a conscious act of intentional recall and recognition is only partially descriptive of memory. Those memories that are out of awareness are of interest, especially emotional memories.

Implicit memory may be involved when there is a behavioral response linked to a past experience that cannot be consciously recollected and in the performance of tasks that do not require conscious recall. This has been most clearly demonstrated in studies in hypnotized subjects who were given posthypnotic suggestions and complied with them without remembering the original request (Kihlstrom and Hoyt, 1990). Similar results have been demonstrated in word association tasks in subjects with amnesia. In both instances, an improvement in task performance was attributed to prior experiences that were not remembered in themselves. Both of these examples illustrate that there may be a dissociation between explicit and implicit memory. This dissociation may be manifest when explicit memory is impaired and implicit memory is spared, as in the experiments with amnesic subjects. Moreover, performance on explicit and implicit memory tasks may affect overall performance. In some experiments, explicit memory but not implicit memory seems to be involved, whereas in others, implicit rather than explicit memory is involved. Therefore, it is likely that implicit and explicit memory effects demonstrate operations of different memory systems in the brain. These systems might include the perceptual representation of experience, procedural memory for skill knowledge, semantic memory for conceptual relations, and the episodic memory of some experiences. In both explicit and implicit memory, memory for prior events may be expressed.

Tobias, Kihlstrom, and Schacter (1992) have studied the relationship between implicit memory and emotional experience. Implicit memory may be expressed through emotional responses as well as in performance on specific perceptual and semantic memory tasks. There are a number of examples of these phenomena: for example, the report of a woman with a phobia for running water. She had no memory of how this response had been acquired until adulthood, when she was visited by an aunt who stimulated a memory of a childhood incident when the woman had strayed away from a picnic and had become trapped under a waterfall. In this instance and in many others, an individual shows a change in an emotional response and in behavior that is attributable to an earlier experience that is not remembered. This dissociation between emotional response and conscious recollection is analogous to the dissociation between implicit and explicit memory.

Experience-based changes in judgments or evaluations, affective responses, and emotional states that occur without explicit memory of the experiences themselves are receiving increasing evaluation in cognitive neuroscience. Examples are amnesia in brain-damaged patients, amnesia in dissociative disorders, hypnotic alterations in emotional state, and what has been referred to as "mere exposure" effects in tests of implicit perception (Zajonc, 1980).

Amnesia Due to Brain Damage

In patients with bilateral lesions of the medial portion of the temporal lobe, which includes the hippocampus and diencephalon, a gross anterograde amnesia occurs such that patients do not remember events that have occurred since the damage happened. For example, when asked to study a list of words and recall them, they show impairments in memory. However, when they are given the stem fragment of a meaningful word, they can demonstrate the same priming effects as normal subjects: They show intact implicit memory. Another example is in prosopagnostic patients, who may demonstrate a deficit in facial recognition following bilateral lesions of the mesial portions of the occipital and temporal cortex. These patients are unable to recognize previously encountered faces as familiar. Still, they may show differential autonomic responses to old and new faces, as measured by skin conductance measures.

Although the responses to faces may not be emotional, the degree of physiologic arousal suggests an emotional response.

Dissociative Amnesia

Amnesia may occur without specific lesions to brain structures in dissociative syndromes (e.g., dissociative amnesia and dissociative identity disorder). In these instances, the patient experiences a loss of autobiographical memory, which may be accompanied by a loss or change in personal identity. The memory loss may be related to a traumatic event that is not available to memory because of the amnesia, yet these patients often display implicit memory for events that are lost to their conscious recollection, and this implicit memory may take the form of an emotional response. A classic case was reported by Janet in 1893. A woman whose drunken husband had been placed on her doorstep was told he was dead as a joke. Subsequently she had no recollection of the event but "froze with terror" when she passed the doorway. Moreover, in dissociative identity disorder, amnesia between personalities is a characteristic feature. Implicit memory may transfer across the multiple personality states, so more than one personality may show strong emotional reactions on an implicit basis. Yet no personality has an explicit memory for those events.

Amnesia and Hypnotic Induction

Hypnotic suggestions alter cognitive function, but may also have emotional and motivational effects, in that emotional states can be altered by hypnotic suggestion. Posthypnotic amnesia has commonly been judged analogous to repression, as described by Freudian theory; however, there may be other explanations, for example, the selective dissociation of explicit and implicit memory: The amnestic subject lacks explicit memory for the suggestion, but experiences emotional arousal as an implicit memory for the posthypnotically suggested behavior. Here, subjects may show implicit memory for the images and respond to the cue without any explicit memory of why they are experiencing the emotion.

Mere Exposure Effects

In a standard implicit memory experiment, the subject is aware of the event at the time it occurs, but fails to consciously recollect that event. For example, Zajonc (1980) has demonstrated what are referred to as "mere exposure effects" for subsequent preference ratings when subjects are consciously unaware of the stimulus during the exposure trials. When subjects were given brief tachistoscopic presentations of irregularly shaped polygons, they later showed preference for the shapes they were exposed to, even though the shapes themselves were consciously recognized at only a chance level. This subliminal "mere exposure effect" has been replicated by others and extended to other judgments. Such preferences reflect implicit perception and memory; they may have implications for subsequent emotional judgments and behavior. In another example, subjects who were exposed subliminally to hostile words later attributed more negative qualities to the pictured target person than subjects who had not received this exposure. Subliminal exposure also has been shown to affect preferences for people's faces and subsequent interpersonal behavior toward them.

All of the above mentioned examples involve changes in evaluative judgment, affective response, or emotional state response in the absence of explicit memory for the experiences themselves. These responses may involve desynchrony among response systems in emotion. In classical animal research on experimental neurosis in dogs, Gantt (1953) observed that the separate components of a conditioned response may be acquired and extinguished at different rates. He noted that these responses may persist for different lengths of time and introduced the term "schizokinesis" to describe them. Subsequently, Lang (1971) suggested a multiple system theory of emotion with several components — physiologic, subjective, and behavioral — which were loosely coupled. When all three systems acted together, intense emotional arousal was experienced, but with mild arousal, he noted, they may be partially independent. Others (Rachman, 1978) have evaluated the therapeutic implications of desynchrony. For example, implosion theory may affect the behavioral component of fear before affecting the physiologic and subjective components. The relationship between desynchrony and dissociation requires continued study.

Additional work is also needed to clarify the relationship between explicit memory and emotion and implicit memory and emotion. It is not easy to identify explicit memory with one component of memory and implicit memory with other components. Tobias, Kihlstrom, and Schacter (1992) point out that the subjective experience of emotion has several components that reflect the individual's awareness of his emotional state, the stimulus that elicited the emotion, and other past encounters with the stimulus. Consequently, it is possible that there may be dissociations within memory components as well as between them.

These authors suggest that the relationship between mood and memory, or the effects of mood on memory, may fall into several general categories. First, there are mood-dependent memory effects, in which retrieval of memory is facilitated by a match between the encoded and retrieved mood states. Second, there may be mood-congruent memory effects, in which the mood at the time of encoding or retrieval facilitates retrieval of affective material that is congruent. Third, there are "resource allocation effects," in which extreme or negative mood states at the time of encoding or at the time of retrieval may impair memory processing. All of these effects have been demonstrated for the study of explicit memory, using standardized tests of recall and recollection.

But how is implicit memory affected by emotional state? One might expect that emotional state would have little effect on implicit memory. For example, in mood-dependent retrieval, a shift in mood state between encoding and retrieval may be analogous to a change in the subject's internal physiologic environment, as is seen with drug-state-dependent memory. A shift in context appears to cause a type of amnesia. Ordinarily, in many forms of amnesia, the most memory loss is evident in the explicit domain whereas the implicit domain seems preserved. If this is the case, implicit memory may transfer over various mood states, although explicit memory may not. Because affect changes the meaning of events but not their perceptual features, mood may be a variable that affects explicit memory.

Yet it is possible that context effects, including mood effects, might have a greater effect on implicit than explicit memory; for example, psychoactive drugs may produce state-dependent memory (i.e., alcohol, amphetamines, barbiturates) and may alter sensory-perceptual processes. Environmental context may alter the processing of perceptual features of events and produce effects that are analogous to modality shifts. Shifts in the environmental context that affect implicit memory may occur that do not affect explicit memory. One must consider the effect of mood on implicit memory. A mood, which is a prevailing emotion, may make the world look darker to people who are sad and brighter to those who are happy. Moreover, mood may serve as a contextual cue and, like other cues, be processed when memories are encoded and influence their retrieval. In research in this area, there is inconsistency in the results of studies of context-dependent memory, perhaps because stronger cues may overshadow weaker ones.

Because of these considerations, implicit memory has recently become a topic for formal research. There was considerable interest in implicit memory effects at the beginning of the century, but it is only recently that they have been investigated again. New studies have assessed mood effects and context effects on implicit memory. Jung's (1974) original experimental "word association studies" should now be considered in the context of implicit memory investigation, using a similar paradigm.

Weingartner, Miller, and Murphy (1977) studied state dependency in the generation of word associations. Subjects were asked to produce the same associated words when in the same mood as on a previous trial. Mathews et al. (1989) studied attentional biases or mood-congruent encoding in anxious subjects with threat-related words and word-stem completions. The clinically anxious patients showed a bias in retrieving threat words in both implicit and explicit conditions, yet the difference was significant only for the implicit memory condition. Here, effects of mood on implicit memory seem stronger than on explicit memory. Tobias and Kihlstrom (1990) studied happy and sad mood, which were musically manipulated at the time of encoding and retrieval. To strengthen the link between the items and mood, the word list contained words with positive and negative affective valence as well as emotionally neutral words. When items were affectively congruent to the encoding mood, that is, the condition where the cue value would be strongest, no mood-dependent memory was demonstrated for explicit memory. However, there was a strong mood-dependent effect in the implicit memory condition, which involved free recall or recall with minimum cues. That is, those subjects who were happy at both encoding and retrieval produced more positive target words than those who were happy at encoding but sad at retrieval. Furthermore, those who were sad at both encoding and retrieval produced more negative words than those who were sad at encoding but happy at retrieval. In this experiment, implicit effects were found even when explicit were not found.

These results suggest differences between mood and other aspects of context. Just as physiologic state and environmental circumstance can be encoded, so mood also can be encoded and serve as a potential cue for memory retrieval. Mood may affect how attention is directed toward the environment and may alter the experienced meaning of events besides serving as a kind of passive background. Consequently, moods, drug states, and environments may have different effects on memory.

The assessment of implicit memory is now focusing on clinically relevant tasks. The experimental literature has focused primarily on perceptual-cognitive tasks that required verbal responses. However, implicit memory research is needed for evaluative emotional responses, in which the subject feels an emotion that has previously been experienced, even though he does not remember the original experience. Implicit memory may be revealed in a wide variety of situations. These may include thought or action that is attributed to a past episode, whether the change resembles the types of perceptual-cognitive tasks that are performed under laboratory conditions or not. For example, if someone who has suffered a violent assault has nightmares or panic attacks and did not experience them before the event, the change in behavior may indicate an implicit memory effect, although the contents of a specific dream may not resemble the specific details of the incident and the event itself is not precisely remembered. As Breuer and Freud (1895) noted, "Hysterics suffer mainly from reminiscences. The subject is not aware of the origin and is unable to recollect the event and does not suspect the causal connection between that precipitating event and the pathological phenomenon."

Modern memory research suggests that what Breuer and Freud referred to as unconscious or repressed memories may now be considered implicit ones. Perhaps a variety of pathological symptoms and not only emotional reactions may involve implicit memory. By considering implicit memory, we may find a new means to integrate psychodynamic insights with current psychological theory, especially in regard to structured memory. Furthermore, the relationships between cognitive, emotional, and motivational processes with psychosomatic interactions may involve similar processes.

AMNESTIC DISORDERS IN CHILDREN

In adults the most common memory disorder is anterograde amnesia, the failure to store new memories, along with variable amounts of retrograde amnesia, the inability to retrieve old memories. These constitute the amnestic syndrome. Acquired forms of the amnestic syndrome do occur in children following head injury or encephalitis, but they are usually associated with other cognitive disabilities and often not specifically emphasized.

Maurer (1992) described a girl who had a stroke *in utero,* with brain lesions involving the temporal lobes. As a child, she showed severe aggressive behavior until the nature of her amnesia was recognized. Through the development of appropriate behavioral strategies that took her amnesia into account, her behavior improved. Her behavioral problems were secondary to her amnesia and the result of an interaction between her memory disability, her environment, and her limited past learning. On the other hand, those who acquire memory problems later in life may have learned to control behavior before the onset of their memory disorders. Therefore, the onset of amnesia in the developmental period may have a different presentation from memory disorders beginning in later life.

There may also be partial amnesias in child-hood. These are generally classified according to the affected domains, for example, as aphasias, agnosias, and apraxias. In addition, more extensive involvement may also occur that involves dysfunction of the lateral frontal lobe. Here again, the presentation in childhood may be as a behavioral problem rather than as a memory disorder.

MEMORY AND DEVELOPMENTAL DISORDERS

Research on memory is pertinent to the devel-opmental disorders. As Maurer (1992) has noted, learning and memory are embedded in one another, as memory provides the means to store and retrieve material and learning uses this information to guide behavior. Problems in attention and memory may be linked in learn-ing disabilities and in attention deficit disorder, where executive function and self-modulation regulate behavior. Whether or not stimulant medication affects memory through enhanced attention is an area of ongoing research. For example, state-bound memory recall has been linked to the use of stimulants. Moreover, Brandys and Rourke (1991) have found differ-ential memory abilities in reading- and arith-metic-disabled children. Other investigators have studied working memory in subtypes of learning-disabled children.

Autobiographical memory has a developmen-tal course and may profitably be studied in chil-dren with autistic disorder who have difficulty describing personal experiences, but may show remarkable memory for factual details. An ani-mal model for autistic disorder involves damage to the hippocampus and amygdala (Mishkin, Malamut, and Bachevalier, 1984). This model does not characterize the whole of autistic disor-der because these monkeys do not have abnormal sensory modulation or the typical hand stereotyp-ies seen in subjects with autistic disorder.

Moreover, the establishment of autobio-graphical memory may require the emergence of affect as a prerequisite. The development of autobiographical memory (Kanner, Rodriguez, and Ashenden, 1972) may be important when considering the emotional development of children with autistic disorder, particularly those who are higher functioning. Finally a person with autistic disorder may respond to drug treatment for an affective disorder but lack self-awareness of the existence of a mood disorder as shown by his failure to report mood symptoms.

In summary, our understanding of the mecha-nisms of memory has been enhanced through advances in neurobiology, cognitive neuro-science, and developmental psychology. The application of this new knowledge offers con-siderable promise for a better understanding of how memory dysfunction may occur in devel-opmental disorders.

REFERENCES

Barth, J. (1992). Once upon a time. *Johns Hopkins Magazine,* June 1992, pp. 33–38.

Bliss, T.V.P., and Lomo, T. (1973). Long-lasting potentiation of synaptic transmission in the den-tate area of the anaesthetized rabbit following stimulation of the perforant path. *Journal of Physiology (London),* 232:331–356.

Brandys, C.F., and Rourke, B.P. (1991). Differential memory abilities in reading and arithmetic-dis-abled children. In B.P. Rourke (ed), *Neuropsy-chological validation of learning disability sub-types.* Guilford Press, New York.

Breuer, J., and Freud, S. (1895). Studies on hysteria. In J. Strachey (ed), *The standard edition of the complete psychological works of Sigmund Freud,* Vol. 2. Hogarth Press, 1955.

Gantt, W.H. (1953). Principles of nervous breakdown in schizokinesis and autokinesis. *Annals of the New York Academy of Sciences,* 56:141–165.

Hebb, D.O. (1949) *The organization of behavior: A neuropsychological theory.* John Wiley & Sons, New York.

Hinton, G.E., and Shallice, T. (1991). Lesioning an attractor network: Investigations of acquired dyslexia. *Psychological Review,* 98:74–95.

_____, McClelland, J.L., and Rumelhart, D.E. (1986). Distributed representations. In D.E. Rumelhart and S.L. McClelland (eds), *Parallel distributed processing,* Vol. 1. Bradford Books/MIT Press, Boston.

Hobson, J.A. (1988). *The dreaming brain.* Basic Books, New York.

Hudson, J.A. (1986). Memories are made of this: General event knowledge and the development of autobiographical memory. In K. Nelson (ed), *Event knowledge: Structure and function in development.* Lawrence Erlbaum, Hillsdale, NJ.

James, W. (1890). *The principles of psychology.* Harvard University Press, Cambridge, MA.

Janet, P. (1893). Continuous amnesia. *Revue Générale des Sciences,* 4:167–179.

Jung, C.G. (1974). *Dreams.* Princeton University Press, Princeton, NJ.

Kandel, E.R., and Hawkins, R.D. (1992). The biological basis of learning and individuality. *Scientific American,* September, 1992, p. 83.

_____, Schwartz, J.H., and Jessell, T.M. (1991). *Principles of neural science,* 3rd ed. Elsevier, New York.

Kanner, L., Rodriguez, A., and Ashenden, B. (1972). How far can autistic children go in matters of social adaptation? *Journal of Autism and Childhood Schizophrenia,* 2:9–33.

Karni, A., Tanne, D., Rubenstein, B.S., Askenasy, J.J.M., and Sagi, D. (1994). Dependence on REM sleep of overnight improvement in a perceptual skill. *Science,* 265:679–682.

Kihlstrom, J.F., and Hoyt, I.P. (1990). Repression, dissociation, and hypnosis. In J.E. Singer (ed), *Repression: Defense mechanism and personality style,* pp. 181–208. University of Chicago Press, Chicago.

Lang, P.J. (1971). The application of psychophysiological methods to the study of psychotherapy and behavioral modification. In A.E. Bergen and S.L. Garfield (eds), *Handbook of psychotherapy and behavior change: An empirical analysis,* pp. 75–125. John Wiley & Sons, New York.

Linton, M. (1975). Memory for real-world events. In D.A. Norman and D.E. Rumelhart (eds), *Explorations in cognition,* pp. 376–404. W.H. Freeman, San Francisco.

_____. (1982). Transformations of memory in everyday life. In U. Neisser (ed), *Memory observed,* pp. 77–91. W.H. Freeman, San Francisco.

Lorenz, K. (1981). *The foundations of ethology,* pp. 70–71, 293. Springer-Verlag, New York.

Lynch, G., and Granger, R. (1992). Variations in synaptic plasticity and types of memory in corticohippocampal networks. *Journal of Cognitive Neuroscience,* 4:189–199.

Mathews, A., Mogg, K., May, J., and Eysenck, M.W. (1989). Implicit and explicit memory biases in anxiety. *Journal of Abnormal Psychology,* 98:31–34.

Maurer, R.G. (1992). Disorders of memory and learning. In I. Rapin and S.J. Segalowitz (eds), *Handbook of neuropsychology: Child neuropsychology,* Vol. 6. Elsevier, New York.

Mishkin, M., Malamut, B., and Bachevalier, J. (1984). Memories and habits: Two neural systems. In G. Lynch, J.L. McGaugh, and N.M.

Weinberger (eds), *The neurobiology of learning and memory.* Guilford Press, New York.

Nelson, K. (1986). *Event knowledge: Structure and function in development.* Lawrence Erlbaum, Hillsdale, NJ.

Pavlides, C., and Winson, J. (1989). Influences of hippocampal place cell firing in the awake state on the activity of these cells during subsequent sleep episodes. *Journal of Neuroscience,* 9:2907–2918.

Piaget, J., and Inhelder, B. (1973). *Memory and intelligence.* Basic Books, New York.

Rachman, S. (1978). Human fears: A three systems analysis. *Scandinavian Journal of Behavior Therapy,* 7:237–245.

Schacter, D.L., and Moscovitch, M. (1984). Infants, amnesics, and dissociable memory systems. In M. Moscovitch (ed), *Infant memory: Its relation to normal and pathological memory in humans and other animals. Advances in the Study of Communication and Affect,* 9:173–216.

Smith, C., and Lapp, L. (1991). Increases in number of REMs and REM density in humans following an intensive learning period. *Sleep,* 14:325–330.

Squire, L. R. (1992). Declarative and nondeclarative memory: Multiple brain systems supporting learning and memory. *Journal of Cognitive Neuroscience,* 4:232–243.

_____, and Zola-Morgan, S. (1991). The medial temporal lobe memory system. Science, 253:1380–1386.

Stevens, C.F., and Wang, Y. (1993). Reversal of long-term potentiation by inhibitors of haem oxgenase. *Nature,* 364:147–149.

Thompson, R.F. (1992). Memory. *Current Opinion in Neurobiology,* 2:203–208.

Tobias, B.A., and Kihlstrom, J.F. (1990). *Effects of mood on implicit and explicit memory.* Paper presented at the annual meeting of the American Psychological Association, Boston. August 14.

_____, Kihlstrom, J.F., and Schacter, D.L. (1992). Emotion and implicit memory. In S. Christianson (ed), *The handbook of emotion and memory. Research and theory,* pp. 67–92. Lawrence Erlbaum, Hillsdale, NJ.

Tulving, E. (1992). Concepts of human memory. In L.S. Squire (ed), *Memory: Organization and locus of change,* pp. 1–31. Oxford University Press, New York.

_____, and Schacter, D.L. (1990). Priming and human memory systems. *Science,* 247:301–306.

Verma, A., Hirsch, D.J., Glatt, C.E., Ronnett, G.V., and Snyder, S.H. (1993). Carbon monoxide: A putative neural messenger. *Science,* 259:381–384.

Weingartner, H., Miller, H., and Murphy, D.L. (1977). Mood-dependent retrieval of verbal associations. *Journal of Abnormal Psychology,* 86:276–284.

Wilson, M.A., and McNaughton, B.L. (1994). Reactivation of hippocampal ensemble memories during sleep. *Science,* 265:676–679.

Winson, J. (1985). *Brain and psyche: The biology of the unconscious.* Doubleday, New York.

_____. (1990). The meaning of dreams. *Scientific American,* November, 1990, pp. 86–95.

Zajonc, R. (1980). Feeling and thinking: Preferences need no inferences. *American Psychology,* 35:151–175.

CHAPTER 10

NEURAL NETWORKS

An artificial neural network is a computer model that is designed to simulate the structure and function of real neurons (Churchland and Sejnowski, 1992). Synaptic plasticity provides the neuroanatomical basis for the modeling of artificial neural networks (networks of artificial neurons), which allow the study of how learning may occur in brain systems.

The brain learns without explicit instructions to create internal representations that make interpretations of imprecise information possible. Neural networks are created by deducing the basic features of neuronal activity and simulating their interconnections (Hinton, 1989, 1992). Computers are then programmed to simulate these features.

Due to limitations of computing power and rudimentary models of neurons, the currently available neural networks are necessarily gross idealizations of real networks. Yet despite their limited approximations, network models are becoming productive in understanding learning and have become particularly useful in rejecting theories about how learning occurs (Rumelhart and McClelland, 1988).

A neural network, like the brain, will recognize patterns, may reorganize data, and most important, learns (Johnson-Laird, 1988). An artificial network is constructed of "units," which are designed to represent neural bodies (Van Camp, 1992). The networks are connected by "links," which represent the axons and dendrites in the brain. A link will carry out calcula-tions by multiplying a unit's output with a weighting factor. This factor is analogous to the "connection strength" of a synapse (Hinton, 1989). The weighted output that is associated with each connection is passed from the link to another unit, which sums up the values passed to it from similar incoming links. When the total input value exceeds a threshold, the unit fires.

Rather than reflecting the geometry of the dendrites and the axons, most artificial neural networks express the electrical output that might occur from a neural system. This output is expressed as a single number, which represents the system's firing rate or activity. It is thought that learning occurs in the brain as changes take place in the degree of inhibition or excitation of one neuron on another, which occurs at the synapse (see Chapter 9).

With the linkages previously described, each unit converts incoming activity that it receives into outgoing activity, which it broadcasts to other units. The conversion takes place in two stages: Initially, incoming activity is multiplied by the weight on that connection and the product is added together with other weighted inputs to produce a quantity, the total input. Second, a unit transforms the total input into output activity, using an input/output function, as shown in Figure 10–1.

As shown in Figure 10–2, the most common artificial neural encoder networks contain three layers of units: an input layer, which is con-

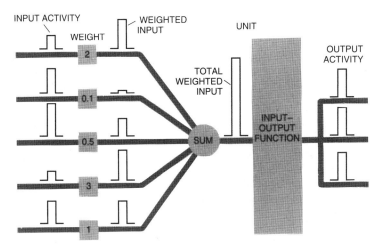

Figure 10–1. *Idealization of a neuron* processes activities, or signals. Each input activity is multiplied by a number called the weight. The "unit" adds together the weighted inputs. It then computes the output activity using an input-output function (from Hinton, 1992).

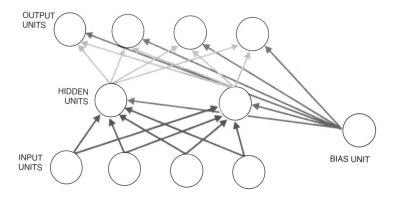

Figure 10–2. *4–2–4 Encoder network* compresses patterns. After a training period, the network accurately reproduces the input by representing the patterns essentially as binary code (as revealed by the hidden units) (from Van Camp, 1992).

nected to hidden units, which are connected to output units. The input units receive raw information; the hidden unit's activity is determined by the activities of the input units and the weight on the connections between input and hidden units. The behavior of the output units then depends on the activity of the hidden units and the weights between hidden and input units.

In real neurons, it is thought that learning occurs through synaptic changes, which occur through modifications in the firing pattern. As the connection strengths change between synapses, the firing pattern of the neural network changes. Similarly, in an artificial network, "learning" occurs when the weighting factors on the links change.

As stated earlier, in an artificial network, there are three types of units: input units, which take information; output units, which send out recognizable or visible signals; and hidden units acting between the input and output units.

These hidden units neither receive direct input from the outside nor produce a visible input.

The selection of weights and thresholds allows the modeling of any logical function. Of particular importance, these networks do not require that you choose the specific weights and thresholds. In Figure 10–3, any weight or threshold could have been used to start.

By repeatedly being shown the pattern of inputs and outputs, a network learns the weights that are necessary to implement the XOR or gate shown in the example. Furthermore, the network can generalize what is learned and, for very large data sets, is able to recognize patterns it has not previously seen.

To avoid changing both weights and thresholds, artificial neural networks often include a biasing unit, which is connected to every unit and allows a threshold to be changed to a weight. In addition, if the output is represented as a sigmoid function, the mathematical calculations are simplified.

Neural networks may be trained in several ways (i.e., supervised learning, reinforcement learning, and unsupervised learning). To create a neural network that performs a specific task, we must choose the connection of the weights to one another and set the weights appropriately. These connections establish whether one unit may influence another, and the weights specify the degree or strength of that influence.

A three-layered network can be taught a particular task by presenting it with training examples, which consist of a pattern of activity together with the desired pattern of activities for the output units. It is then determined how closely actual output matches desired output. Subsequently, the weight of each connection is changed so that the network produces a better approximation. Various methods are used to train networks. One of the simplest is the back propagation algorithm (Rumelhart, Hinton, and Williams, 1986; Crick, 1989).

With back propagation, the network needs to be taught by a teacher; however, humans learn most things without teachers. For example, children learn to understand sentences and interpret visual scenes without direct instructions. Conse-

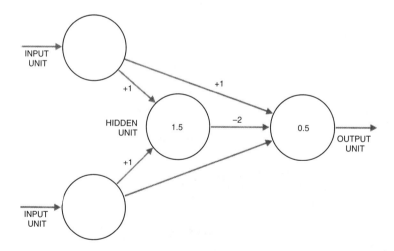

Figure 10–3. *Artificial Neural Network* shown here represents an "exclusive or" (XOR) gate: The output unit fires only if an input unit is presented with a 1. The numbers along the connections are weights, and those inside the units are threshold values. In the figure, if one of the input units is presented with a 1 and the other with a 0, the input to the hidden unit is $(1 \times 1) + (0 \times 1) = 1$. Because this value is less than that of the threshold value (1.5) of the hidden unit, the hidden unit will not fire (its output will be 0). The overall value to the output unit shown will be $(1 \times 1) + [0 \times (-2) + (0 \times 1) = 1]$. Because this is greater than the threshold, the output unit will fire. It should be noted that not all input units connect to hidden units. This artificial network is an exclusive gate where the output activity only fires if the input unit is presented with a 1. Numbers shown along the connections are weights and those inside the circles are threshold values (from Van Camp, 1992).

quently, developing a network that can learn appropriate internal representations without a teacher is important. Several general-purpose, unsupervised procedures have been developed that can adjust weights in networks appropriately. These unsupervised learning algorithms are classified according to the representations they create. In some instances, such as in principal component methods, hidden units cooperate and the representation of an input pattern is distributed across all of them. On the other hand, in competitive methods, the hidden units compete and representations of input are localized in single hidden units that are selected. Recently, more powerful approaches have been developed that lie between the extremes of purely distributed and purely localized representations.

It is thought that the brain uses what are known as *population codes,* in which information is represented by a whole population of active neurons. It has been demonstrated that in the monkey brain, to move the eyes, the total required movement is encoded by the activities of a whole population of cells, each of which represents a different movement. An eye movement, then, corresponds to the average of all of the movements encoded by active cells. In this experiment, if some brain cells were anesthetized, the eye moved to the point associated with the average of the remaining active cells. These *population codes* may be used not only for eye movements but also to encode faces. In both instances, the brain must represent entities that vary among many different dimensions. For the face, multiple points are needed in multidimensional space of possible faces so that any face can be represented by activating all of the cells that encode similar faces. The *population coding* approach is important because it may work when some neurons are damaged. The loss of a random subset of neurons may have little effect on the average of that population's activity.

Neural network models have been applied to address brain/behavior relationships. For example, a neural network model has been used to study distortions in processing regarding either excessive randomness of activity or excessive pruning of neuronal connections. Other models have been applied to the study of physiologic effects of catecholamines at the cellular level. Such physiologic effects can be simulated in a neural network, which can be used to account for the influence of stimulant drugs on cognitive function. This has led to models being developed to study cognitive deficits in schizophrenia in regard to dysfunction of dopaminergic neuromodulation of the prefrontal cortex. Another area in which neural network models have been applied is in the study of sleep. Modulation of individual units in a neural network model results in changes in the processing of sequences that resemble the changes in cognition that occur during dreaming. Neural network models can also be used to study language development and to study acquired dyslexia. These studies involve constructing a neural network model, which is trained to interpret wordlike inputs and then damaged (Hinton and Shallice, 1991). Following damage, the pattern of errors produced may mimic aspects of the kinds of errors found in patients with brain dysfunction. As a result, the model may potentially account for patient errors and allow new hypotheses to be directly tested. Though in its infancy, the neural network provides a simulation of dysfunctional brain systems and may offer models for understanding them more completely.

REFERENCES

Churchland, P.S., and Sejnowski, T.J. (1992). *The computational brain.* MIT Press/Bradford Books, Boston.

Crick, F. (1989). The recent excitement about neural networks. *Nature,* 337:129–132.

_____. (1992). Neurons for computers. *Scientific American,* 267:145–151.

Hinton, G.E. (1989). Connectionist learning procedures. *Artificial Intelligence,* 40:185–234.

_____, and Shallice, T. (1991). Lesioning an attractor network: Investigations of acquired dyslexia. *Psychological Review,* 98:74–95.

Johnson-Laird, P.N. (1988). *The computer and the mind.* Harvard University Press, Cambridge, MA.

Rumelhart, D.E., and McClelland, J.L. (1988). *Explorations in parallel distributed processing: A handbook of models, programs and exercises.* MIT Press, Boston.

_____, Hinton, G.E., and Williams, R.J. (1986). Learning representations by back propagating errors. *Nature,* 323:533–536.

Van Camp, D. (1992). Neurons for computers. *Scientific American,* 267:170-172.

CHAPTER 11

CONSCIOUSNESS

Consciousness is at the center of the study of both objective and subjective experience; to experience existence is to be conscious (Flannagan, 1992). *Consciousness* refers to a particular capability found in living systems, whereas *awareness* refers to the experience of exercising consciousness in a particular situation. Attention is linked to consciousness and refers to the control the organism or environment can exert over the direction of consciousness in the selection of the contents of awareness (Tulving, 1985). Until recently, consciousness was discussed primarily in psychological or functional terms (Dennett, 1991; Edelman, 1989; Jackendoff, 1987; Johnson-Laird, 1988) but was not considered by cognitive science and neuroscience because methods were unavailable to approach it.

This chapter provides a background for the study of consciousness and reviews recent developments. It considers consciousness from an evolutionary standpoint, discusses various concepts and levels of consciousness, reviews cognitive approaches and the links of consciousness to attention, considers consciousness and memory (especially working memory), outlines clinical situations in which consciousness is affected, and summarizes recent thoughts on the neurobiology of consciousness.

EVOLUTION OF THE NEOCORTEX

To consider consciousness, we must begin with its basis in evolution. The emergence of consciousness is linked to the development of the neocortex, which is composed of a sheet of neurons in the dorsal forebrain that originated between 160 and 300 million years ago and is unique to mammals (Allman, 1990). The neocortex is present in all mammals and may well have been present in mammal-like reptiles that lived between 160 and 240 million years ago (Carroll, 1988).

Development of the neocortex required evolutionary changes in the regulation of both neuronal proliferation and migration to produce additional cortical layers. The early precursor of the neocortex in amphibians may correspond to the dorsolateral cortical region. Thalamic inputs into the dorsolateral region may retain their primitive connections to cellular layers in the transformed neocortex. This new thalamic input is topographically organized to form the basis for the spatially ordered maps of vision, somatothesis, and hearing in the cortex.

The neocortex has multiple layers of neurons, each with specific inputs and outputs. Those structures related to the neocortical system that may be linked to consciousness include the neocortex, the thalamus, and the basal ganglia.

A large portion of the neocortex is dedicated to the topographic representation of the senses, such as vision, touch, and hearing. The olfactory cortex, the hippocampus, and the reptilian "general" cortex show similar neuronal layering but do not contain topographical maps.

The true receptive field of neocortical maps extends beyond the perceptual aspects of the sensory stimulus and is mapped by the interaction of stimuli presented outside the classical receptive field with stimuli presented within it. These large, nonclassical receptive fields are ideally suited to perform spatially integrative functions needed for perceptual constancies of color, motion, and space and the discrimination of figures from the background. Long-term perceptual representational memory involving the special senses (e.g., vision) may be embedded within these topographically mapped cortical areas. Perceptual representational memory depends on spatial location and is shown in priming experiments.

The neocortex's involvement in the extraction of figures from an ambiguous sensory world requires substantial computation. The topographical organization of the neocortical maps is well suited to extract figures from background and may indeed be the reason that the neocortex is topographically organized. Once the figure is resolved, it may be permanently stored, at least in part, in these mapped regions. Storage would enable rapid resolution of structures in the environment, even when relevant features are ambiguous.

The development of the neocortex in mammals requires a secure and protected environment and constant body temperature. Infant mammals depend on adults partly because of their lack of ability to thermoregulate. Thermoregulation is needed so that energy can be devoted to growth. Maternal care, shelter, warmth, and milk, provided through lactation, provide for the dependent young. MacLean (1990) has emphasized that nursing, audiovocal communication, and play are the basic features that distinguish mammals from reptiles.

During their period of dependency, infant mammals' play behavior may be crucial to the development of the neocortex. Playful interactions with the environment may provide the initial training for neocortical networks that eventually will enable the animal or growing child to localize events, to identify and to adapt to the environment (Allman, 1990). For the child, this playful interaction persists into adulthood. The interface of play with REM sleep activity may be crucial to the full establishment of neocortical networks during development.

Direct connections from the thalamus to the cingulate region may allow the limbic brain to be connected to the prefrontal cortex. This connection of the limbic system and cortical regions may be critical for parental behavior. The mammalian parent inhibits aggressive impulses toward the young, although reptilian species do not. This capacity to inhibit aggression, and as MacLean (1990) says, "to look with feeling" may be the basis of empathy. One might hypothesize that empathy is the first form of consciousness that accompanies inhibition of aggression toward one's own young. Thus, "defending consciousness" may have been a first form of social consciousness within the nest. Therefore, consciousness might have its origins in the early mammalian species that defend their young from the attack of predators. This recognition of self-sameness in other members of the species may have allowed the evolution of the family. If this is the case, then the evolution of consciousness is deeply tied to the early linking of affect and cognition.

Perhaps from this first empathetic concern, other aspects of consciousness subsequently emerged. Reflective consciousness (i.e., the capacity to think about one's thoughts and experiences) is a later human development.

CONCEPTS OF CONSCIOUSNESS

Consciousness "is a state of awareness of the self and the environment" (Fish, 1967). Sims (1988) suggests that it is best used as an adjective because a person does not possess consciousness, but is a conscious being. Consciousness is not separable from what one is conscious of; that is, it implies knowing something or being directed toward understanding something. Clinically, it refers to an inner awareness of experience, a potential intentional response, and an experience of a conscious self. On the other hand, unconscious refers to a lack of inner existence or experience. The term "unconscious" (Sims, 1988) refers to three situations in which there is no subjective experience: first, in brain disease, where a person may be on a classified continuum from normal consciousness to coma; second, in sleep, where there is a continuum from wakefulness to deep sleep (the alert person may be aware of only parts of the environment because there is also a continuum of vigilance from a specific object of awareness to total unawareness) third, in those processes that cannot be observed through introspection. Each of these processes are out of awareness.

LEVELS OF CONSCIOUSNESS

Vigilance, lucidity, and self-awareness (Sims, 1988) are all aspects of consciousness. Vigilance is on a continuum with drowsiness (Chapter 6). It may be linked to anxiety or to the basic affects. It may be heightened with interest, pleasure, anger, or fear and reduced during boredom and depression. These changes may be most evident in the cognitively impaired or brain-damaged person.

The sensorium (consciousness or full awareness of internal and external events) may be clear or clouded. Clouding refers to a slight impairment of consciousness on the alertness–coma continuum. With clouding, intellectual function (e.g., attention, concentration, recognition, judgment, speech, and planned action) may be impaired.

Consciousness of the self is an emerging capacity that accompanies alertness and awareness. In psychiatric disorders, there is an impairment in self-awareness in regard to the ability to distinguish the "I" from the "Not I" (Jaspers, 1963). Jaspers outlines four characteristics of self-awareness: (1) the feeling of awareness of activity (carrying out an activity provides an awareness of carrying it out); (2) an awareness of unity (I am one person, not many); (3) an awareness of identity (continuity of being one person all the time); and (4) an awareness of the boundaries of the self (distinguish myself from the outside world, which is not self).

Self-awareness may be expressed as self-concept and self-image. Self-concept refers to conscious abstract awareness of one's self, whereas the body image refers to physical aspects and those that are not in awareness (Sims, 1988). Developmental phases of self-awareness and differentiation from the environment (ages 1 to 3), the emergence of an externally derived self-image and establishment of a social role (ages 4 to 10), the reestablishment of the body image at puberty (ages 11 to 14), and the establishment of mature roles of social self in adolescence are described in Chapter 15.

CONSCIOUSNESS AND MEMORY

Remembering is a conscious experience; to remember is to be consciously aware of past events. Primary memory (James, 1890) is identified with consciousness, and the rehearsal of an idea is a conscious process; activated memory is conscious.

In considering consciousness, working or short-term (a few seconds) and very short-term (a fraction of a second) memory may be the most pertinent. Working or short-term memory is limited in the number of items it may hold at one time — approximately seven — yet the storage potential of memory is far greater than this. An ambiguous event may have only one interpretation at a time in consciousness, and generally tasks are carried out one at a time. Still, affectively linked implicit memories may lead to automatic behavior and parallel processing. Because consciousness is linked to the executive function of attention, it has the capacity to inhibit automatic responses generated through perceptions and affects that are linked to implicit memory. Furthermore, information processing may occur out of awareness such that solutions subsequently become available to consciousness.

Long-term episodic memory apparently is not necessary for consciousness, because those with brain injury who may not be able to lay down new episodic memory are conscious.

Tulving (1985) links the three basic memory systems — procedural, semantic, and episodic — to three kinds of consciousness: anoetic (non-knowing), noetic (knowing), and autonoetic (self-knowing). Anoetic consciousness, which is characteristic of procedural memory, is temporally and spatially bound to the current situation. This form of consciousness registers perceptions, internally represents them, and allows behavioral response to internal and external aspects in the present. Noetic consciousness is the characteristic of semantic memory. It allows one to be aware of and cognitively process objects, events, and the relations among objects and events, when these objects and events are absent. This allows flexible action upon symbolic knowledge of the world. Noetic consciousness accompanies information being entered into and retrieved from semantic memory. It may be associated with "involuntary memory" when experience comes into awarenesses without our conscious choice.

Autonoetic consciousness may be correlated with episodic memory and is necessary to remember personally experienced events. To remember an event, one is aware of it as part of one's own past existence. This form of consciousness gives the phenomenological quality to remembrance and distinguishes it from other forms of awareness (e.g., perceiving, thinking, imagining, or dreaming).

Tulving (1985) studied case N.N., who had profound amnesia for personal events before and after a closed head injury. N.N. cannot recall a single personal event or incident from his past. His knowledge of the past has an impersonal quality, as does his knowledge of other aspects of the world, yet his language skills and general knowledge skills are intact. His awareness of chronological time is intact, but his awareness of subjective time is severely impaired. This patient lacks autonoetic consciousness and has severely impaired episodic memory. His difficulty lies in the ability to "apprehend and to contemplate extended subjective time." His case suggests that amnesia may be characterized by an abnormality in consciousness as well as in the memory of past events. Tulving emphasizes the distinction between knowing and remembering so that the prior occurrence of specific events is meaningful. People do make judgments about the accuracy of their performance when asked about memories. People can know something happened by remembering the event as their own experience. He suggests that episodic memory has subjective certainty that leads to more effective action in the present and better planning for the future. Understanding consciousness and its emergence from the brain as consciousness of self is the major challenge in the study of consciousness.

COGNITIVE APPROACHES TO CONSCIOUSNESS

In *The Computer and the Mind* Johnson-Laird (1988) emphasizes a computational model and suggests that the brain is organized as a hierarchy of parallel processes with an operating system that directs them and corresponds to the conscious mind. In this model, the conscious mechanism expresses the results of computations that occur in the brain but not how they take place. No specific brain area is designated as the location of this processing. He considers self-reflection and self-awareness in his analyses.

On the other hand, in *Consciousness and the Computational Mind* Jackendoff (1987) suggests that consciousness is associated with intermediate levels rather than with the highest levels of the brain. In reaching this conclusion, he considers the language system, the visual system, and music.

Both Johnson-Laird and Jackendoff place emphasis on consciousness and working memory. Both authors discuss a serial process, perhaps analogous to attention, on top of the parallel processes. These models suggest a neuroscience analysis that considers both attention and working memory.

Even though consciousness has been defined and its disorders have been classified phenomenologically with increasing reliability, many questions remain unanswered. The most important of these is, "How can living physical bodies in the physical world produce consciousness?" (Dennett, 1991). This is the question that the cognitive sciences now attempt to address. Dennett asks, "How can a combination of electrochemical events lead to profound experience? Events in the brain just occur as processes occur in other organ systems. Yet experienced events are conscious; it is some body's experience."

Crick and Koch (1990) state that one of the functions of consciousness is to "present the results of underlying computations." These computations involve an attentional mechanism, which temporarily binds neurons together by synchronizing their oscillations. Dennett (1991) inquires to whom the computations are presented. He suggests that computations are presented to working memory, where they lead to further computations that guide behavior, inform verbal reports, and double back recursively to offer new input to working memory. But where does consciousness occur in the brain? (the question of the neuroscientists), What functions does it perform? (the question of the cognitive psychologists), and How are these functions performed without a separate entity, mind? (Dennett's question).

Dennett's solution (1991) is to offer his *multiple drafts model of consciousness*, which posits that all varieties of perception, thought, or mental activity are completed in the brain as "multitrack processes of interpretation and elaboration of sensory inputs." Consequently, information entering the nervous system is under continuous "editorial revision." These editorial processes take place over fractions of a second, during which time additions, incorporations, and amendments to them may occur. Still, we do not experience those processes that take place in the retina, auditory system, or skin, but we experience the products of many of these processes—limited individual representations—which may become more complex in form. In Dennett's view, feature detection takes place only once and is spatially and temporally distributed such that fixed new contents are precisely located in time and space. These contents may or may not become conscious. There is no single stream of consciousness, but multiple channels, which operate in parallel and, according to Dennett, create multiple drafts for action.

These narrativelike sequences have been described as scripts and stories. Through them temporal sequences are represented. Yet the underlying neural architecture is not a blank slate, but depends on experience, and structures are built up as a result of the brain's interaction with the world. There is competition among the many concurrent events in the brain, but one narrative becomes dominant and is experienced. In this way, conscious events may emerge from scripts and narratives that are initially out of awareness but become linked to affect and reach consciousness.

This multiple drafts model, which focuses on narrative scripts, is complex, and because the study of consciousness is new, complex analyses of introspection may be premature. Still, the study of consciousness is important because the major mental disorders are disorders of consciousness. Subcortical experiences come into the sensorium and enter awareness, and thus become conscious. An investigation of consciousness requires the identification of specific processes that come into consciousness.

A NEUROBIOLOGICAL THEORY OF CONSCIOUSNESS

Although we are aware of the results of both perceptual and memory processes, as noted earlier, we lack access to the processes that lead to this consciousness. Mental processes must be associated with active neuronal processes. However, we do not know whether different aspects of consciousness (e.g., pain and visual awareness) use the same or different mechanisms. Experiments in higher mammals may be relevant to the study of mechanisms involved in consciousness. Language in primates should not be essential for consciousness, yet language may enhance consciousness. Although animal studies do not assist with self-referential consciousness or self-consciousness, similar mechanisms might be involved. Consciousness may involve forms associated with emotion, sensory experience, pain, thinking, etc.

Crick and Koch (1990) suggest that consciousness can be approached at the neuronal level and depends on short-term memory and serial attention processes. They speculate that attention establishes a firing of neurons in a "semi-oscillatory way" that imposes temporary global unity "on neurons in different brain regions." Such oscillation would activate working (short-term) memory.

BRAIN REGIONS INVOLVED IN CONSCIOUSNESS

Consciousness occurs in the alert state and possibly in REM sleep, where dreams have some attributes of consciousness. Among brain regions, conscious operations most likely occur in the neocortex and possibly in the paleocortex, because local brain damage may remove aspects of consciousness (e.g., in agnosias). The hippocampus is not essential to consciousness, but hippocampal activity does reach consciousness. Areas of the hindbrain, such as the cerebellum, may not be essential. However, regions linked to the neocortex (e.g., the thalamus and basal ganglia) may be necessary. Consciousness may be linked to a more extensive "cortical system."

Moreover, an intact corpus callosum, the massive fiber bundle that connects the two cortical hemispheres, may be necessary for full consciousness. Investigations of persons who have lesions of the corpus callosum may also be relevant to the establishment of consciousness. In subjects with split brains, the left side of the brain, for right-handed people, is not aware of the activity in the visual system taking place on the right side, although a normal person is aware of both sides. These split-brain findings suggest that some information that is associated with consciousness can move through the normal corpus callosum. With the exception of some emotional states, the transferred information cannot be transmitted from one side of the cortex to the other by subcortical pathways, which remain intact.

Individuals with cortical blindness also may demonstrate a degree of consciousness (Stoerig and Cowey, 1989). They may point accurately to the positions of objects in their blind visual field, even though they deny that they see anything. The pointing is voluntary, and the individual is aware of the direction to which he is pointing. The existence of "blind sight" is of interest in regard to the neural pathways that are involved in consciousness because it may help us to understand which are involved. Still, it is possible that the visual signal is present but so weak in these patients that it escapes awareness, although it may be adequate for gross discriminations.

Consciousness does seem to require neuronal activity, so it may be correlated with a subset of neurons firing in the cortical system, yet consciousness may take different forms depending on the parts of the cortex that are involved. It also is possible that there are one or a few basic underlying mechanisms. It is not clear which neurons are involved, whether they are of a particular neuronal type, whether there is anything particular about their connectivity, and whether there is anything special about how they fire.

If there is a basic mechanism for consciousness that is similar in different parts of the brain, particularly in various parts of the neocortex, then one sensory system, such as the visual system, might be investigated as a model (Crick and Koch, 1990). The visual system is similar in man and higher primates and would be easier to study in regard to consciousness than more complex aspects of consciousness, such as self-awareness. This basic visual awareness has been referred to as "bare awareness." Visual awareness requires that relevant neurons in many cortical areas cooperate in a unified form of activity. In primates (e.g., in monkeys) there are many specific visual areas in the neocortex, perhaps as many as two dozen. These areas are connected in several

hierarchies, and the processing within any one of these areas involves largely parallel processing. Moreover, there are back projections and cross connections between cortical areas and from the cortex back to the thalamus.

In addition, visual input has specific connections. For example, the output from the retina projects through the lateral geniculate nucleus to the primary visual cortex. In the visual cortex, neurons may respond to simple features, such as the edge of an object, and occupy a small part of the visual field. On the other hand, neurons in higher cortical areas respond to more complex features, such as aspects of faces, so their receptive fields are larger. Different cortical areas may respond to different features. Some cells are specialized for motion or depth, others for shape and color, and still others for bodily position in space. A coherent visual picture most likely emerges from cooperative activity between these regions.

CONVERGENCE ZONES

Damasio (1989) tested patients with brain lesions and suggested the study of convergence zones, cortical areas that at any moment may respond to different levels of organization. Crick and Koch (1990) suggest that the neuronal correlates of convergence zones may be neurons or subsets of neurons that back-project.

Damasio (1989) suggests that the brain binds entities and events by multiregional activation from the convergence zones. Therefore, many cortical areas take part at any moment and at different levels. He suggests that synchronous activity in these various cortical areas is coordinated by feedback projections from the convergence zones. It is possible that these convergence zones exist in several places in the brain, such as the thalamus, the claustrum, the inferior temporal region, and areas related to higher levels of the motor system that may be involved in visual awareness. How awareness is correlated with neocortical levels in the visual system is not known, but it may be linked through particular brain regions that are involved with attention.

THE BINDING PROBLEM

How neurons temporally become active as a unit has been designated the *binding problem*.

Because objects are not only seen but also heard and felt, binding must extend across different sensory modalities.

The experience of perceptual unity indicates that the brain binds or links together in a coherent way neurons that are actively responding to various characteristics of a perceived object. In an interpersonal encounter, neurons would respond to facial motion, color characteristics of the face, the words that were being elicited, and possibly memory traces that may be associated with the recognition of the face. All of these activities would need to be bound together to jointly generate the perception of the face of the specific person.

There may be several types of binding, so those neurons responding to a drawn line may bind to a particular set of points; such binding may be constitutionally determined. Other types of binding may be needed to recognize familiar objects, such as letters of the alphabet. This binding would be frequently repeated to generate a learned response. On the other hand, binding may be neither constitutionally determined (e.g., visual) nor learned (e.g., reading), but responsive to novel events. To respond to novelty, neurons that are activated most likely are not strongly bound together. An adaptive response to novelty would entail rapidly arising binding. Such binding would be transitory and have considerable potential capacity to adapt to new events.

Transient binding would require an attentional mechanism that would allow attention to move in a serial fashion from one point to another. This rapid attention must be very fast and must move through different spatial scales. What reaches visual awareness may be the result of this rapid attentional step. This would indicate that attention and awareness are tightly bound to one another. Here, the results of attention would become conscious, but the attentional mechanisms themselves would remain out of awareness.

WORKING MEMORY AND CONSCIOUSNESS

Awareness must also be associated with iconic memory and short-term, or working, memory. Iconic memory (Coltheart, 1983) stores information at a precategorical level much like the simple visual capacity that leads to orientation or movement. Iconic memory has a large capacity and decays quickly, perhaps in half a second or less. On the other hand, working memory (Baddeley, 1986) may last for several seconds, but also has a limited capacity, perhaps up to seven items. It is different for different modalities and may be involved in abstract representation. Short-term memory can be prolonged through rehearsal; it may be the form of memory that is activated in the binding process to consciousness. Although we do not know the location of iconic and working memory, both are likely distributed throughout specific cortical areas such that auditory events are stored in auditory areas and visual events in visual areas. To highlight the importance of working memory and consciousness, there is no report of a person who is conscious but has lost all forms of short-term (working) memory.

CRICK-KOCH THEORY

Having reviewed the various elements that may be important in the establishment of consciousness, using visual awareness as a model, Crick and Koch (1990) ask how these speculations might be brought together. Their view is as follows: For visual awareness, objects in the visual field must give rise to appropriate responses in designated cortical areas. Visual attention would then select one of these objects at a particular location. This may take place through the topographical maps mentioned earlier that may code for conspicuous locations in the visual field. Once a location is selected, probably as a result of its conspicuousness, the information must be referred back to an individual feature map. The system, then, must produce neurons that oscillate together to produce a representation of the object attended to. To be affected, the involved neurons must be synchronized, perhaps at specific oscillation frequencies. The results of these underlying computations with attention are temporally bound together. The binding may lead to "working awareness" (Crick and Koch, 1990). When binding has occurred, this information would then be placed in working memory.

The essential features of visual awareness include running short-term memory, the transient iconic form, and working memory, which lasts for a longer period of time.

Information about single objects would be distributed in various parts of the brain, but there has to be a way to establish temporary unity on the neurons that are involved. This may be achieved through the very fast attentional mechanism. This mechanism would concentrate on one object at a time, choosing by "a winner take all" process those objects that are the most pertinent. Unity would involve neurons firing together in semisynchrony. This firing would activate the needed parts of the working memory system. Although the neuronal basis of this memory system is not known, it is most likely that it is non-Hebbian and involves transient alterations in synaptic strengths. In this neuronal activity in the visual system, much does not reach full awareness. Some activity out of awareness corresponds to computations that are needed to arrive at the best interpretation of incoming information that is compatible with stored categorical information. Apparently, it is this best interpretation that we become aware of.

Consciousness is rich in information, although much of it is retained only briefly. The systems of consciousness move rapidly from one object to another, although they can handle large amounts of information coherently and instantaneously. These abilities to switch rapidly and handle large amounts of information, when combined with very brief memory systems, make consciousness seem unfathomable. The brain is far more complex than computers, none of which can mimic the complex, rapidly changing, and highly parallel activity of the brain. Future research on consciousness, using models such as visual awareness, require better understanding of the neuronal basis of attention and very short-term memory. Crick and Koch (1990) suggest that one model might be to study visual input when a percept changes, even though visual input is constant. Such approaches should be pursued and neurobiological theories constructed that combine molecular neurobiological and clinical imaging approaches.

SUMMARY

Visual awareness and consciousness in general bind to information briefly and switch rapidly from one object to another. Consciousness may handle a very large amount of information in a coherent way in a single moment and combine with very transient memory systems. Its complex, rapidly changing, and parallel organization is unique to the human brain.

We are only beginning to develop theories of consciousness and investigate how physical events that take place while we think and act relate to subjective sensations. The study of waking consciousness will ultimately move to an investigation of consciousness of self. It has been suggested that consciousness emerges without intentionality from brain functions as a "change from quantity," the activation of 10^{12} profusely interconnected neurons, into "a new quality," that of self-experience or self-observation (Fischer, 1987). The neurobiological approach outlined in this chapter is a functional one that defines a person as being conscious of his or her identity as the experiencing subject across different experiences. Although not currently definable in terms of neurobiology, it is the experiencing person who remains the subject at the center of the investigation of consciousness.

REFERENCES

Allman, J. (1990). The origin of the neocortex. *Seminars in the Neurosciences,* 2:257–262.

Baddeley, A. (1986). *Working memory.* Oxford University Press, Oxford.

Carroll, R.L. (1988). *Vertebrate paleontology and evolution.* W. H. Freeman, New York.

Coltheart, M. (1983). Iconic memory. *Philosophical Transactions of the Royal Society of London, B,* 302:283–294.

Crick, F., and Koch, C. (1990). Toward a neurobiological theory of consciousness. *Seminars in the Neurosciences,* 2:263–275; 138:1–25.

Damasio, A.R. (1989). The brain binds entities and events by multiregional activation from convergence zones. *Neural Computation,* 1:123–132.

Dennett, D. (1991). *Consciousness explained.* Little, Brown, Boston.

Edelman, G.R. (1989). *The remembered present.* Basic Books, New York.

Fish, F. (1967). *Clinical psychopathology.* John Wright, Bristol, U.K.

Fischer, R. (1987). Emergence of mind from brain: The biological roots of the hermeneutic circle. *Diogenes,* 138:1–25.

Flanagan, O. (1992). *Consciousness reconsidered,* p. 220. MIT Press, Cambridge, MA.

Jackendoff, R. (1987). *Consciousness and the computational mind.* MIT Press, Cambridge, MA.

James, W. (1890). *The principles of psychology.* Harvard University Press, Cambridge, MA.

Jaspers, K. (1963). *General psychopathology.* (trans. J. Hoenig and M.W. Hamilton from the German 7th ed., 1963). Manchester University Press, Manchester, UK.

Johnson-Laird, P.N. (1988). *The computer and the mind.* Harvard University Press, Cambridge, MA.

MacLean, P. (1990). *The triune brain in evolution: Role in paleocerebral functions.* Plenum Press, New York.

Sims, A. (1988). *Symptoms in the mind: An introduction to descriptive psychopathology.* Bailliere-Tindall, W.B. Saunders, Philadelphia.

Stoerig, P., and Cowey, A. (1989). Wave length sensitivity in blindsight. *Nature,* 342:916–918.

Tulving, E. (1985). Memory and consciousness. *Canadian Journal of Psychology,* 26:1–12.

PART III

THE DEVELOPMENTAL PERSPECTIVE

The developmental perspective emphasizes maturation of the brain in the context of social experience, the environmental interface. During development, the mind and brain are considered as a unit, and its maturational process requires a facilitating environment. Although there have been longstanding debates regarding the impact of nature and nurture, development is the outcome of their union. In this sense, mind and brain are two ways of talking about the same thing, so what is going on in the brain helps understand what is going on in the mind, yet it must always be remembered that there is plasticity in development and that experience shapes the brain. Debates over nature and nurture have led to philosophical positions that emphasize either innate processes or psychosocial experiences. A developmental perspective views both as coming together and interacting. As development progresses with the emergence of consciousness and a sense of self, developmental task mastery becomes a critical concern.

The developmental perspective draws on evolutionary biology and the emergence of species-typical behavior. This approach to development is outlined in the first chapter of this part, which deals with ethology (Chapter 12). The chapter begins with a discussion of the evolution of species-typical behavior and indicates that there is a genetic predisposition to perform certain behaviors and to learn certain things. The full expression of species-typical behavior requires an average, expectable environment that produces similar experiences for individual members of a species. When the environmental provision is met, experience-expectant neuronal systems (Greenough and Black, 1992) may undergo synaptic pruning, leading to the preservation of those systems that are most important for social adaptation.

Ethology deals with the biology of behavior, describes the form and function of behavior (the four why's) throughout development, and makes comparisons among different species. The chapter on ethology describes the differences between behavioral, psychological, and ethological approaches and provides an ethological understanding of the mechanisms of behavior. Some terms used in ethology are *sign stimulus, innate releasing mecha-*

nisms, sensitive periods, attachment, dominance/submission hierarchy, working models, and *continuity and discontinuity in development* (Bowlby, 1969; Lorenz, 1982).

The second chapter in this part titled "Cognitive Development," emphasizes socioemotional development based on cognitive developmental theory and research. The cognitive view moves from ethology through its extensions into "working models" and views of cognition that are facilitated by sociocultural experience.

The third chapter in this part deals with emotion expression and regulation. In doing so, it addresses motivational issues from a developmental point of view and the expression of early feeling states with an emphasis on the self-conscious emotions. In addition to fear, sadness, anger, joy, surprise, and disgust, the self-conscious emotions of embarrassment, guilt, and shame are powerful factors in motivation. Consideration of emotion must take into account the beginnings of affective contact with others and the importance of affective attunement (Stern, 1985). Affect is modulated in development through play, which gives context and provides a means of mastering basic emotions.

The fourth chapter in this part addresses the self system, which emerges with consciousness and utilizes the social cognitive mode. The chapter begins with a discussion of the social self as originally proposed by William James (1890) and discusses object relations, attachment, cognitive, and motivational aspects of the self. It culminates in the establishment of a sense of personhood.

The fifth chapter in this part deals with the evolution of language and the development of representational abilities. Both pretend-play and the development of a narrative mode are described. Through the use of the imagination, affect is regulated and temperamental traits may be channeled as personality develops, perhaps through the mediation of cognitive scripts.

The sixth and final chapter of this part discusses temperament and personality. It reviews the current status of temperament (Goldsmith et al., 1987; Kohnstamm, Bates, and Rothbart, 1989) and its relationship to personality and personality trait disorder.

REFERENCES

Bowlby, J. (1960). *Attachment and loss.* Vol. 1, *Attachment.* Basic Books, New York.

Goldsmith, H.H., Buss, A.H., Plomin, R., Rothbart, M.K., Thomas, A., Chess, S., Hinde, R.A., and McCall, R.B. (1987). Roundtable: What is temperament? Four approaches. *Child Development,* 58:505–529.

Greenough, W.T., and Black, J.E. (1992). Induction of brain structure by experience: Substrates for cognitive development. In M.R. Gunnar and C.A. Nelson (eds), *Developmental behavioral neuroscience. The Minnesota Symposia on child psychology,* 24:155–200.

James, W. (1890). *The principles of psychology,* Vol. 1. Henry Holt, New York.

Kohnstamm, G.A., Bates, J.E., and Rothbart, M.K. (1989). *Temperament in childhood.* John Wiley & Sons, New York.

Lorenz, K.Z. (1982). *The foundations of ethology. The principal ideas and discoveries in animal behavior.* Simon and Schuster, New York.

Stern, D. (1985). *The interpersonal world of the infant.* Basic Books, New York.

CHAPTER 12
ETHOLOGY

Ethology is derived from the Greek *ethos,* meaning "habit" or "manner." A developmental ethologist describes the form and function of behavior and traces its development during the life span of the individual (ontology) and from the evolutionary history of the species (phylogeny). Just as comparative anatomists and physiologists investigate bodily function, the ethologist compares behavior between species, noting that it is influenced by both environmental and cultural influences. Because behavior and bodily form have coevolved, a modern view of ethology is that there is a genetic predisposition to perform certain behavior patterns and learn specific things. Experience is needed to a greater or lesser degree to establish the form of behavior and its behavioral context. Ethological studies lead to a better understanding of how one's unique genetic endowment interacts with the interpersonal environment.

From a developmental perspective, ethology addresses the emergence of an inner life by studying behaviors that are rooted in our biological and evolutionary past. Many unique human behavioral features, such as social ranking, territoriality, and incest avoidance, may have origins in our primate heritage. Although both Meyer and Freud emphasized the role of early experience in development (Bowlby, 1988), systematic research using their formulations has proven difficult. However, developmental research, using an ethologically based theory of socioemotional bonding, has been more successful in predicting later outcome. These recent studies in child development emphasize working models and utilize an ethological vantage point to understand how mental experience is acquired and integrated. Patterns of behavior are as characteristic to a species as is physical morphology, and the ritualization of behavior leads to identifiable cultural patterns as we move from animal to human ethology.

This chapter reviews the history, definition, scope, basic aims, methodology and concepts of ethology, the origins of sociability, patterns of attachment, emotional bases of attachment behavior, attachment and working models during development, and the relationship of ethological studies to developmental disorders.

HISTORY

Although observations and classifications of animal and human behavior were recorded in antiquity by Aristotle and Plato, modern investigations of animal behavior began in the earlier part of this century, as naturalists began to study animals in their natural environments and experimental psychologists conducted animal studies in the laboratory. With Pavlov's (1927) discovery of conditioned reflexes, the possibility of empiric experimentation following the exact sciences was introduced into the behavioral sciences. Pavlov's conditioning experiments in his laboratory led to the development of animal models of psychopathology, as exemplified in the experimental neurosis he produced in dogs—work that was continued by Gantt (1944). Other laboratory-based experiments established the behavioral view, which emphasized the consequences of behavior and led to the formulation of the *Law of Effect*, which postulates that a behavior that is followed by a satisfying state of affairs will be strengthened, whereas one that is followed by an annoying state of affairs will be weakened (Thorndike, 1898). The behavioral view was further developed by Skinner (1938), who conducted laboratory studies of discrete and easily measured behavior in individual subjects over time. His investigations changed the focus of explanations for behavior from stimuli and classical conditioning to consequences and emphasized a form of conditioning he called "operant." Skinner's approach has had its greatest impact in the development of the treatment approach known as behavior modification.

In contrast to the experimental psychologists, the ethologists studied animal behavior in naturalistic settings and emphasized that animals evolve not only morphologically but also behaviorally to survive and reproduce. The roots of ethology lie in evolutionary biology and the work of Darwin, his predecessors, and active investigators in this century. The best known of the latter are the founders of modern ethology, Konrad Lorenz (1981), Niko Tinbergen (1951), and Karl von Frisch (1953), who were awarded the Nobel prize in 1973 for their seminal understanding of the roots of animal behavior. Lorenz (1977, 1981) and Tinbergen (1951) clarified the term "instinct," which previously had been used to describe innate behavior.

Looking at behavioral manifestations, Lorenz and Tinbergen demonstrated that phylogenetic adaptations determine behavior in both animals and in man. The phylogenetic approach incorporates evolution into the study of behavior by emphasizing the possibility that some behavior, through phylogenetic adaptation, may be genetically programmed. This suggests that not only physical morphology but also motivational and behavioral tendencies may have their origin in the fitness or adaptive function of the evolutionary past.

Classical ethological studies have investigated and described animal behavior in the wild, emphasized the natural setting as essential when the adaptive function of behavior was being stud-

ied, and addressed the survival value of behavior. In recent years, a neo-Darwinian synthesis has emerged that takes into account a model based on the interaction of genes and environment. For humans, that environment incorporates culture (including symbolic language), defined as the man-made part of the environment, and maintains that the capacity for culture grew out of natural selection (Darwin, 1871).

Bowlby (1969, 1973, 1988) has extended the study of ethology in his investigations of attachment, loss, and separation in childhood, and Eibl-Eibesfeldt (1989) has emphasized human ethology in his anthropological studies. Bowlby's biological attachment theory (1969), subsequently elaborated by Ainsworth (1969, 1973), perceives the mother-child bond as a predetermined phylogenetic adaptation that leads to the subsequent development of personalized relationships. Robert Hinde (1987) has highlighted the role of ethological methods in the study of social communication. Recently, ethologists have moved from the study of intact animals in their natural settings and have added experimental modifications to the natural environmental setting. In the neurosciences, neuroethology (Hoyle, 1984) has emerged with the aim of examining neurophysiological events related to innate behavioral acts in a variety of behaviors exhibited by various animals. MacLean (1985) has taken an evolutionary view in his neuroanatomic investigations of the effects of brain lesions on complex species-typical behavior.

As ethologists have moved from the natural setting to experimental environments, fitness rather than survival value (Betzig, 1989) has been emphasized, particularly as they address abnormal development in animals who have apparent or potential fitness failures (Suomi, 1985). Here, animal models have been suggested for pathological conditions in man. Animal models of psychopathology have been identified by Harlow and Zimmermann (1959) and Suomi (1985), using ethological approaches.

The phylogeny of behavior assumes comparisons between species and addresses natural selection. In the past, much emphasis has been placed on "survival of the fittest" by emphasizing sexual and aggressive aspects of behavior (Darwin, 1872), based on studies carried out in often crowded, tropical settings. Others

(Kropotkin, 1989) have emphasized mutual aid, "shared helpfulness," or cooperation in evolution, particularly for those species who live in sparsely settled environments. Still others (Calvin, 1990) have suggested that climatic changes alternating between ice ages and global warming have led to fluctuations in selection and have required substantial adaptations in the brain.

The reciprocity of aggressive and sexual motivation has been studied in individuals and in groups, leading to investigation of the biological and social origins of altruism and aggression in childhood (Zahn-Waxler, Cummings, and Iannotti, 1986). Kinship patterns have been emphasized as family groups have been investigated using the methods of ethology. Hinde (1987) has emphasized that the study of capacities for social perception, mutual understanding, and social skills require not only investigation of the mother-infant relationship but also the study of interpersonal relationships with peers.

DEFINITION

Human ethology is defined as the biology of human behavior (Eibl-Eibesfeldt, 1979). Included in its scope are morphology, ecology, genetics, phylogenetics, developmental biology, sociobiology, and physiology. In ethology, the methods of these fields are adapted to the study of man (Eibl-Eibesfeldt, 1979). Principal concerns of the ethologists deal with the functional aspects of behavior (e.g., exploratory, shelter seeking, care eliciting, care giving, sexual, mimicking, combative) and the role of these behaviors in adaptation. Tinbergen (1963) includes the following within the definition of ethology: (1) the investigation of behavioral causation through investigation of physiological mechanisms that underlie specific behaviors; (2) the survival value or fitness function of behavior; (3) the evolution or phylogenetic history of behavior (phylogenetic adaptations); and (4) the ontogeny of behavior over a given individual's life history. Research into these four areas has expanded considerably in the past 30 years. Investigations of behavioral causation have been undertaken by neuroethologists (Hoyle, 1984) who have turned their attention to basic causation through the study of cellular mechanisms of behavior in a variety of species from a one-celled gastropod, Aphysia, to insects, birds, and primates. Among neuroethologists, there may be differences in focus, with some emphasizing fixed action patterns of behavior (units of behavior characterized by their unvarying form and their independence of environmental stimuli) that occur in invertebrates, e.g., stereotypical marching of immature locusts, the leap of the grasshopper (Hoyle, 1984), and other more complex brain mechanisms, such as those involved in complex aggressive and courtship displays (MacLean, 1973, 1985).

For a biologist, behavior has evolved and is in ongoing evolution. Behavior is a product of, and contributes to, natural selection; both genetic and environmental changes reflect themselves in behavior. Although behavior must be well described and understood before proceeding to nonobservable causal mechanisms, ethologists also view humans as cultural beings who have evolved and are naturally selected for the degree of "adaptative modifiability" present in their behavior.

THE ROOTS OF BEHAVIOR

The ethologist must ask, How has behavior evolved? How do we trace gradual divergences in social behavior throughout evolution? We cannot use fossils as evidence because fossils do not behave, but we can classify behavior by making comparisons among species and looking for similarities. Species-specific behaviors have evolved just as anatomical structures have evolved. To make comparisons, both similarities that may be seen in primates and convergences for certain functions that are seen in other species must be considered (e.g., bats' wings and walking forelimbs). How do we approach the animal roots of behavior in man? Tinbergen (1963) suggests that first we ask how, and if, man is unique from other creatures. Bodily function and the structure of organs, including nerve cells, are generally not unique; man's uniqueness resides in his behavior. The structure that may function uniquely in man is the brain as it relates to behavior.

The scope of human ethology includes not only animal-like patterns in human behavior but also similarities or convergences in humans when compared to animals. One must understand cultural patterns of behavior and their evolution. In studying cultural patterns, the perspective is on their role in establishing overall fitness. Human ethological studies have turned to mother-infant interaction, sex-related behaviors, aggression, territorial behavior, and utilization of territory. Cultural patterns are considered for each form of behavior.

BASIC AIMS AND METHODOLOGY

The ethologist seeks to understand how successful interaction with the environment takes place to survive, reproduce, and develop competence. The emphasis is on adaptation (e.g., feeding, avoiding predation, finding a mate, raising young).

The method of study in ethology is an indirect one, as true similarities are distinguished from convergences. Description of human behavior requires a disciplined language. In ethology, adaptation is investigated through producing an ethogram, which provides a comprehensive description of all *functional* units of behavior for the species being studied. For each unit, the physiological and environmental factors that regulate it, its phylogenetic origins, its ontology in the individual, and its adaptive or fitness function are established (Zumpe and Michael, 1990). The goal is to understand factors that influence motivation or emotional state, how these factors create a predisposition to behave in certain ways, and how such predispositions are communicated to others.

Early ethological studies were carried out in fish and birds and focused on inborn (innate) behavior, leading to the misunderstanding that ethologists focus only on innate or unlearned behavior. Modern ethological studies emphasize genetic predispositions to perform certain behavior patterns and to learn certain things that interact with experience to shape the form of behavior and the context of its occurrence.

Ethological description in all species starts with the construction of an ethogram, or behavior profile, as described by Zumpe and Michael (1990). These behavioral descriptions take place in natural settings and focus on discrete behavioral units, such as movements and gestures (e.g., walking, running, feeding, speech use, and facial expressions), particularly as they occur in natural settings. Animal studies

describe behavior but not its intention. In constructing a human ethogram, problems arise in the description of objective and subjective states and in the interpretation of dysfunction. In describing human behavior, movements are often described differently than in animals — e.g., she walked up the hill; he looked at her. Then there are descriptions of moods (e.g., the person appears happy or sad,) and descriptions of movements (e.g., the child hid from her; the goal was to win the game), but there are also mixed descriptions of human behavior (e.g., he was annoyed when she frowned at him).

In constructing an ethogram, observations are made in a natural environment and all behavioral sequences are recorded, including postures, movements, facial expressions, and vocalizations. These may be recorded as general categories (e.g., aggression) and/or broken down into smaller functional units (e.g., teeth baring, piloerection, and extended claws). This is followed by a determination of adaptive behavior that involves analyzing chains of "who does what to whom" in order to designate the relationship between the behavior-eliciting situation, the specific behavior, and the effects of that behavior. The next step is to determine ontogeny — to discover the time of first appearance of the behavior during the individual's life time and to record any subsequent changes in form and function. The following aim is to determine phylogeny — to establish if the behavior pattern occurs in closely related species, is present in geographically isolated populations, develops in individuals who are isolated from conspecifics since birth, and has any specific morphological and/or physiological correlates. Final physiological and environmental regulation is established by determining the effects of changing one variable while holding others constant.

Ethological questions include descriptions of characteristic behaviors, the functions of these behaviors, and how they can be modified, as well as what the limitations are on their modifiability (McGuire and Fairbanks, 1977). One asks, What are environmental, genetic, and physiological determinants? What environmental events are of particular importance in establishing and maintaining behavior? Why are some behaviors less modifiable than others?

Ethologists have focused on species-typical behavior in animals, so the human ethologist must identify the species-typical behaviors in humans. Tinbergen (1963) suggests that "adaptative hereditary changes" are accompanied by "a new type of evolution," a psychosocial or cultural evolution, or social transmission, based on accumulated transfer of knowledge or behavioral patterns. Individual adaptation requires individual experience. One must wonder how much change has occurred genetically and structurally since Cro-Magnon times.

Modern human characteristics are the result of the evolved flexibility of the organism, which makes new learning possible with the rapid "accumulation of transferred knowledge." Humans differ in the extent that they can learn. This allows the accelerating accumulation of information over the generations to be transferred to new generations. But how unique is this learning to humans? Acculturation learning does occur in chimpanzees, who, for example, can learn to open a coconut after watching another animal carry out this activity or learn other activities from a parent. However, observational learning occurs from mother to infant and not from just anyone in the troop. Moreover, observational learning occurs from those higher in the dominance hierarchy to those who are lower in the hierarchy, yet, in regard to new behaviors, the young often transmit to the older: Typically, mothers learn from their offspring, and the males in a troop are the last to acquire a new trait. In humans, learning occurs from superiors, but perhaps less well from those one does not respect. Far more information is needed in regard to psychosocial learning in humans. Transfer from one generation to another may occur in animals, including nonrational learning — e.g., ducks avoided an area where the previous generation had experienced foxes (Lorenz, 1981). This avoidant behavior was carried on to later generations although fences had been erected and the next generation had no experience of foxes. Nonrational avoidance mechanisms as well as adaptive traits can be carried over from one generation to the next through social learning. Wilson and Sober (1994) suggest that "the construction of social structures" in humans affects fitness differences within groups and might effect natural selection at the group level.

Ethological constructs used, such as dominance, attachment, and territoriality, are not theories. For example, dominance does not explain behavior but describes interactions in certain situations. Experimental alteration of characteristics of the physical or social environment may include deprivation strategies to gather information on the effects of experience on behavior or experimental drug use to investigate modification of behavioral traits. Observations are carried out to evaluate (1) proximate factors (close in space, time, order, or meaning) that may be causally eliciting behavior; (2) the function of the behavior in regard to adaptability (survival and reproduction); and (3) limits on behavior (plasticity or behavior modifiability). A biological focus addresses physiological factors or species-typical patterns that could be missed in a learning theory model, or social interactive factors that could be pertinent in psychodynamic approaches. The evolution of behavior is complex, and behavioral patterns may be multiply determined. These determinants could interact with one another to inhibit or facilitate behavior. Moreover, patterns of behavior could evolve together (mosaic evolution). This leads to a more complex analysis that acknowledges that genetic, environmental, physiological, and learning aspects frequently have to be present simultaneously to generate the behavioral response.

Human ethological research has particularly focused on nonverbal and verbal communication, aggression (territoriality and conflict management), mechanisms of bonding, and aspects of social structure (gender roles, rank order, and incest taboos) (Eibl-Eibesfeldt, 1979, 1989).

A basic question is how biological inheritance has influenced social behavior. One point of comparison of behavior is that of animal and human rituals. Patterns of maternal care and the physical appeal of infants are important for bonding in animals. Social rituals are present in bird species and in mammals, e.g., a bird (the wingless cormorant) returns to the nest to his mate and is only allowed to remain if he brings a twig. Offering nest material seems to have a function of appeasement. Gift passing as a ritual is a common practice in humans. Another example of a ritual is mutual feeding in animals and humans. Mouth feeding is seen in humans; Eibl-Eibesfeldt (1989) suggests that it was the ultimate source of the kiss. The function of this behavior seems to be similar in anthropoid apes (gorillas, chimpanzees) and in humans. The differences among species suggests that these are analogues that serve similar functions but have a different evolutionary origin. Because mouth or "kiss" feeding is seen in humans and may be found in anthropoid apes (Eibl-Eibesfeldt, 1989), it may be homologous, that is, similar in structure and descended from a common ancestral form.

BASIC CONCEPTS

Analogies and Homologies

Studies of nonprimates and primates may be of help in understanding human behavior both as behavioral analogies and homologies. If similarities in comparable characteristics of two species emerge from a common ancestral form, the resemblance is referred to as "homology." However, if the similarity is the consequence of independently developed adaptation to similar environmental contingencies, the term "analogy" is used. The term "phyletic homology" has been used to describe genetically transmitted characteristics, and the term "homologies of tradition" has been used if the feature is culturally transmitted (Eibl-Eibesfeldt, 1989).

Fixed Action Patterns

Fixed action patterns (the old term was "instinctive movement") are units of behavior characterized by "unvarying form and independent of environmental input." They are genetically coded and are not modified by experiences. Sign Stimuli are the innate releasing mechanisms that release this unvarying pattern. Environmental input may only affect a fixed action pattern if it serves as the Sign Stimulus. Rather than reflex chains, they are patterns of behavior—e.g., flight in birds develops with maturation (Provine, 1981). Walking in human infants depends on the coordination of fixed action patterns that are functional before the maturation of the musculoskeletal system, which is needed for complete expression. Walking, climbing, and hanging movements are seen in premature infants, and full-term infants at 6 weeks may show spontaneous kicking that mirrors the time sequence of the adult walking cycle (Thelen, Bradshaw, and Ward, 1981).

A common phylogenetic basis for a pattern of behavior is suggested when the pattern has an identical form and function in different, but related, species; for example, the sequence of stereotyped movements of the head, face, and mouth seen in human infants and neonatal primates in searching for the nipple. Similar patterns of behavior have been noted in components of greeting, courtship, and aggression in humans in geographically remote settings, and in deaf and blind children who demonstrate facial expressions of emotion, such as smiling, laughing, and crying. These develop without an opportunity for imitation or learning (Eibl-Eibesfeldt, 1989).

Conflict Behaviors

Conflict behaviors are elicited during simultaneous exposure to conflicting stimuli that must be responded to quickly. They are postures, movements, facial expressions, and vocalizations that are produced by the simultaneous activation of two or more incompatible behavioral tendencies. For example, initial approaches between conspecifics may be associated with potentially conflicting behavioral patterns and emotional responses. Greeting rituals may be derived from concurrent and competing tendencies to approach or to withdraw. The ritual may serve to reduce activation of two or more conflicting approach/withdrawal tendencies. For example, approach-avoidance conflict may arise in a shy child when a stranger enters the home. The child's desire to meet the new person is in conflict with the tendency to withdraw from unfamiliar situations. Such responses may be basic to motivational conflicts in both animal and human species. Tinbergen and Tinbergen (1972) suggest motivational conflict in children with autistic disorder when they are approached socially. Although Wing and Ricks (1976) take exception to their views in autistic disorder, the ethological methods they describe may be applicable in other settings.

Conflict behaviors that are elicited with motivational conflict (i.e., the activation of two incompatible behaviors) include intention movement, redirected behavior, displacement activity, vacuum activity, alternation, compromise, and ambivalence. Intention movement is demonstrated when a behavior is seen in an abbreviated form and not in its full expression; for example, a hungry bird arrives at a food source along with a higher-ranking bird. The availability of food elicits approach, but the rival's presence suggests avoidance. In this situation, one may observe intention movements of escape, such as stretching of the neck and tail movements. Another example is that of a student who turns in his chair as if to get up when challenged to answer a question posed by his teacher. The movement sequence of getting up from his desk is suppressed because of fear, or possibly due to respect for the higher-ranking teacher. Here, the intensity needed to perform the behavior may not be sufficient for its completion, or there may be competing tendencies that interfere with its full expression. Such behaviors may occur out of awareness.

Redirected movement or behavior occurs when two conflicting stimuli are simultaneously aroused, such as aggression and soothing behavior. An aggressive display may be redirected from a person, for example, hitting the wall rather than another person. Redirected aggression may be demonstrated in early courtship in a number of species, including primates (Zumpe and Michael, 1979). When aggression is not redirected, the pattern of courtship may break down. However, joint redirection of aggression by both partners toward a third party may enhance bonding.

Displacement activity is another form of conflict behavior. These are low-priority maintenance behaviors, such as self-grooming (i.e., adjusting hair or clothing at times of stress), that are not appropriate to the social context. It has been suggested that these patterns of behavior become disinhibited when there is a mutual, but total, inhibition of two high-priority behaviors, such as attack and flight, neither of which is an option appropriate to the situation.

Vacuum activity is behavior that occurs in the absence of a normal eliciting stimulus, as if the individual were responding to a hallucination of the usual eliciting stimulus. In this instance, the tendency to perform a behavior is intense following prolonged inhibition of the behavior or prolonged absence of the eliciting stimulus. Animals who are restricted in activity, such as a dog that has been kept inside for a prolonged period of time, may bark at nonexistent intruders when released to go out. Lorenz (1981) used the term *auf Leerlauf,* more correctly translated as "in neutral," after observing his tame starling, raised on boiled eggs, suddenly move to the ceiling and go through feeding movements with a nonexistent fly.

Alternation is another activity pattern that occurs when one, then another, of the competing behavior tendencies briefly overrides the other such that alternation occurs between two appropriate responses, for example, rapid alternation between an approach response and a withdrawal response.

Compromise formation is seen when a behavior is performed that is appropriate to both conflicting behavioral tendencies. This can be illustrated by a conflict about eating high-calorie sweets versus abstinence; the compromise might be to eat a low-calorie snack.

Finally, *ambivalence* is demonstrated when intention movements that are appropriate to each of the two conflicting responses are combined into a single pattern. Postures and facial expressions that suggest ambivalence between the responses may be seen when aggression-motivated and flight-motivated behavior are concurrently elicited. For example, one may observe various presentations of aggression and fear in the facial expressions and body postures of a dog who is threatened. Ambivalence about contact with another person might also be noted in a social gathering when initial eye contact with another guest is initiated from a distance by raising of the eyebrows and smiling, followed by turning the head away and gaze aversion when further contact is not desired.

Ritualization

Lorenz (1981) pointed out that rituals perform the functions of communication, channeling aggression, and producing cohesion of pairs. In the course of evolution, many conflict behaviors have become ritualized into behavioral displays (display behaviors) to allow rapid responding and clearer communication of intent, for example, the eyebrow flash accompanied by a smile on greeting, bowing, the salute, and kissing rituals. These ritualized activities are often seen as behavioral rehearsals, as in play fighting. Ritualizations are characterized by stereotypy, typical intensity, associated morphological specialization, threshold changes, and motivational changes. A ritual shows a similar form within a species and is stereotyped and inflexible. When the form is constant over a range of drive intensities, it is said to have a *typical intensity,* which ordinarily follows the intensity of the underlying motivation. Its standardization and typical intensity reduce the chances of the signal being misunderstood when it is performed, thus making it highly adaptive. For example, when two people first see one another, there is a rapid raising and lowering of the eyebrows, the "eyebrow flash," which is accompanied by a smile. This is seen in all cultures, is ritualized, and has a typical intensity. Eibl-Eibesfeldt (1989) reported a duration of approximately 0.3 seconds and the maximal raising of the eyebrows for about 0.16 seconds. Ritualization may be enhanced by prominent morphological features, such as prominent eyebrows in humans, tail feathers in birds, and by features, such as antlers in stags, that enhance the signal value. Because of the importance of eye signals in social nonverbal communication, the face is normally scanned in primates. Finally, eyebrow position conveys information about emotional state (e.g., anger or sadness).

Neuroethologists have documented that the anatomical basis of these facial displays is in the superior temporal sulcus in those primates who show selective response to faces (DeSimone, 1991; Harries and Perret, 1991; Perret and Rolls, 1983). Damage to this region may lead to prosopagnosia (lack of ability to recognize faces). MacLean (1973) has shown that lesions in the inferior segment of the globus pallidus eliminates sexual and aggressive displays in squirrel monkeys.

The threshold for ritualizations may vary such that more intense stimulation may be needed for its expression, or a ritual may be lost only to be restored in hybrids. The motivation leading to a ritual display may also change from one species to another. For example, a display focused on ritualized redirected aggression may become incorporated into a courtship display such that, as in rhesus monkeys, redirected threats may become sexual invitation displays (Zumpe and Michael, 1979).

Other patterns of display are the dominance hierarchies. In wolves, dominance hierarchies are terminated when the loser shows a submissive posture by offering its throat and thus

inhibiting attack. In humans, cultural rituals, such as bowing, kneeling, or head lowering, may have similar functions. Aggression is also ritualized in humans and animals through patterns of combat and particular aggressive displays.

Signals that have a communicative base must relay their information to specific targets. Patterns of movement become simplified and accentuated in evolution as signals, with rhythmic repetition. In humans, these become apparent in courtship rituals used in mate selection.

Innate Releasing Mechanisms

There are innate predispositions to carry out patterns of behavior, such as ritual displays and conflict behaviors, and there are also predispositions to respond to specific stimuli (Zumpe and Michael, 1990). Here, the issue is the biologically given basis for receiving stimuli. There are key environmental stimuli or releasers, and the performance that is elicited is thought to require an "innate releasing mechanism." Examples of releasers are potentially dangerous aspects of the environment; for example, in the visual cliff experiment, the infant hesitates when a precipice is covered by a glass plate until signaled by the mother. This human response is based on simple cues from the mother, such as eyebrow position, movement, and social dominance.

An exaggeration of a feature that normally elicits a response may act as a supranormal stimulus and be more effective than the naturally occurring one in eliciting a response. For example, the characteristics of the young of many species that are perceived as more attractive are the rounded head and the shorter distance between the eyes and lower jaw, resulting in an enhanced probability of a caregiving response. On the other hand, exaggerations of the infant schema in cartoon character drawings and in human dolls and models are rated as more appealing than a more "natural infant."

IMPRINTING, SOCIAL BONDING, ALTRUISM, AND EMPATHY

A comparative approach to behavioral ethological concepts has begun to assist in understanding the genetic bases of behavior. Such an approach may provide new insights into human motivation and a clearer framework for understanding nonverbal communication, particularly in infants and children. The evolution of biological systems moves more slowly than cultural evolution. Imprinting, attachment, and bonding are universal and species-typical patterns of behavior and are examples of areas where fruitful comparative research has occurred.

Imprinting

The modern concept of imprinting was formulated by Lorenz (1935) from his studies of birds (ducklings and goslings). Lorenz described imprinting as a specialized form of early learning and an example of an innate predisposition to acquire specific information. Ducklings and goslings have an innate following response. Surrogate objects, such as a stuffed cube, a hen, or a person, can elicit the following response. If the object is followed for a while, the bird becomes imprinted on that object and the readiness to follow other objects disappears (Eibl-Eibesfeldt, 1989). Imprinting is characterized by irreversibility and a sensitive period when imprinting information can be acquired before being put to use. It is specific, and the information is retained for life.

Neuronal changes have been reported following imprinting that demonstrate a genetic-environmental interface. Imprinting leads to a reduction in the number of spines on the dendrites of neurons involved in processing the imprinted stimulus. Because these spines contact other neurons, there is a corresponding reduction in interneuronal connections. When domestic chicks were imprinted to follow a pure tone, a reduction in dendritic spines of 45% in the auditory area was found in the forebrain of these chicks in contrast to nonimprinted controls. Moreover, when the imprinting was to the natural call of the hen, a 27% reduction was demonstrated in the same neuronal type (Wallhausser and Scheich, 1987). Through these neuronal changes, the neurons became irreversibly tuned for the perception of specific stimuli (i.e., the call). Reductions of synaptic connections in the chick and other birds distinguishes imprinting from other forms of learning, which are generally related to increases in interneuronal connections (Eibl-Eibesfeldt, 1989). Imprinting may take place

well before the behavioral patterns have matured. This is found with sexual imprinting. Object imprinting has been demonstrated in hand-raised jackdaws and parakeets, who have been found to be sexually imprinted on humans when they mature despite lack of exposure to humans since early life and having been raised only with conspecifics. Following such early exposure, jackdaws prefer humans and court them as sexual partners (Eibl-Eibesfeldt, 1989). In humans, inhibition against sexual attraction to members of the opposite sex may occur if both sexes have grown up together in the same home.

Social Bonding, Altruism, and Empathy

In mammals, the social bond is established through early attachment behavior that makes mutual aid possible. The importance of mutual aid in evolution (Kropotkin, 1989) is drawing support from studies in ethology and neuroethology. In the neo-Darwinian framework, which focuses on fitness, it has been hard to account for altruism, which places the fitness of the society over that of the individual. The emphasis on the production of progeny does not necessarily guarantee fitness. As one moves from insects to humans, the number of progeny produced decreases substantially. In sociobiology, altruistic care is aimed at survival of the young and continuation of one's own genes. Simon (1990) considers that the neo-Darwinian emphasis on fitness accounts only for this reciprocal altruism — behavior that is usually reciprocated — and therefore has no net effect on fitness. He suggests that being receptive to social influence (docility) also contributes to fitness and may be selected. The cost of this receptivity may be the loss of an individual for the maintenance of group fitness when sociability is selected. The selection for cooperativeness in a group may have as its outcome the production of some individuals who are altruistically self-sacrificing. This may occur most often in kinship group selection. It is their sacrifice that saves the group and contributes to species survival even though certain individuals are lost. In evolution, adaptability of the species may ultimately be selected, and altruism may well be an important aspect of this selection process. These views on group and kin selection are highly controversial in sociobiology, where it is argued that if all selection is at the gene level and genes propagate themselves at other genes' expense, what is the selective advantage of behavior that leads to others' genes surviving at the expense of one's own (Wilson, 1975)? Genetic roots for receptivity to social influence have not been identified. Donald (1991) suggests that consideration of altruism at the human level must take into account the cognitive dimension of human evolution. This includes the emergence of advanced representational abilities and memory systems that allow the reconfiguration of mental architecture and the capacity to understand another's perspective.

On the other hand, MacLean (1990) approaches altruism and empathy by emphasizing the relationship of brain evolution and behavior. He suggests that the capacity to "look with feeling" (empathy) evolves in mammalian evolution. In tracing the origins of empathy, MacLean (1985) has investigated the evolutionary origins of species-typical behavior in reptiles and mammals. Reptiles follow daily routines and show territorial defense. They establish a home base but do not show mother-infant attachment. An analysis of reptilian behavior suggests that basic territorial patterns, including attachment to place, are essential to species survival. MacLean (1985) suggests that in the evolutionary transition from reptiles to mammals, several changes take place that facilitate mother-infant contact and interpersonal bonding. Among the most important is the establishment of audiovocal contact with maternal responsiveness to the infant's separation call. To hear the infant's separation call, a new step in mammalian evolution is required that involves the development of the bones of the inner ear. Two small bones of the jaw joint of the earlier mammal-like reptile, the articular and the quadrate, become the malleus (hammer) and the incus (anvil) (Romer, 1966). This evolution of the ossicles in the inner ear and the development of the auditory system allows the cry of the newborn to be heard. Concurrently, the descent of the larynx into a new position is of evolutionary significance in that it allows vocalization and the production of the separation cry.

Lesion studies in squirrel monkeys and in hamsters (MacLean, 1985) suggest that three linked evolutionary events underlie attachment, bonding, and the establishment of social skills. These are audiovocal contact (the separation call); nursing and the milk let-down reflex, which may be linked to the separation call; and the emergence of play behavior in apes and humans, which provides a means to develop social skills. With these changes, contact can be maintained vocally, feeding can occur in a secure setting, and interpersonal learning can begin, first through imitation, then through play, which facilitates social learning. According to MacLean, the brain regions that become linked developmentally for this to occur are the limbic system, the striatal complex, and the cingulate cortex.

Looking with feeling requires a further evolutionary adaptation linking the visual system with the prefrontal cortex and the limbic, or emotional, brain and may provide a neuroethological basis for empathy. Such internally derived experiences may be necessary for an individual's identification with the feelings of others. Perhaps this awareness is a prerequisite to develop a sense of concern for others in addition to oneself and, ultimately, a sense of responsibility for planning for their future as members of a family (MacLean, 1990). Dawkins (1989, p. 200) suggests that it may be possible that a unique quality of man is the "capacity for genuine, disinterested [non-selfish] altruism." He notes that humans potentially have the power to defy the selfish genes of their birth through the use of conscious foresight to imagine the future.

THE ORIGINS OF SOCIABILITY

The ontogeny of individual development becomes progressively important as one moves up the phylogenetic tree and the number of offspring produced decreases. The study of individual development leads to the study of the development of relationships in human and animal behavior. In considering the origins of behavior, we consider not only features that are uniquely present in humans, but also their phylogenetic origins. An ethological viewpoint is ultimately one that addresses the animal roots of human behavior in evolution. Through identifying these roots, animal studies can be utilized that may shed light on human problems. There are risks of cross-species generalization, so caution is needed when comparisons are made.

Eibl-Eibesfeldt (1989) suggests that several evolutionary steps may have been necessary for the evolution of sociability. Perhaps the earliest form is seen in the congregation of fish into swarms for protection against predators. This is followed in evolution by pair bonding, which requires partner proximity and compatibility. Because physical contact is not necessary for fertilization, the emergence of sociability may begin initially with physical contact, as in some deep sea fishes when the male adheres to the female. The next step bonding occurs when there is a behavior fixation on the sexual partner. Initially, proximity may be to a specific location, and later to a compatible partner. The presence of that specific partner may become necessary for certain behaviors to occur. This has been reported in songbirds, in which duet singing may only be satiated in the partner's presence, or the triumph ceremony of the Greylag geese, which occurs only in the presence of a partner (Eibl-Eibesfeldt, 1989). In these instances, proximity is necessary for behavior to occur, but the evolution of social contact requires the mammalian evolution of nursing, the separation call, and play as previously noted. (MacLean, 1985). With the emergence of parent- offspring vocal signals and infant visual appeal, affectionate responses may have first emerged. Parental care is a turning point in behavioral evolution. The next turning point is individual bonding between mother and infant. Here, parents and young seek one another's proximity and will defend the bond between them against any intervention, and strangers will be ignored. Early identification of the young takes place with a repertoire of infant signals that lead to an innate response from the mother and a reciprocal response from the young. Mothers respond to distress or isolation calls, and some species use olfactory cues to recognize their young.

In some species, bonding may occur during a brief "sensitive period." For example, mother goats who remain with their kids for five minutes after birth and then are separated for one hour will respond when the kid is returned, but if they are separated immediately for one hour after birth, the kid is treated as a stranger. The peptide oxytocin may be a mediator of this brief "sensitive period" (Eibl-Eibesfeldt, 1989).

In humans, the decisive evolutionary event is the establishment of bonding. Parental care

and mutual aid provide the origins of sociability. Sexuality, territorial defense, and fear of predators, although important, are not adequate as preadaptations for sociability. The intensity of early mother-infant bonding was investigated by Harlow and colleagues (Harlow and Zimmermann, 1959) who studied orphaned rhesus monkeys reared on surrogate mothers. They found that breaking the attachment bond through separation led to behavior symptoms that were similar to those described in hospitalized infants and children (Bowlby, 1969; Robertson, 1958; Spitz, 1946). Suomi and Harlow (1972) subsequently studied the social rehabilitation of isolate-reared monkeys. They demonstrated that the basis of affection is contact comfort (a secure base).

Infant rhesus macaques when isolated from their mothers show phases of agitation, protest, withdrawal, despair, and detachment similar to those seen in human infants. Moreover, in monkeys, the mother-infant relationship, effects of isolation, and infant responses to the environment depend on characteristics of the mother or mother-surrogate (Mason and Capitanio, 1988), mother-infant feedback (Hinde, 1983), food availability, and the social setting. The degree of behavioral disruption produced by social isolation is proportional to the age that the isolation occurs and its duration. Isolation from birth has greater effects than isolation after some mother or peer-aged contact. Six months of isolation has greater impact than three months. If the monkey is isolated for 12 months, complete resocialization is essentially impossible. Although monkeys isolated for shorter periods of time can be rehabilitated and may be difficult to distinguish from their socially reared counterparts, rehabilitated monkeys do not fully develop social strategies when competing for resources nor do they appear to perceive social relationships and respond appropriately to social cues in these situations (Anderson and Mason, 1978).

With severe isolation, both infant monkeys and humans show self-hugging, self-sucking, and self-biting. In addition, they show stereotypical movements, such as rocking, and they react to others with inappropriate fear and aggression. Socially isolated rhesus mothers failed to show normal mothering behavior and neglected their infants (Kraemer, 1985).

Physiologically, there is failure to thrive in isolated rhesus infants, and immune compromise is apparent. Moreover, anatomical and neurochemical changes have been demonstrated in the brains of monkeys who were socially isolated for the first 9 months of life when they were autopsied as adolescents at 19 to 24 years of age (Martin et al., 1991). The autopsied monkeys who were socially isolated had, during their development, shown persistent stereotyped movements, self-directed behaviors, and maladaptive psychosocial behavior (Sackett, 1972). Because the striatum undergoes changes in neurotransmitters and in neurotransmitter receptors during normal development in the postnatal period prior to achieving an adult pattern of organization (Graybiel et al., 1981), this brain region was examined. Studies of the brains revealed that the chemoarchitecture of the striatum showed selective alterations when compared to control animals, suggesting regional vulnerability. These findings are consistent with social isolation affecting the postnatal maturation of neurotransmitters in some brain regions (Martin et al., 1991). The abnormal motor and psychosocial behavior may be related to sensory/social deprivation, leading to alterations in the peptidergic and dopamine systems in the basal ganglia.

Spitz (1946) demonstrated the effects of early sensory and social deprivation on infant development in his classic paper on anaclitic depression, where he found not only failure to thrive but also increased infant mortality. Subsequently, Bowlby (1973, 1988) used an ethological orientation to investigate the establishment of the bond between mother and infant by addressing its biologic origins as he sought to understand the severity of the distress that children experience when separated from their mothers. His work in children is based on ethological studies of bonding in birds and mammals, in which strong bonds between parents and offspring are observed. He concluded that attachment and bonding have evolved as universal protective mechanisms for the young. Bowlby (1988) suggests that an ethological approach posits that such emotionally significant bonds between individuals (1) have basic survival functions; (2) can be understood by assuming a cybernetic system with a biological

basis in each partner whose goal is to maintain proximity between infant and parent during development; (3) lead to working models at the level of the mind, of one's self, of others, and of the patterns of interaction between them; and (4) suggest pathways of developmental progression rather than specific phases of fixation during development or of regression in times of stress. The way these bonds form from child to parent and parent to child have major developmental consequences in later life.

ORGANIZATION OF ATTACHMENT AND BONDING

In ethological theory, the tendency to make social bonds is present from the beginning of life. Such bonds are not derived from the need for food, sex, or dependency but are protective and basic to careseeking or in caregiving. Their formation requires accessibility to the adult; a secure base is essential to attachment and, once established, leads to exploration. Exploration involves leaving that close proximity; play and peer contact remove the young from accessibility to parental care, but the secure base is returned to at times of threat. The secure base in humans is maintained throughout childhood and adolescence, and, as the child matures, the time away that can be tolerated becomes greater— from half days at age 3, to weeks or months in adolescence. Bowlby (1988) proposed that analogous to physiological models of homeostasis, attachment behavior is a form of environmental homeostasis regulating distance and accessibility. It is activated by fear of harm or the need for care when tired or hungry; it is relieved by reunion with the caregiver, which provides reassurance and comfort. These control systems themselves are sources of activity, making theories of drive or psychic energy obsolete. A failure to respond causes stress reactions in infants, separation anxiety in the younger child, and possibly the experience of betrayal in the adolescent. An attachment relationship inhibits aggressive behavior— changes that may be neurochemically modulated.

The attachment system is most efficient in interacting with the person whom the child feels is the most likely to respond. A failure in response by the family caregiver causes stress and may be traumatic. Attachment is based on reciprocity of care-eliciting behavior in the child with caregiving by the parent. Caregiving is complementary to attachment behavior. Altruistic care of the young promotes survival of offspring and one's own genes. Thus, ethology emphasizes altruism and sociability.

As a consequence of early experiences, a child increasingly develops internal working models of relationships as attention and memory emerge with maturation. These working models allow the simulation and planning for future events in the real world. They allow the child to plan behavior for the future, so by 5 years of age, children's working models may have evolved to include awareness of caregivers' own interests, moods, and intentions. Each of these is considered by the child in planning. The parents develop complementary working models of the child to themselves. Some working models are in constant use; others may be automatized in memory and operate largely out of awareness over long periods of time.

PATTERNS OF ATTACHMENT

The theoretical work of Bowlby (1969) and the methodological contributions of Mary Ainsworth and colleagues (1978, 1985a, 1985b) have provided a means to test the quality of mother-infant attachment and to extend these observations to better understand the antecedents, stability, construction, and long-term sequelae of patterns of attachment. Ethology, evolutionary biology, control systems theory, and insights from contemporary cognitive developmental psychology have provided a framework to investigate the long-term implications of the parent-infant bond. The initial work on attachment theory emphasized the quality of the caregiver's response to the infant's cues for proximity and help and the role of attachment in forming personality. Ainsworth extended Bowlby's work by emphasizing the importance of security or insecurity in the attachment relationship and devised a methodology for testing secure and insecure attachment — i.e., the Strange Situation procedure (Ainsworth et al., 1978). This paradigm has become the primary means for assessing the security of infantile attachments by infant developmental researchers. The research on attachment has been extended to

evaluate the representational aspects of attachment relationships in children and adults, cross-cultural influences on the functioning of the attachment system, and the role of temperament in the establishment of attachment.

Four basic patterns of attachment have been reliably described (Ainsworth, 1985a, 1985b; Ainsworth et al., 1978; Main, Kaplan, and Cassidy, 1985; Main and Stadtman, 1981; Main and Weston, 1981). Which pattern develops depends on treatment by the parental figure and the child's responsiveness. These patterns of attachment were identified using the Strange Situation paradigm developed by Ainsworth et al. (1978). The Strange Situation procedure is a semistandardized, easy-to-use, and easily scorable means to identify infants who are securely or insecurely attached to their caregivers. In the Strange Situation procedure, differences in attachment security are evaluated by creating conditions with gradually escalating stress that activate the infant's attachment behavior system. The Strange Situation paradigm is a seven-episode procedure, which lasts 21 minutes, in which various social changes are observed to occur in an experimental play room setting while the infant is playing with toys. These changes include a stranger's presence or absence and the caregiver's departure and return in addition to other social events. The infant's response to the caregiver is directly observed, and the reunion response is particularly emphasized to classify them as either securely attached (Group B), insecure-avoidant (Group A), insecure-resistant (Group C) (Ainsworth et al., 1978) and "insecure-disorganized" (Main and Hesse, 1990; Main, Kaplan and Cassidy, 1985; Main and Solomon, 1986).

If the pattern of attachment is secure, it is likely to be associated with healthy development and lead to socially competent behavior. In this instance, the parent is available, is sensitive to the child's signals, and is appropriately and lovingly responsive when the child needs protection. An insecure or anxious pattern may emerge if there is uncertainty as to the parent's availability or responsiveness. Because of this uncertainty, attachment is potentially insecure and the child is prone to experience separation anxiety, a form of anxiety that is associated with anxious attachment, (i.e., anxious-resistant or anxious-ambivalent attachment). With insecure attachment, there is anxiety about exploration and about moving away from the secure parental base. Separation anxiety is unlike other forms of anxiety in that it may be terminated by contact with the parent. However, with an anxious attachment, in which the parent is alternatingly available or unavailable, the child experiences uncertainty and separation anxiety is enhanced. Experiences of uncertainty and potentially of abandonment or threats of abandonment may lead to chronic anxious attachment. Moreover, a punitive parent may use threat of abandonment, leading to insecure attachment, as a means of control. A third pattern of attachment, insecure or anxious-avoidant attachment, occurs when the child, through experience, learns to expect to be continuously rejected and has no confidence of being helped. This pattern of constant rejection may lead to compulsively self-reliant behavior in individuals and may be a precursor for delinquency as the individual attempts to survive without the support of a caregiver. Finally, children with the insecure-disorganized form of attachment are fearful of their caregiver. They may be unable to use their caregiver as a secure base and may be socially inhibited. Winnicott (1958) described disturbances in interpersonal relations as characteristic of children with an antisocial tendency. Children who exhibit the antisocial tendency continually seek attention but do so in an inappropriate or antisocial way, such as through stealing or social disruption.

Patterns of attachment persist through time and may be predictive of later behavior. Main, Kaplan, and Cassidy (1985) reported that the pattern of attachment to the parent at 12 months persisted with few exceptions at 6 years. Sroufe (1983) found that the pattern of attachment in infancy at 12 months was predictive of behavior in a nursery school group at age 3½ years. In this study, the children with a secure pattern at 12 months were described by teachers as cooperative, resourceful, and able to socialize well with other children. Those with an early anxious attachment were described as attention-seeking, hostile, and lacking in spontaneous emotionality. The anxious-resistant group were described as tense, easily frustrated, impulsive, and often passive. Follow-up studies are in progress to see the impact of early attachment difficulties at later phases of development.

Once patterns of attachment are established, they tend to persist; the patterns tend to be self-perpetuating. The securely attached child is easier to care for and less demanding. The anxious-ambivalent or anxious-resistant child tends to whine and cling, and the anxious-avoidant child tends to be bad-tempered and often bullies others. Vicious behavioral cycles may emerge from these interactions.

Although patterns are likely to persist, they do not necessarily do so. During the early years of life, the stability of the attachment depends on the consistency of the relationship. Not only may the mother-child and father-child pattern differ, but if a parent treats a child differently, the pattern may change. Stability of attachment cannot be simply attributed to temperament (Sroufe, 1985). Ainsworth et al. (1973) found that placid newborns may become anxious and demanding if their mothers are rejecting and insensitive. As a child grows older, the pattern of attachment and of personality features becomes more resistant to change.

There is a tendency to impose earlier patterns of attachment experience and the working models of self onto new relationships and to persist in these patterns despite "the absence of fit" (Bowlby, 1988). This "transference" of patterns of relating to new situations supports an object relations or interpersonal view of psychoanalytic theory rather than the classical form. This model considers internal models of the self and of psychological bonding as interactional models between individuals. Studies of attachment lead to questions about continuity and discontinuity in development. They also suggest that attachment and subsequent internal working models may be studied in developmental disorders.

Expanded Applications of Attachment Theory

New classification schemes are being developed to clarify the diversity of patterns of attachment functioning and new ways of assessing attachment in the Strange Situation paradigm and outside it (Gardner et al., 1986; Thompson, Connell, and Bridges, 1988; Waters and Deane, 1985). Moreover, attachment theory and research is being applied in clinical situations (Belsky and Nezworski, 1988), including studies of parent-child relations in the preschool years (Greenberg, Cicchetti, and Cummings, 1990) and in children at older ages (Main and Cassidy, 1988). More recent views of attachment present attachment relationships as being continuously constructed and reconstructed during development, and confirm many long-standing assumptions about the formative importance of attachment relationships but question other assumptions (Thompson, 1991).

The bulk of the research on the antecedents of attachment security has focused on the maternal behavior that leads to security and attachment. Additional research is needed to specify more clearly which maternal behaviors foster either secure or insecure attachment, but previous studies have confirmed that maternal behavior significantly influences attachment security, as predicted. Other contributors to attachment include the father's involvement in caregiving and the parental satisfaction with the marital relationship (Easterbrooks and Goldberg, 1984; Goldberg and Easterbrooks, 1984), socioeconomic stress as it affects family relationships (Vaughn, Gove, and Egeland, 1980), and the infant's temperamental characteristics, which may affect the parental response in the Strange Situation paradigm (Thompson, Connell, and Bridges, 1988). These studies of attachment would suggest that infants are affected by their broader environment and not simply the emotional relationship provided by the mother. Notably, the father's role, socioeconomic stresses, and cultural norms for child care affect the construction of attachment bonds (Thompson, 1991).

Another factor that is undergoing evaluation is the stability of the attachment relationship. Initial studies showed substantial test-retest stability; however, subsequently, when children from lower-income homes, in addition to those from middle-income homes, were studied, the proportion of infants whose attachments were stable ranged from 48% to 96% over 6- to 8-month intervals during the second year of life (Lamb et al., 1985). The changes in stability may be linked to changes in caregiver relations, which are affected by more life stresses, particularly in low-income settings. However, in middle class settings when living conditions change for the family that affect the mother-

infant interaction, the security of attachment is also affected. Stability of attachment, then, reflects the dynamic conditions in early life between parent and infant as well as the ongoing accommodations that must be made as children grow. The best predictions of later behavior, based on attachment status, take into account the consistency in support by the parental figure over time. In regard to outcome at later ages, the security of attachment has some predictive value if there is consistency in caregiving. Supportive parental care in infancy, if maintained, may facilitate sociability, prosocial behavior, and social competence at later ages. However, when caregiving conditions show significant change, this continuity may not be evident. Behavioral continuity results from the interaction of the child in relation to others over time, and current caregiving influences are as important as early ones. Secure attachment requires consistent caregiving conditions to maintain earlier behavioral patterns.

Since Bowlby's (1969) original description, current thinking in evolutionary biology has shifted from emphasizing a single optimal behavioral pattern regulating attachment processes, the secure pattern, that is adapted to a particular style of parental caregiving behavior — sensitive parenting — to viewing organisms as being able to utilize a variety of conditional strategies depending on their life circumstances. Hinde (1982) has suggested that different patterns of infant behavior may be adaptive in different caregiving contexts and in relationship to differences in the type of maternal care provided. These expanded observations suggest greater flexibility and plasticity in the attachment systems and greater diversity in their origins. The plasticity of attachment behavior systems indicates that early intervention may be effective because an insecurely attached infant or child may not necessarily remain so.

EMOTIONAL BASES OF ATTACHMENT BEHAVIOR

Emotion has long been considered an important part of the attachment system. Emotional processes were regarded by Bowlby (1969) as a major component of the appraisal process through which attachment behavior is initiated, monitored, and finally terminated. In fact,

Sroufe and Waters (1977) indicated that the "set goal" of the attachment behavior system is the infant's sense of emotional security with the caregiver.

The major controversy in relation to emotion and attachment has focused on individual variations in emotional arousal and its regulation, and how this contributes to attachment security. Thompson (1990) has evaluated variations in emotional dynamics during the Strange Situation testing and emphasizes the intensive and temporal fluctuations of emotional behavior that may relate to the regulation of distress during the testing. Attachment classifications (A, B, C) must take into account the quality and intensity of distress during a separation episode in the testing paradigm. An insecure-avoidant infant may show relatively little separation distress, which is slow in onset and short in duration, whereas an insecure-resistant infant may produce intense distress, which is difficult to soothe, and the securely attached infant may take a middle ground. Variability in emotional reaction does not link directly to a secure or insecure attachment, but emotionality does motivate parental behavior and the individual response that is provided.

Investigations of emotionality in attachment have been extended to Down syndrome, in which similar responses linking distress intensity in mother-directed contact seeking were seen (Thompson et al., 1985), yet in Down syndrome an association between distress and resistant behavior was apparent, suggesting that the affectively more subdued member of the Down syndrome group with poor emotional regulation showed heightened distress, which provoked angry as well as positive contact from the parent. Thus, poor regulation of emotion may have a negative impact on the parent, although emotionality itself stimulates an expected parental response. Thompson (1991) has found that individual differences in emotional behavior are more consistent throughout the Strange Situation testing than are differences in social interactive behavior. This suggests that emotional behavior may reliably identify individual differences in socioemotional reactivity. In this study, emotional reactions predicted later social behavior toward the mother. Emotional reactions and their regulation may assume a major role in the subsequent

reorganization of an infant's social behavior in Strange Situation testing. If an infant behaved with a consistent emotional response over time when retested in the Strange Situation, consistency in social behavior was also apparent. However, those infants who were unstable in their emotional responses from one occasion to the next did not show consistency in social behavior. Consequently, emotional reactions have an important role in predicting social behavior within the Strange Situation. The author points out that temperament in itself is probably not the source of the organizational role of emotionality in his studies.

In the Strange Situation, the infants' emotional reactions tended to be regulated by seeking emotional cues from their caregivers, that is, from social referencing (Klinnert et al., 1983). When strangers entered the room, infants would look at the parent's face for emotional cues, and these cues may have contributed to regulation of emotion. In this way, parents and infants both contribute to emotional self-regulation to organize attachment in the Strange Situation. Emotional processes, then, govern attachment behavior and are multiply determined and dynamic. They show a flexible accommodation to changing conditions and contingencies. The roots of attachment processes and emotion regulation are important in flexible adaptation to new and changing situations.

Emotional constructs seem to play a central role in the function of attachment systems. In children with atypical development, problems in emotion self-regulation may play an important role in the establishment of secure attachment.

ATTACHMENT AND WORKING MODELS

The role of mental representational features has been emphasized by Bretherton (1987), and by Main, Kaplan, and Cassidy (1985), who portrayed attachment as not only a behavioral system but also a conceptual system that governs social relations throughout life. These authors suggest that through the history of interactions with the caregiver, an infant generates a rudimentary conceptual representation of the attachment figure. These representations have been referred to as "working models" that form the basis for secure and insecure attachment by the end of the first year of life and are maintained to guide subsequent behavior at later ages. These representations of significant relationships may be stored and operate outside conscious awareness, leaving them prone to stability over time. Such consistent, long-term models may not only affect the parent-child relationship but also be carried on as caregiving tendencies to the next generation, as the child internalizes the role of caregiver and of the one being cared for (Sroufe and Fleeson, 1986).

If attachments may be described as internalized conceptual models, then individual differences in attachment security may lead to social expectations that differ from those of the caregiver. Working models suggest expectations by children of a caregiver's responsiveness and accessibility to them. Thompson (1991) suggests that by the end of the first year of life, early primitive representation regarding a caregiver's behavior may have become consolidated as it is relevant to the infant's security and support.

Another aspect of the representational theory considers whether a mother's quality of care for her infant is related to her own representations of her life experience as a child. Several studies (Main and Goldwyn, 1984; Main, Kaplan, and Cassidy, 1985; Ricks, 1985) have suggested that a mother's representations of her own experiences of childhood care relate to her infant's security of attachment at the end of the first year of life. These authors suggest that attachment as internalized representations provide working models for both the caregiver and the infant receiving care and that these models may be maintained and reproduced in caregiving roles in later life. In reviewing parents' memories of early experiences of care, particularly recollections of security and comfort and fears of abandonment and separation, they found that, overall, an infant's attachment status bore a relation to the parents' conceptualization of attachment-related issues, including their own acceptance or rejection as children and their self-esteem. Although the parents' reports are a recollection of memories of their childhood, these recollections are the source of the parents' contemporary working models of attachment as it relates to their own children. These findings suggest the importance of examining how a secure or insecure parent-infant attachment does affect an adult's representations of attachment-related experiences. Just as sensitive parenting facilitates security in a child, a child who is securely attached may also affect parents' perceptions of their own parenting ability, their self-esteem, and perhaps their reflections on their own earlier experience. Thus, the behavior of the infant or child may affect the parents' own beliefs. In this sense, attachment demonstrates mutually reinforcing influences between parents and offspring that persist over time as long as there are not major changes in family relationships.

The relationship between attachment in infancy and at school age is receiving continued emphasis (Cassidy, 1988; Cassidy and Main, 1985). These studies emphasize the continuity in functioning based on the working model hypothesis of internalized representations. If infants do construct working models of their caregivers that result in secure or insecure attachment, such working models might exert an ongoing influence on how children cope with attachment concerns at later ages.

Measures of 6-year-olds' thoughts about separation-related experiences and their behavioral responses to separation and reunions with parents were evaluated by Main and Cassidy (1988), who found moderately strong relationships between attachment status in the first year of life and attachment behavior at age 6. To assure consistency in family circumstances, the sample was optimized by excluding families who had been separated or divorced and those in which the child had a major separation from the parent. Additional research is necessary to evaluate the influences that normally lead to change as well as stability in children's attachment systems. This requires a focus on families in which there are interruptions of familiar interaction patterns within the home through changes in life circumstances. Such studies must address representations of attachment when family changes, such as divorce, separation, and remarriage, occur.

DEVELOPMENTAL CHANGES IN ATTACHMENT RELATIONS

Investigations of attachment in adults and in the 6-year-old sample relied on the same constructs used in work with infant attachment (i.e., perception of parental acceptance, responses to separation and reunion, and feelings about rejection and inaccessibility).

An important issue in the study of attachment during development is that, at certain times, conflict between parents and offspring may be important to facilitate independence (Trivers, 1974, 1985). In infancy, weaning is an example of a conflict area, psychological individuation is an example during the toddler years, and issues of independence that arise in school-aged and adolescent children are also examples. Resistant behavior by the child toward the parent may not indicate insecurity and, in fact, may be adaptive.

Bowlby (1969) has discussed the developmental aspects of attachment in the context of the "goal-corrected partnership." Increasingly, the child is capable of viewing the parents' goals and plans from the parental perspective and may participate in the process of creating joint arrangements for regulating proximity and other attachment-related concerns. The goal-corrected partnership is facilitated by the emergence of language and new conceptual abilities. Inferences about adults' behavior, better understanding of relationship roles, and the use of language to communicate, reflect on feelings, and maintain self-control have developmental salience. As the child grows older, these developmental accomplishments facilitate joint negotiation of issues related to attachment. Therefore, in assessing attachment at older ages, the new conceptual and representational skills of a child must be considered. Security issues as they relate to attachment remain important but change as the nature of parent-child interaction becomes more sophisticated and multifaceted. As the child matures, attachment representations must consider the meaning of relational security at different ages.

Overall, the construction and reconstruction of early social attachments is a flexible process. The infant plays an active role in early life, as does the child in later life, in the construction of attachment relationships through developing expectations of that relationship and exercising affective self-regulation. The interaction of the child's developing relational and representational abilities with the changing social environment leads to the construction and reconstruction of social attachments. With this viewpoint, one may be optimistic about both normal develop-

ment and development in children with developmental disorders because there is an inherent flexibility in early social relationships (Thompson, 1991). An infant with early difficulty in emotion regulation or an infant with insecure attachment may respond to an appropriate psychosocial intervention. Early internal representations may be modified because our concepts of ourself and of others as social partners develop gradually and are subject to multiple influences.

APPLICATION OF ETHOLOGY TO DEVELOPMENTAL NEUROPSYCHIATRY

Brain Damage and Social Behavior

An ethological approach in developmental neuropsychiatry utilizes the ethogram or behavior profile but must also consider the impact of brain dysfunction on behavior. Processing of social information in both humans and nonhuman primates depends on intact limbic structures, particularly the amygdala and the orbital frontal cortex, with which the amygdala is connected. The analysis of data on single-neuron studies in monkeys who observed the action of other monkeys supports a neural basis for social representation. The study of how social representations are formed (i.e., the biology of social representation and understanding) is essential. Human social cognition is plastic, and social judgments may change, particularly as a result of cultural learning and experience. Still, plasticity in social representation occurs and is critical.

Damage to the limbic frontal lobes, especially the orbital frontal lesion, may result in lack of appreciation for social rules. Damasio, Tranel, and Damasio (1990) found that damage to orbital and lower mesial frontal lobes resulted in a patient's having the incapacity to make appropriate social judgments in real life. It was thought that the patient failed to accurately assess the character or motivations of other persons.

In macaque monkeys, lesions of the amygdala, orbital frontal cortex, and temporal pole induced experimentally also produce altered social behavior. Behavioral changes noted include decreased aggression, social withdrawal, and failure of internal behavior. The existence in an animal model of neural activity that encodes the apparent purpose or emotional state of another indicates there may be a definable neural substrate for a brain module that involves social understanding. Furthermore, the fact that a monkey may complete logical tests in social domains but not in nonsocial ones further supports the evolutionary origin and primacy of social cognition or social understanding. Brothers (1990) has investigated responses from single cells in rhesus monkeys and found that these cells may be highly specific as parts of ensembles of cells that respond to social behavior. It has been suggested that there are brain cells that socially respond to viewer-centered, common-object-centered, and goal-centered activities (Perret and Rolls, 1983). For example, brain cells that respond to hand-object interactions, cells selective for particular actions on objects, and goal-centered neurons have been described. When the experimenter moved away from a monkey toward a door, cells were activated, suggesting the social significance of being left alone. Finally, neurons are selective for visual features, such as limb movements of body parts. Perhaps movement might be initially encoded, then subsequently encoded for the direction of movement or type of action, expressive content, or goal-directed behavior in social interactions. Brothers suggests that neurons appear to code for higher level aspects of others' activities as well as basic interactions.

Brothers and Ring (1992) suggest that not only are mental representations, such as the appearance of a face, drawn from sensory input, but concurrently the cognitive capacity for representing minds is independent. There is a phylogenetic or evolutionary system that recognizes affective displays and, in humans, assigns recognition to social behavior. From the evolutionary point of view, a premium may be assigned to the individual who can accurately attribute qualities—such as helpful, trustworthy, or untrustworthy—to others. These characteristics may be developed sufficiently that they are maintained even when procedural memory is lost but social memory or emotional memory is maintained.

Attachment and Developmental Disabilities

An understanding of infant bonding is especially important in mental retardation syndromes, such as Down syndrome, where the infant's ability to recognize social cues may be limited. Despite this, intense social contact with the parent has been shown to facilitate bonding (Cytryn, 1975)

in this and other mental retardation syndromes. Attachment and bereavement do take place, although the bereavement response is often not adequately appreciated. The development of anxious attachment and compulsive self-reliance in children with developmental disorders who have abnormal early interpersonal contact may also occur. Preattachment behaviors involving vocalization, motor movement, and social awareness may be problematic or even lacking in children with language disorders, cerebral palsy, or autistic disorder. In pervasive developmental disorder, social perplexity is characteristic and avoidance of social contact may interfere with early bonding, yet parents generally become strongly attached to their child with an autistic disorder despite the child's limited responsiveness.

Whether or not children with autistic disorder develop attachment early in life has been of particular interest in regard to attachment research. Shapiro et al. (1987) studied 36 children, ages 30 to 63 months, with diagnoses of Pervasive Developmental Disorder, Autistic Disorder, Pervasive Developmental Disorder Not Otherwise Specified, Developmental Language Disorder, and a matched group of children with mental retardation. Using the Ainsworth Strange Situation paradigm, which was modified for this study, these authors found that children with Pervasive Developmental Disorder did demonstrate attachment behavior that was not significantly different from the attachment behavior seen in younger children who were not developmentally delayed. Sixty-four percent of children with developmental disorders showed behavioral change on separation, and 44% demonstrated negative mood change. The quality of the attachment was not correlated with the diagnosis or with developmental quotients, mood change, or behavior change. Affective display on separation correlated with security of attachment, but this was not statistically significant.

Hermelin (1984), beginning with the observation that children with autistic disorder not only do not attend to people but also have limited contacts with objects, has reviewed their perception, language, and thinking. She notes that initially studies in autistic disorder were cognitive in nature, because methods to study cognitive functions were better developed than those used for noncognitive functions. Nonetheless, the association between cognitive deficits and social abnormalities remains unanswered, as stated earlier. Tinbergen and Tinbergen (1972) attempted to utilize an ethological approach in autistic disorder but did not fully appreciate the brain dysfunction found in the syndrome. Despite this, their observations on motivational conflict and on applying ethological methods to a developmental disorder are of importance. Wing and Ricks (1976) suggest that ethological methods might be used to study the "perceptual and cognitive bases of social recognition and possible impairment of these functions in children with autistic disorder." An "ethological approach" has been applied by others, and a beginning has been made in studying the perceptual and cognitive bases of social recognition in autistic disorder, addressing proxemics, attachment, aggression rituals, social reciprocity, and working models (theory of mind).

Studies of attachment and bonding in childhood continue to illuminate our understanding of developmental disorders and have led to considerable progress. Kraeplin (1971) said that "it will be necessary to search for the roots and the manifestations of our inner lives everywhere — in the souls of children, of primitive men, of animals. Furthermore, it will be necessary to establish to what degree lost emotions of the individual and the phylogenetic past are reborn in illness." This chapter emphasizes how far we have come along this path.

REFERENCES

Ainsworth, M.D. (1969). Object relations, dependency and attachment: A theoretical review of the infant-mother relationship. *Child Development,* 40:969–1025.

———. (1973). The development of infant-mother attachment. In B.M. Caldwell and H.N. Ricciuti (eds), *Child development research,* pp. 1–95. University of Chicago Press, Chicago.

———. (1985a). Patterns of infant-mother attachments: Antecedents and effects on development. *Bulletin of the New York Academy of Medicine,* 61:771–791.

———. (1985b). Attachments across the life span. *Bulletin of the New York Academy of Medicine,* 61:792–812.

———, Blehar, M.C., Waters, E., and Wall, S. (1978). *Patterns of attachment: Assessed in the strange situation and at home.* Lawrence Erlbaum, Hillsdale, NJ.

Anderson, C.O., and Mason, W.A. (1978). Competitive social stragegies in groups of deprived and experienced rhesus monkeys. *Developmental Psychobiology,* 11:289–299.

Belsky, J., and Nezworski, T.M. (eds). (1988). *Clinical implications of attachment.* Lawrence Erlbaum, Hillsdale, NJ.

Betzig, L. (1989). Rethinking human ethology: A response to some recent critiques. *Ethology and Sociobiology,* 10: 315–324.

Bowlby, J. (1969). *Attachment and loss.* Vol. 1, *Attachment.* Basic Books, New York.

———. (1973). *Attachment and loss.* Vol. 2, *Separation.* Basic Books, New York.

———. (1988). Developmental psychiatry comes of age. *American Journal of Psychiatry,* 145:1–10.

Bretherton, I. (1987). New perspectives on attachment relations in infancy: Security, communication and internal working models. In J.D. Osofsky (ed), *Handbook of infant development* (rev. ed.), pp. 1061–1149. John Wiley & Sons, New York.

Brothers, L. (1990). The social brain: A project for integrating primate behavior and neurophysiology in a new domain. *Concepts in Neuroscience,* 1:27–51.

———, and Ring, B. (1992). A neuroethological framework for the representation of minds. *Journal of Cognitive Neuroscience,* 4:107–118.

Calvin, W.H. (1990). *Ice age climates and the evolution of intelligence.* Bantam Books, New York.

Cassidy, J. (1988). Child-mother attachment and the self in six-year-olds. *Child Development,* 59:121–134.

———, and Main, M. (1985). The relationship between infant-parent attachment and the ability to tolerate brief separation at six years. In J.D. Call, E. Galenson, and R.L. Tyson (eds), *Frontiers of infant psychiatry,* Vol. 2, pp. 132–136. Basic Books, New York.

Cytryn, L. (1975). Studies of behavior of children with Down's syndrome. In E. J. Anthony (ed), *Explorations in child psychiatry,* pp. 281–287. Plenum Press, New York.

Damasio, A.R., Tranel, D., and Damasio, H. (1990). Individuals with sociopathic behavior caused by frontal damage fail to respond automatically to social stimuli. *Behavioural Brain Research,* 41:81–94.

Darwin, C. (1871). *The descent of man.* John Murray, London.

———. (1872). *The expression of emotions in man and the animals.* John Murray, London.

Dawkins, R. (1989). *The selfish gene.* Oxford University Press, New York.

DeSimone, R. (1991). Face-selective cells in the temporal cortex of monkeys. *Journal of Cognitive Neuroscience,* 3:1–8.

Donald, M. (1991). *Origins of the modern mind: Three stages in the evolution of culture and cognition.* Harvard University Press, Cambridge, MA.

Easterbrooks, M.A., and Goldberg, W.A. (1984). Toddler development in the family: Impact of father involvement and parenting characteristics. *Child Development,* 55:740–752.

Eibl-Eibesfeldt, I. (1979). Human ethology: Concepts and implications for the sciences of man. *The Behavioral and Brain Sciences,* 2:1–57.

———. (1989). *Human ethology.* Aldine de Gruyter, New York.

Gantt, H. (1944). *Experimental basis for neurotic behavior.* Harper, New York.

Gardner, W., Lamb, M.E., Thompson, R.A., and Sagi, A. (1986). On individual differences in Strange Situation behavior: Categorical and continuous measurement systems in a cross cultural data set. *Infant Behavior and Development,* 9:355–375.

Goldberg, W.A., and Easterbrooks, M.A. (1984). Role of marital quality in toddler development. *Developmental Psychology,* 20:504–514.

Greenberg, M.T., Cicchetti, D., and Cummings, M. (eds). (1990). *Attachment in the preschool years: Theory, research, and intervention.* University of Chicago Press, Chicago.

Graybiel, A.M., Ragsdale, C.W. Jr., Yoneoka, E.S., and Elde, R.P. (1981). An immunohistochemical study of enkephalins and other neuropeptides in the striatum of the cat with evidence that the opiate peptides are arranged to form mosaic patterns in register with the striosomal compartments visible by acetylcholinesterase staining. *Neuroscience,* 6:377–397.

Harlow, H.F., and Zimmermann, R.R. (1959). Affectional responses in the infant monkey. *Science,* 130:421–432.

Harries, M.H., and Perret, D.I. (1991). Visual processing of faces in temporal cortex: Physiological evidence for a modular organization and possible anatomical correlates. *Journal of Cognitive Neuroscience,* 3:9–24.

Hermelin, B. (1984). Thoughts and feelings. *Australian Autism Review,* 10–19.

Hinde, R.A. (1982). Attachment: Some conceptual and biological issues. In J. Stevenson-Hinde and C. Murray Parkes (eds), *The place of attachment in human behavior,* pp. 60–76. Basic Books, New York.

———. (1983). Feedback in the mother-infant relationship. In R.A. Hinde (ed), *Primate social relationships,* Section 6.2. Sinauer Associates, Sunderland, MA.

———. (1987). *Individuals, relationships, and culture: Links between ethology and the social sciences.* Cambridge University Press, New York.

Hoyle, G. (1984). The scope of neuroethology. *The Behavioural and Brain Sciences,* 7:367–412.

Klinnert, M.D., Campos, J.J., Sorce, J.F., Emde, R.N., and Svejda, M. (1983). Emotions as behavior regulators: Social referencing in infancy. In R. Plutchik and H. Kellerman (eds), *Emotion: Theory, research, and experience,* Vol. 2. *Emotions in early development,* pp. 57–86. Academic Press, New York.

Kraemer, G.W. (1985). Effects of differences in early social experience on primate neurobiological development. In M. Reite and T. Field (eds), *The psychobiology of attachment and separation,* pp. 135–161. Academic Press, New York.

Kraepelin, E. (1971). Annual Reports, 1966–71, Max Planck Institute for Psychiatry, p. 7. Munich, Germany.

Kropotkin, P. I. (1989). *Mutual aid: A factor in evolution.* Black Rose, Montreal.

Lamb, M.E., Thompson, R.A., Gardner, W.P., and Charnov, E.L. (1985). *Infant-mother attachment.* Lawrence Erlbaum, Hillsdale, NJ.

Lorenz, K. (1935). Der Kumpan in der umwelt des vogels. *Journal of Ornithology,* 83:137–413.

———. (1977). *Behind the mirror. A search for a natural history of human knowledge.* Methuen, London.

———. (1981). Introductory history. In *The foundations of ethology. The principal ideas and discoveries in animal behavior,* pp. 1–12. Simon and Schuster, New York.

MacLean, P. (1973). *A triune concept of the brain and behavior.* University of Toronto Press, Toronto.

———. (1985). Brain evolution relating to family, play, and the separation call. *Archives of General Psychiatry,* 42:405–417.

———. (1990). *The triune brain in evolution: Role in paleocerebral functions.* Plenum Press, New York.

Main, M., and Cassidy, J. (1988). Categories of response to reunion with the parent at age 6: Predictable from infant attachment classifications and stable over a 1-month period. *Developmental Psychology,* 24:415–426.

———, and Goldwyn, R. (1984). Predicting rejection of her infant from mother's representation of her own experience: Implications for the abused-abusing intergenerational cycle. *Child Abuse and Neglect,* 8:203–217.

———, and Hesse, E. (1990). Parents' unresolved traumatic experiences are related to infant disorganized attachment status: Is frightening and/or frightened parental behavior the linking mechanism? In M. Greenberg, D. Cicchetti, and M. Cummings, (eds), *Attachment in the preschool years,* pp. 161–182. University of Chicago Press, Chicago.

_____, and Solomon, J. (1986). Discovery of an insecure-disorganized/disoriented attachment pattern: Procedures, findings and implications for the classification of behavior. In M. Yogman and T.B. Brazelton (eds), *Affective development in infancy,* pp. 95–124. Ablex, Norwood, NJ.

_____, and Stadtman, J. (1981). Infant response to rejection of physical contact by the mother: Aggression, avoidance and conflict. *Journal of the American Academy of Child Psychiatry,* 20:292–307.

_____, and Weston, D.R. (1981). The quality of the toddler's relationship to mother and to father: Related to conflict behaviour and the readiness to establish new relationships. *Child Development,* 52:932–940.

_____, Kaplan, K., and Cassidy, J. (1985). Security in infancy, childhood and adulthood: A move to the level of representation. In I. Bretherton and E. Waters (eds), *Growing points of attachment theory and research,* Monographs of the Society for Research in Child Development, 50, Serial No. 209 (1–2), 66–104. University of Chicago Press, Chicago.

Martin, L.J., Spicer, D.M., Lewis, M.H., Gluck, J.P., and Cork, L.C. (1991). Social deprivation of infant rhesus monkeys alters the chemoarchitecture of the brain: I. Subcortical regions. *Journal of Neuroscience,* 11:3344–3358.

Mason, W.A., and Capitanio, J.P. (1988). Formation and expression of filial attachment in rhesus monkeys raised with living and inanimate mother substitutes. *Developmental Psychobiology,* 21:401–430.

McGuire, M.T., and Fairbanks, L. (1977). Ethology: Psychiatry's bridge to behavior. In M.T. McGuire and L.A. Fairbanks (eds), *Ethological psychiatry: Psychopathology in the context of evolutionary biology,* pp. 1–40. Grune and Stratton, New York.

Pavlov, I.P. (1927). *Conditioned reflexes.* Oxford University Press, London.

Perret, D.I., and Rolls, E.T. (1983). Neural mechanisms underlying the visual analysis of faces. In J.P. Ewert, R. R. Capranica, and D.J. Ingel (eds), *Advances in vertebrate neuroethology,* pp. 543–566. Plenum Press, New York.

Provine, R.R. (1981). Development of wing-flapping and flight in normal and flap-deprived domestic chicks. *Developmental Psychobiology,* 14:279–291.

Ricks, M.H. (1985). The social transmission of parental behavior: Attachment across generations. In I. Bretherton and E. Waters (eds), *Growing points in attachment theory and research.* Monographs of the Society for Research in Child Development, Serial No. 209, 211–227, University of Chicago Press, Chicago.

Robertson, J. (1958). *Young children in hospital.* Tavistock Publications, London.

Romer, A.S. (1966). *Vertebrate paleontology.* University of Chicago Press, Chicago.

Sackett, G.P. (1972). Isolation rearing in monkeys: Diffuse and specific later behavior. *Colloques internationaux du C.N.R.S.* 198:61–110.

Shapiro, T., Sherman, M., Calamari, G., and Koch, D. (1987). Attachment in autism and other developmental disorders. *Journal of the American Academy of Child and Adolescent Psychiatry,* 26:480–484.

Simon, H.A. (1990). A mechanism for social selection and successful altruism. *Science,* 250:1665–1668.

Skinner, B.F. (1938). *The behavior of organisms.* Appleton-Century-Crofts, New York.

Spitz, R.A. (1946). Anaclitic depression. An inquiry into the genesis of psychiatric conditions in early childhood. *Psychoanalytic Study of the Child,* 2:313–342.

Sroufe, L.A. (1983). Infant-caregiver attachment and patterns of adaptation in preschool: The roots of maladaptation and competence. In M. Perlmutter (ed), *Minnesota Symposium in Child Psychology,* Vol. 16. University of Minnesota Press, Minneapolis.

_____, and Fleeson, J. (1986). Attachment and the construction of relationships. In W.W. Hartup and Z. Rubin (eds), *Relationships and development,* pp. 51–71. Lawrence Erlbaum, Hillsdale, NJ.

_____. (1985). Attachment classification from the perspective of infant-caregiver relationships and infant temperament. *Child Development,* 56:1–14.

_____, and Waters, E. (1977). Attachment as an organizational construct. *Child Development,* 48:1184–1199.

Suomi, S. (1985). Ethological approaches to psychiatry: Animal models. In H.I. Kaplan and B.J. Sadock (eds), *Comprehensive textbook of psychiatry,* pp. 226–236. Williams & Wilkins, Baltimore.

_____, and Harlow, H.F. (1972). Social rehabilitation of isolate-reared monkeys. *Developmental Psychology,* 6:487–496.

Thelen, E., Bradshaw, G., and Ward, J.A. (1981). Spontaneous kicking in month-old infants: Manifestation of a human central locomotor program. *Behavioral and Neural Biology,* 32:45–53.

Thompson, R.A. (1990). Emotion and self-regulation. In R.A. Thompson (ed), *Socioemotional development. Nebraska Symposium on Motivation,* Vol. 36, pp. 383–483. University of Nebraska Press, Lincoln, NE.

_____. (1991). Construction and reconstruction of early attachments: Taking perspective on attachment theory and research. In D.P. Keating and H.

Rosen (eds), *Constructivist perspectives on developmental psychopathology and atypical development*, pp. 41–67. Lawrence Erlbaum, Hillsdale, NJ.

_____, Cicchetti, D., Lamb, M.E., and Malkin, C. (1985). Emotional responses of Down syndrome and normal infants in the Strange Situation: The organization of affective behavior in infants. *Developmental Psychology*, 21:828–841.

_____, Connell, J.P., and Bridges, L. (1988). Temperament, emotion, and social interactive behavior in the Strange Situation: An analysis of attachment system functioning. *Child Development*, 59:1102–1110.

Thorndike, E.L. (1898). *Animal intelligence; An experimental study of the associative processes in animals*. The Macmillan Company, New York.

Tinbergen, N. (1951). *The study of instinct*. Clarendon Press, Oxford.

_____. (1963). On aims and methods of ethology. *Zeitscrift fur Tierpsychologie*, 20:410–433.

Tinbergen, E.A. and Tinbergen, N. (1972). Early childhood autism: An ethological approach. In *Advances in Ethology: Beihefte zur Zeitshrift fur Tierpsychologie*, 10:1–53.

Trivers, R.L. (1974). Parent-offspring conflict. *American Zoologist*, 14:249–264.

_____. (1985). *Social evolution*. Benjamin-Cummings, Menlo Park, CA.

Vaughn, B.E., Gove, F.L., and Egeland, B. (1980). The relationship between out-of-home care and the quality of infant-mother attachment in an economically disadvantaged population. *Child Development*, 51:1203–1214.

Von Frisch, K. (1953). *The dancing bees*. Harcourt Brace Jovanovich, New York.

Wallhausser, E., and Scheich, H. (1987). Auditory imprinting leads to differential 2-deoxy-glucose uptake and dendritic spine loss in the chick rostral forebrain. *Developmental Brain Research*, 31:29–44.

Waters, E., and Deane, K.E. (1985). Defining and assessing individual differences in attachment relationships: Q-methodology and the organization of behavior in infancy and early childhood. In I. Bretherton and E. Waters (eds), *Growing points in attachment theory and research*. Monographs of the Society for Research in Child Development, 50, Serial No. 209, 41–65. University of Chicago Press, Chicago.

Wilson, E.O. (1975). *Sociobiology: The new synthesis*. Harvard University Press, Cambridge, MA.

Wilson, D.S., and Sober, E. (1994). Reintroducing group selection to the human behavioral sciences. *Behavioral and Brain Sciences*. 17:585–654.

Wing, L., and Ricks, D.M. (1976). The aetiology of childhood autism: A criticism of the Tinbergen's ethological theory. *Psychological Medicine*, 6:533–543.

Winnicott, D.W. (1958). The antisocial tendency. In D.W. Winnicott (collected papers), *From pediatrics to psychoanalysis*. Hogarth Press, London.

Zahn-Waxler, C., Cummings, E.M., and Iannotti, R. (1986). *Altruism and aggression: Biological and social origins*. Cambridge University Press, New York.

Zumpe, D., and Michael, R.P. (1979). Relation between the hormonal status of the female and direct and redirected aggression by male rhesus monkeys (Macaca mulatta). *Hormones and Behavior*, 12:269–279.

_____, and _____ (1990). Ethology and human behavior. In A. Stoudemire (ed), *Human behavior: An introduction for medical students*, pp. 241–260. J.B. Lippincott, Philadelphia.

CHAPTER 13

COGNITIVE DEVELOPMENT

The human species is distinct because of the richness of its cognitive processes. Cognition refers to the use or handling of knowledge (Gregory, 1987). It is linked to perception in the application of knowledge-based processes to make sense out of sensory signals as they are neurally encoded. Cognitive processes are linked to memory, particularly to working memory, as individual events assume meaning and generalizations are drawn from particular circumstances to facilitate adaptation. Gregory (1987) suggests that the word "cognition" may be related to *gnomon* — the shadow-casting rod of a sun dial, which provides knowledge of time by casting shadows. Human cognition is unique in its time sense in that it allows for learning based on past experience and planning based on the capacity to anticipate a personal future.

This chapter considers cognition from a developmental perspective and reviews traditional cognitive developmental approaches and recent developments in cognitive developmental theory.

DEVELOPMENTAL PERSPECTIVE

From a developmental perspective, the development of intelligence over the life span is of particular importance. Although intelligence is difficult to define, there is broad agreement on two features. Intelligence involves the capacity first, to learn from experience, and second, to adapt to one's environment (Sternberg and

Powell, 1983). In considering intelligence, both general intelligence and the development of multiple special skills in specialized domains, such as verbal ability and visuospatial ability, must be taken into account. Psychologists involved with test construction and measurement have tested children's abilities on a wide range of tasks that intercorrelate, and by using statistical methods, have suggested the importance of a broad underlying category of general intelligence, or "G." Tests have also been developed to measure more specific domains of cognitive functioning. Developmentally, both the growth of general intelligence and of special skills are important. General measures of overall intelligence have been found to predict performance on a variety of adaptive tasks, yet the study of general intelligence has also demonstrated that people who show inferior performance on one type of task are not necessarily inferior on other types of tasks. Domain-specific skills are also important, because some individuals perform well on some tasks and poorly on others. Moreover, those physical and psychosocial factors that influence the development of verbal skills may differ from those that influence visuospatial skills. By adulthood, verbal abilities are primarily subserved on the left side of the brain, whereas the visuospatial abilities primarily involve the right side.

Intelligence has been viewed both as a continuous and as a discontinuous process. Developmentally, different processes are important in cognition at different times during development. The use of different brain systems for learning during different times of development suggests a discontinuity in intellectual development between the early infancy period and middle childhood. Developmental studies have demonstrated that the interconnections between different skills vary at different ages. For example, during the first year of life interest in perceptual patterns makes a major contribution to cognitive abilities. However, verbal abilities are major contributors subsequently. Evidence consistent with discontinuity in intellectual development is found in studies of infant scores on developmental assessments, where a weak correlation is shown between cognitive skills in the first two years of life and IQ measured in later childhood (McCall, 1979). Studies of genetic influences on intelligence also support discontinuity, in that genetic influences on early cognitive measures are weak, but are much stronger for intelligence when assessed for older children (Plomin, 1986). Finally, the family environment for preschool children between ages 2 and 5 apparently has a greater effect on intelligence than it does in infancy (Rutter, 1985).

Others (Bornstein and Sigman, 1986) have shown that discontinuity in intellectual development is influenced by which specific cognitive skills are being evaluated in infants. Infant coping with novelty does predict later intelligence in that infants who are curious about novel stimuli tend to show the highest IQ results later. For example, infants who rapidly lose interest in familiar stimuli but regain interest when engaged with a new stimulus tend to show higher IQ levels in later life. A correlation of 0.5 has been recorded using methods that assess response to novelty at 6 months with IQ at school entry, whereas there is almost no correlation using standardized test scores. These results suggest that intellectual development in infants needs to be viewed in the context of their interest and curiosity about their surroundings in addition to standardized testing and that there may be less discontinuity in general intelligence than previously considered (Rutter and Rutter, 1993).

COGNITIVE DEVELOPMENTAL THEORIES

Developmental differences in intelligence are most strikingly shown in the stages of intellec-

tual growth. Clinical psychological testing approaches, or psychometrics, have emphasized the increase in children's cognitive abilities as they grow older. Following the development of the standardized general intelligence test, Piaget (1952), Vygotsky (1978, 1987), and Werner (1948; Werner and Kaplan, 1963) are the developmental theorists who have addressed cognitive development most specifically.

Piaget's Theory

Piaget's interest in cognitive growth was initially stimulated by his curiosity about why children at a particular age gave the same wrong answers to standardized questions. This led him to investigate cognitive development from the perspective of how children come to know (genetic epistemology). Piaget observed children's approaches to problem solving and talked to them about how they solved particular problems. His emphasis was on the styles of cognitive performance rather than on the levels of cognitive achievement. Utilizing this approach, he suggested that there are several successive developmental periods.

The first is the *sensorimotor period,* which occurs in the first two years of life. Here, before children have mental representation ability, the approach to learning is by trial and error. This is followed by a phase referred to as *"preoperational thinking,"* where the child is able to construct internal representations. These are demonstrated in language or make-believe play at a time when learning is perceptually dominated. Children in the preoperational phase do not formulate rules or concepts. Around ages 5 to 7, Piaget describes the next stage, that of *concrete operations,* as primarily characterized by an ability to acquire rules that allow the child to make deductive inferences. Concurrently, he suggests, children become able to appreciate others' points of view and understand the significance of rules in social situations and in competitive games. Finally, there is the stage of *formal operations,* which is initiated at the beginning of adolescence and is accompanied by an ability to engage in abstract manipulation of propositions, to formulate hypotheses, and to make deductions.

Inhelder (1968) in her book *The Diagnosis of Reasoning in the Mentally Retarded* applied Piaget's stages to mentally retarded persons and concluded that there were arrests in the development of cognition such that profoundly mentally retarded persons (IQ<25) did not regularly progress beyond sensorimotor mental functioning, severely mentally retarded persons (IQ 25 to 40) achieved early preoperational levels, and moderately mentally retarded persons (IQ 40 to 55) reached later preoperational abilities. Finally, the mildly mentally retarded (IQ 55 to 70) only developed concrete operational abilities.

In Piaget's view, the child functions as a scientist who solves problems, and development progresses as the child manipulates his or her environment and then actively works to develop more rational, logical, and abstract modes of thought. The importance of maturation in the child's experience in his or her physical and social environments was recognized by Piaget. However, the child's own internal activities and self-regulatory processes are crucial in his theory of intellectual development. Intelligence functions to assist the child to adapt to the environment, and movement from one stage of intellectual development to the next results from the child's actively working toward adaptation through processes referred to as *"equilibrium."* Equilibrium for Piaget involves three phases. First, the child's mode of thought must be adequate to confront or adapt to the challenges of the environment; when this occurs, the child is in a state of equilibrium. In transitions from one stage to the next, disequilibrium occurs due to shortcomings in the child's mode of thought when new challenges that are beyond the child's cognitive level occur. Faced with these challenges, the child attempts to restore equilibrium through the processes of assimilation, or modification of the environment to fit existing cognitive structures, and accommodation, the changing of one's own cognitive structures to fit the new environmental challenge. Taken together, assimilation and accommodation result in a higher level of thought, which allows the child to reach mastery and adapt and move to the next stage of development to restore equilibrium. The equilibrium model was developed to explain how structural change takes place from one stage to the next and to describe how competence for specific reasoning develops.

Current Perspective on Piaget

Much of Piaget's original research has been revised as it has been systematically tested. His view that the child is an active agent in learning and the importance of this activity in cognitive development continues to be emphasized. Infants do actively scan their environment, choosing patterned over nonpatterned stimuli and novel over familiar stimuli. Older children, through their questions and comments, constantly construct schemes of what they know and try to fit their new knowledge to these schemes. The role of imitation and mastery in learning has been demonstrated for both children and animals. On the other hand, the suggestion that development follows a series of discrete stages that are followed in an unvarying order has been revised (Brainerd, 1978; Case, 1985). There is more flexibility in development than is suggested by Piaget's approach. Still, the establishment of cognitive structures is an important aspect of cognitive performance. Specific cognitive processes seem to underlie how children deal with cognitive problems, and these structures change qualitatively as well as quantitatively with increasing age.

Although the specifics of cognitive structure that were proposed by Piaget have not been substantiated by empirical research, the majority of neo-Piagetian and other cognitive theorists acknowledge the general notion of underlying or deep structures (Demetriou and Efklides, 1987; Sternberg and Powell, 1983; Gelman and Baillargeon, 1983). One model (Pascual-Leone, 1987) emphasizes units of mental attentional capacity and suggests that qualitative changes in style of thought depend on quantitative increases in these units. Another theorist, Case (1987), accepts that there is quantitative change but indicates that several informational processes are needed to regulate cognitive performance.

Piaget's (1952; Inhelder and Piaget, 1958) investigations dealt primarily with genetic epistemology and did not focus specifically on the role of the social world in providing structure to reality and in helping the child to make sense of it. The main line of Piaget's approach emphasized how the child invented operations to understand physical reality, and these were presented in broad, logical categories rather than addressing specific features of a problem.

Although he did discuss social roles, particularly in relationship to peer interactions in middle childhood, Piaget did not emphasize how children's interactions with companions contributed to their cognitive development. Instead, he placed considerable emphasis on the cognitive development of the solitary and curious child. Piaget provided detailed descriptions of the states differentiating children's thought at various ages rather than specifying the mechanisms responsible for levels of development. Case seeks to unite Piagetian and information processing theories of development. He recognizes automatization and biologically based increases in working memory with maturation as essential in increasing the capacity to process information (Case, 1985). He suggests that cognitive growth results from changes in the amount of information that can be retained in working memory (short-term) and in the acquisition of certain central conceptual structures.

THE SOCIOCULTURAL CONTEXT OF COGNITIVE DEVELOPMENT

Vygotsky's Theory

Vygotsky's (1978) methodological and theoretical orientation focused on development and historical change. Like Piaget, Vygotsky viewed the child as an active organism that worked to overcome impediments in the environment through problem solving. He studied cognitive growth in children by creating obstacles or providing alternative routes to complete tasks. He observed children as they encountered these obstacles and used aids to solve problems. By challenging them with difficult tasks, he could observe the children studied as they developed new skills. Vygotsky emphasized the importance of play, as did Piaget, and suggested that play creates opportunities for children to try new behaviors and master environmental challenges as they use their imagination to facilitate their own development. Vygotsky (1978, p. 56) suggested that "development proceeds not in a circle but in a spiral, passing through the same point at each revolution while advancing to a higher level."

Vygotsky emphasized *internalization* as an important mechanism for cognitive growth rather than equilibrium, as had Piaget. He suggested that not only does language reflect thought, but thought comes into existence through language. He further suggested that children internalize their speech, and the child's words to adults become the child's words to himself or herself and his or her own thoughts. Vygotsky emphasized those aspects of development that proceed from the social context to the individual, whereas Piaget seems to stress the aspects of development that emerge from the individual in relation to a social environment. In Vygotsky's approach, the process of internalizing social activity, such as language, leads to higher cognitive development. His approach, which focuses on the crucial role of the child's proximal environment, emphasizes individual differences and that development reflects the dynamic relations between the child and his or her particular environment, which differ among individuals and across time for the same person, whereas Piaget's developmental stages emphasize problem-solving abilities that apply universally across cultures.

The role of language is particularly important in Vygotsky's view, and he assigned a planning function to speech that anticipated the interest and attention currently placed on metacognitive skills — i.e., those involved in planning, monitoring, and evaluating performance on intellectual tasks (Sincoff and Sternberg, 1989). He proposed that development proceeds from early to later stages as a result of internalization of culturally produced sign systems, such as speech, writing, and number systems. He observed that in early speech development, speech accompanies the child's actions and reflects the variability of problem solving among children. Subsequently, speech moves more and more toward the beginnings of the process such that it comes to precede action rather than being a running commentary on action. In this way, it comes to function as an aid to a plan that has been conceived but not yet accomplished. Inner speech guides, determines, and dominates the course of action so that the planning function of speech joins the existing functions of language to reflect the external world (Vygotsky, 1978, p. 28).

With his emphasis on language, Vygotsky spoke of the crucial importance of instruction to facilitate cognitive growth and viewed intelligence as a capacity that benefits from instruction. He suggests that learning creates a *"zone of proximal development"* wherein the course of intellectual development may be followed. The zone of proximal development was described by Vygotsky (1978, p. 86) as the distance between the actual developmental level as determined by independent problem solving and the level of potential development that might be reached through problem solving under adult guidance or in collaboration with peers who are more capable. The capability of children with equal levels of mental development to learn under a teacher's guidance varies. Vygotsky emphasized that consciousness emerges out of the interaction of higher mental processes with the tool of language (Bruner, 1987, p. 3; Vygotsky, 1987).

Werner's Theory

Werner (1957) believed that development represents a "systematic, orderly sequence of events consisting of two general dimensions." The first is the pattern of different developmental levels (or stages), the second is what form development takes — i.e., is it a smooth process from one stage to the next or an abrupt transition between qualitatively different stages? The process of development involves both the organism (the mechanisms that are involved in that change) and the developmental processes (the nature of the changes that occur through ontogenesis). Werner introduced the orthogenetic principle, which provides a foundation for all developmental processes. The *orthogenetic principle* states that "whenever development occurs, it proceeds from a state of relative globality and lack of differentiation to a state of increasing differentiation, articulation, and hierarchic integration" (Werner, 1957, p. 126). Werner suggested that the developmental process progresses from a global whole to discrete yet integrated systems (uniformity versus multiformity). Moreover, he described development as smooth or discontinuous (continuity versus discontinuity) in its course of change, as the extension of a general group of individual thrusts (unilinearity versus multilinearity), and as being fixed and stable, or adaptive and mobile (fixity versus mobility) (Salkind, 1985, p. 234).

For Werner (Werner and Kaplan, 1963), the mechanisms of cognitive growth, differentiation, and hierarchization are not different from mechanisms responsible for the development of the nervous system and other biological processes. Rather than emphasizing equilibrium or internalization, Werner highlighted the increasing differentiation and specialization of mental capacities and abilities, the increasing ordering, grouping, and subordination of capacities and abilities (Sincoff and Sternberg, 1989). Rather than progressing through a series of stages, development proceeds as new capacities emerge and separate out from older, more global and general capacities. Stage-related theories of development imply that once a child reaches a certain level of functioning, he or she does not revert to previous modes of thought. Werner suggests that previous modes of thought are accessible even after the differentiation of abilities occurs. The lower level then develops as an integral part of a more complex organization wherein the higher processes dominate the lower ones. Werner used a comparative approach and studied the mental life of normal children, children in primitive societies, and children with psychotic disorders. His interest in cognitive growth has considerably influenced recent developmental theorists as they evaluate developmental processes.

Recent Developments in Cognitive Development Theory

The mechanisms of cognitive development suggested by Piaget's findings are often difficult to replicate, particularly in regard to the ages when children master specific tasks. Moreover, children differ in their understanding and acquisition rates of related concepts. The mode of thought characteristic of a particular stage does not necessarily apply across many types of tasks and problems. Piaget was primarily interested in universal patterns of development rather than in intellectual differences among children of the same age. Moreover, he emphasized cognitive competence rather than cognitive performance. Vygotsky did recognize and emphasize the importance of individual differences in development, but his tasks are difficult to operationalize and test. Many of his core concepts are plausible but are difficult to define in a way that they can be systematically investigated. For example, the processes involved in internalization are difficult to assess because they involve a series of transformations. Finally, Werner's emphasis on differentiation and hierarchical mechanisms provides a global approach that also is difficult to define and to operationalize for specific testing.

Despite the difficulty in operationalizing their specific approaches, these three theorists have stimulated considerable interest in understanding cognitive development. More recent cognitive studies have drawn on their models but use different techniques, such as information processing methodologies and computer simulation. Fischer (1980) proposed a stage theory of skill learning in which the child's thinking develops through the activation of five transformational rules. Siegler (1981, 1984, 1991) has introduced an information processing account of development of intellectual skills that stresses the importance of encoding and strategy implementation. Sternberg (1984, 1985) has suggested a three-part theory of the development of intelligence that emphasizes the relations among the child's internal information processing components, his or her experience, and his or her environment. Keil (1981, 1984) emphasizes the importance of domain-specific knowledge structures and representations. He asserts that development proceeds through general, all-purpose cognitive processes that restructure specific knowledge. Keil's work suggests constraints on development that limit a child's cognitive competence, which may have educational implications. He proposes that humans, as biological organisms, have developed specialized "mental organs" that they have come to use through the course of evolution to solve problems in their physical and mental world.

Two general categories of constraints are organismic and domain-related (Sincoff and Sternberg, 1989). Organismic constraints may be both age-related and cognitive. Those stage theorists (Piaget and Vygotsky) who specify that cognitive abilities are linked to specific age ranges impose age-related constraints that limit the rate and type of development from infancy to adolescence. Cognitive constraints refer to differences in the rate of intellectual growth in childhood as distinct from adulthood. In addition, the functional capacity of the child's working, or short-term, memory provides constraints on cognition with age (Case, 1974 and Chi, 1976). Those theorists concerned with

knowledge emphasize domain-related limitations, that is, limitations in acquiring knowledge within a cognitive domain, such as mathematics. For example, Sternberg (1984) suggests that there may be constraints within a domain of knowledge when novelty is introduced. A child who is skilled in multiplication or division may have difficulty when fractions are introduced, but once understood, information processing becomes automatized and the domain-related constraint created by novelty vanishes. Thus, limited knowledge in a specific domain constrains cognitive development, and cognitive growth consists of overcoming these constraints through acquiring new knowledge and reorganizing it. Carey (1985) emphasizes the emergence of new knowledge structures from the reorganization and expansion of older ones.

Thus, current theories of cognitive growth continue to evaluate older theories and to emphasize new approaches based on new knowledge of the cognitive sciences. Current areas of emphasis are the organizing principles in development, specific cognitive processes (executive processing and nonexecutive processing), the role of knowledge in cognitive growth, how individual differences arise, the issue of context (the role of experience in intellectual development and the role of specific environments on development), and constraints on development (organismic constraints and domain-related constraints) (Sincoff and Sternberg, 1989). The problem of cognitive growth requires an integration of each of these approaches. Such integration must take into account motivation and social cognition (Fiske and Taylor, 1984). Sincoff and Sternberg (1989) suggest a heuristic model, shown in Figure 13–1, to integrate each of these considerations. Although other models might be proposed, cognitive growth involving information processing of experience requires continual acquisition and reorganization of knowledge. Both participation in early life events and interpretation of these events are crucial to cognitive growth. In the figure, the interactions shown involve information processing, experiences, and knowledge.

As shown in the figure, metacognitive processes include planning, self-monitoring, and self-evaluation to govern nonexecutive processes. These include information that is perceived, encoded, and stored in working memory; organized and compared with older information through combination and comparison; and synthesized to provide a response. This allows the acquisition and reorganization of procedural knowledge and declarative knowledge in memory. (Procedural knowledge derives from procedural memory of the sequence of steps required to accomplish a task, i.e., production rules. Declarative knowledge refers to factual information.) Moreover, executive functions utilize the output from other modules, such as the phonological module, which is involved in language. Working memory constrains information processing because its usable capacity for short-term storage determines the extent and nature of information processing. However, with more efficient processing, the demands placed on memory are reduced. More efficient processing may occur as automatization of familiar responses takes place, which increases the operational efficiency of working memory. With practice dealing with repeated experiences and similar types of problems, processing becomes faster and more efficient.

The child's cultural and social environment plays an important role in determining experiences—not only the types of experiences but also the value placed on them. The processing of experiences leads to reorganization as new knowledge is acquired (Siegler, 1991). Siegler's model of strategy construction implies the automatization of processing—linking experience and knowledge so that automatized information is directly retrieved rather than actively reprocessed. Finally, the figure shows that knowledge or absence of knowledge about types of problems may influence feelings about those problems and either facilitate or inhibit motivation for continuing to seek out more experience for information processing. Although the diagram separates information processing from motivation, it may not be possible to clearly separate cognitive and affective systems as shown.

Cognitive growth proceeds from an interaction between a child's experience and processing its information content. Rapidly increasing stores of procedural and declarative knowledge contribute to further growth and denote the level of the child's development. With cognitive growth, knowledge from various domains is acquired and organized. As children grow older, their intellec-

tual skills become more distinct and are applied not only to academic problem solving but also to interpersonal problem solving (social cognition) and to the discrimination of affective states. Individual differences may emerge that result from differences in experiences, educational background, and practice experience in a variety of problem areas and lead to different knowledge bases for each individual child.

Cognitive growth is dynamic in nature, and various developmental mechanisms will assume importance at different points in time, as indicated earlier. Metacognitive processing refers to those executive functions that guide problem solving and intellectual activity through planning, monitoring, and evaluating performance on specific cognitive tasks. The ability to assemble higher levels of executive control over behavior and problem solving characterizes cognitive change with increasing age. Thus, metacognitive processing assumes greater importance for older children than younger ones, as the former spend more time planning solutions to problems, whereas younger children utilize nonexecutive processing to a greater extent in knowledge acquisition and reorganization. Metacognitive abilities are important in the regulation of cognitive performance and are not available to very young children. It is debatable whether these abilities begin as a qualitative change that emerges in an all-or-none manner and spans all cognitive domains. An alternative is that they may be content-driven and context-specific, so individual children may vary in the extent to which these skills are available, depending on the type of tasks performed and the context in which the task must be accomplished. Still, cross-cultural studies do demonstrate that broadly similar cognitive progress does occur in different cultures and that maturational processes most probably play a key role in ongoing cognitive development. In addition, experience plays an important role in cognitive growth for comprehensive knowledge in a specific domain to be acquired—i.e., experience is more important in how knowledge is reorganized when little is known about a domain than when a larger knowledge base has been previously consolidated. The rate and extent of the acquisition of knowledge and its reorganization may be more substantial during childhood and adolescence because it is during these years that

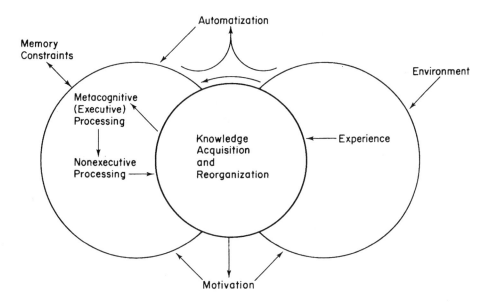

Figure 13–1. A heuristic model for integrating the theoretical considerations necessary for understanding cognitive growth. In this figure, interactions between the child's information processing and his or her experiences lead to continued acquisition and reorganization of knowledge. The figure is shown as a Venn diagram to emphasize the interactions among the child's information processing, experiences and knowledge (from Sincoff and Sternberg, 1989).

knowledge structures are first organized and consolidated (Sincoff and Sternberg, 1989). Being exposed to large amounts of information as language is acquired may be necessary for these knowledge structures to adequately develop. To facilitate cognitive growth, each of the interacting systems shown in the figure must be considered.

Sternberg and Powell (1983) have reviewed information processing models, suggesting seven key features: (1) the knowledge base, (2) the range of cognitive processes available, (3) memory capacity, (4) strategies employed, (5) efficiency of representations of information, (6) process latencies and difficulties; and (7) executive control. These authors indicate that the range of cognitive processes available changes with age so that metacognitive skills, which allow comprehension of second- and third-order relationships, do not develop until early adolescence. Moreover, as children grow older, they tend to use more comprehensive strategies that take account of more available information. Mastery of more difficult tasks are also

accomplished with increasing age, as is the executive control ability to think about one's own thinking to decide how to approach a problem.

Overall, intellectual development apparently involves the growth of increasingly sophisticated executive control strategies, the emergence of the ability to comprehend higher-order relationships, more thoroughness in information processing, and greater flexibility in the use of various strategies to account for and process more information. Cognitive development presumes the emergence of specific cognitive skills based on proposed underlying structures.

Domains of Thinking

Moreover, cognitive processes may differ depending on the domain of thinking involved and the specifics of the task context. Recent studies in cognitive development have shifted their focus to consider advances in skills and knowledge in particular domains in addition to increases in general cognitive capacity (Feldman, 1980; Fischer, 1980; Rogoff, 1982; Siegler, 1981). From this perspective, cognitive development involves the enhancement of skills and knowledge in particular domains rather than simply increased general capacity. Recent research in cognitive development focuses on the definition of specific problems and the goal structures of the particular skill being developed. The topics addressed include language and the development of academic skills, such as reading, writing, and mathematics, which have been considered to be separate from basic cognitive processes, such as attention and memory. Research efforts focused on this view of cognitive development have focused on analysis of task requirements and descriptions of the transformations in thinking that take place as part of the learning of particular skills. Using these approaches, the study of cognitive development is tied more to specific cognitive performances without assuming that the skills and problems of thinking are inherent.

Context is given a central position in cognitive development, and cognitive developmental sequences are defined in terms of the efforts made by the child along with the domain of the particular problem being approached. This definition of cognition limits the consideration of context to the structure or features of the task involved or the domain of knowledge being approached. This more extensive view of cognition and context suggests that task characteristics and cognitive performance may be viewed in regard to the goal of the activity and its interpersonal and sociocultural context. Here, the purpose of thinking is that it leads to effective action. Activities are goal-directed, and the goals are defined socially and culturally.

The types of problems that are solved, the knowledge resources, and effective solutions are viewed as situated in a social matrix of values and purposes. The individual uses cognition based on sociocultural definitions of the problems to be solved. Solutions to problems occur in social situations, which define the problems and offer learning opportunities based on social interaction. In this regard, children act as "apprentices in thinking" (Rogoff, 1990) and are active in their efforts to learn from observing and participating with peers and adults as they develop skills to handle culturally defined problems and build from their mastery to construct new solutions. Children's cognitive development is then embedded in the context of social relationships; children take an active role in making use of social guidance. Yet social guidance takes place in many settings, so the child's participation is not necessarily perceived by the child as instructional, although interactional learning occurs. Differences in the goals for development vary among cultures as children use companions and adults for learning through explanation, discussion, modeling, joint participation, and active observation. Rogoff (1990) refers to this as guided participation in describing the sociocultural learning process. Guided participation involves children and their caregivers and peer companions in joint processes to build bridges from their present understanding to reach new understanding. Children's participation in activities is arranged and structured with gradual changes based on new capacities as the child matures. Intersubjectivity is basic to guided participation. Intersubjectivity emphasizes the active nature of thinking and problem solving rather than considering cognition as the passive possession of information. The child explores and solves problems rather than simply acquiring skills or memories.

In summary, cognitive development specifically addresses problem solving and the integration of mental processes. It includes remembering, planning, and categorizing as parts of problem solving and includes cognitive processes that have sometimes been referred to as skills, such as writing and calculating, and processes involved in reaching interpersonal goals, such as constructing narratives and using others for help in reaching goals (Rogoff, 1990). A goal-directed approach to cognition integrates cognitive, affective, and social processes to reach those goals as Vygotsky (1987) pointed out when he wrote that "thought . . . is not born of other thoughts. Thought has its origin in the motivating sphere of consciousness, a sphere which includes our inclinations and needs, our interests and impulses, and our affect and emotion. The affective and volitional tendency stands behind thought. Only here do we find the answer to the final 'why' in the analysis of thinking."

REFERENCES

Bornstein, M.H., and Sigman, M.D. (1986). Continuity in mental development from infancy. *Child Development*, 57:251–274.

Brainerd, C.J. (1978). The stage question in cognitive developmental theory. *Behavioral and Brain Sciences*, 1:173–213.

Bruner, J. (1987). Prologue. In R.W. Rieber and A.S. Carton (eds), *The collected works of L.S. Vygotsky*, Vol. 1, *Problems of general psychology*, p. 3. Plenum Press, New York.

Carey, S. (1985). *Conceptual change in childhood.* MIT Press, Cambridge, MA.

Case, R. (1974). Mental strategies, mental capacities, and instruction: A neo-Piagetian investigation. *Journal of Experimental Child Psychology*, 18:372–397.

––––––. (1985). *Intellectual development: Birth to adulthood.* Academic Press, Orlando.

––––––. (1987). The structure and process of intellectual development. *International Journal of Psychology*, 22:571–607.

Chi, M.T.H. (1976). Short-term memory limitations in children: Capacity or processing deficits? *Memory and Cognition*, 4:559–572.

Demetriou, A. and Efklides, A. (1987). Experiential structuralism and neo-Piagetian theories toward an integrated model. *International Journal of Psychology*, 22:679–728.

Feldman, D.H. (1980). *Beyond universals in cognitive development.* Ablex, Norwood, NJ.

Fischer, K.W. (1980). A theory of cognitive development: The control and construction of hierarchies of skills. *Psychological Review*, 87:477–531.

Fiske, S.T., and Taylor, S.E. (1984). *Social cognition.* Random House, New York.

Gelman, R., and Baillargeon, R. (1983). In J.H. Flavell and E.M. Markman (eds), *Cognitive development* (Vol. 3 of *Mussen's handbook of child psychology*, 4th ed.) John Wiley & Sons, New York.

Gregory, R.L. (ed.) (1987). *The Oxford companion to the mind.* Oxford University Press, New York.

Inhelder, B. (1968). *The diagnosis of reasoning in the mentally retarded.* John Day, New York. (originally published in 1943).

––––––, and Piaget. J. (1958). *The growth of logical thinking from childhood to adolescence.* Basic Books, New York.

Keil, F.C. (1981). Constraints on knowledge and cognitive development. *Psychological Review*, 88:197–227.

––––––. (1984). Mechanisms of cognitive development and the structure of knowledge. In R.J.

Sternberg (ed), *Mechanisms of cognitive development.* W.H. Freeman, New York.

McCall, R.B. (1979). The development of intellectual functioning in infancy and the prediction of later IQ. In J.D. Osofsky (ed), *Handbook of infant development*, pp. 707–741. John Wiley & Sons, New York.

Pascual-Leone, J.A. (1987). Organismic processes for neo-Piagetian theories: A dialectic casual account of cognitive development. *International Journal of Psychology*, 22:531–570.

Piaget, J. (1952). *The origins of intelligence in children.* W.W. Norton, New York.

Plomin, R. (1986). *Development, genetics and psychology.* Lawrence Erlbaum, Hillsdale, NJ.

Rogoff, B. (1982). Integrating context and cognitive development. In M.E. Lamb and A.L. Brown (eds), *Advances in developmental psychology*, Vol. 2. Lawrence Erlbaum, Hillsdale, NJ.

––––––. (1990). *Apprenticeship in thinking: Cognitive development in social context*, p. 17. Oxford University Press, New York.

Rutter, M. (1985). Family and school influences on cognitive development. *Journal of Child Psychology and Psychiatry*, 26:683–704.

––––––. and Rutter, M. (1993). *Developing minds: Challenge and continuity across the life span.* Basic Books, New York.

Salkind, N.J. (1985). Organismic model: Orthogenesis and dialectics. In N.J. Salkind (ed), *Theories of human development*, p. 225. John Wiley & Sons, New York.

Siegler, R.S. (1981). Developmental sequences within and between concepts. *Monographs of the Society for Research in Child Development*, 46 (2, Serial No. 189):1–70.

––––––. (1984). Mechanisms of cognitive growth: Variation and selection. In R.J. Sternberg (ed), *Mechanisms of cognitive development.* W.H. Freeman, New York.

––––––. (1991). *Children's thinking.* Prentice Hall, Englewood Cliffs, NJ.

Sincoff, J.B. and Sternberg, R.J. (1989). The development of cognitive skills: An examination of recent theories. In A.M. Colley and J.R. Beech (eds), *Acquisition and performance of cognitive skills*, pp. 19–60. John Wiley & Sons, New York.

Sternberg, R.J. (1984). Mechanisms of cognitive development: A componential approach. In R.J. Sternberg (ed), *Mechanisms of cognitive development.* W.H. Freeman, New York.

––––––. (1985). *Beyond IQ: A triarchic theory of human intelligence.* Cambridge University Press, Cambridge, MA.

––––––, and Powell, J.S. (1983). The development of

intelligence. In P.H. Mussen (series ed) and J.H. Flavell and E.M. Markman (volume eds), *Handbook of child psychology,* 3rd ed., Vol. 3. John Wiley & Sons, New York.

Vygotsky, L.S. (1978). *Mind in society: The development of higher psychological processes.* Harvard University Press, Cambridge, MA.

_____. (1987). Thinking and speech. In R.W. Rieber and A.S. Carton (eds), *The collected works of L.S. Vygotsky* (transl. N. Minick). Plenum Press, New York.

Werner, H. (1948). *Comparative psychology of men-tal development.* International Universities Press, New York.

_____. (1957). The concept of development from a comparative and organismic point of view. In D.B. Harris (ed), *The concept of development,* pp. 125–148. University of Minnesota Press, Minneapolis.

_____, and Kaplan, H. (1963). *Symbolic formation: An organismic-developmental appraoch to language and the expression of thought.* John Wiley & Sons, New York.

CHAPTER 14

EMOTION EXPRESSION AND REGULATION

Darwin (1872), in his classic text *The Expression of the Emotions in Man and Animals,* documented the innateness and universality of facial expression of emotion and suggested that there is a universal repertoire of emotional expression. He believed, and it is now widely accepted, that there is a consensus in various cultures as to the meaning of emotional expression. Although rooted in our mammalian heritage, human emotional expression shows a greater range and considerably more plasticity than that of other species. The study of emotions is a key to understanding human motivation and adaptation. The emergence of emotion in evolution is of importance in the development of emotional bonds and in the study of temperament and personality development. The term "affect" is used to describe a pattern of observable behaviors that express subjectively experienced feeling states based on emotion. Normal affective expression is shown by variability in facial expression, voice tone, and expressive hand and body movements.

In the study of emotion, consideration must be given to how emotions are displayed or expressed through bodily activities (e.g., facial expression and postures signifying emotion). The next consideration is how emotions are regulated, inhibited, or controlled. Is emotion a direct outcome of brain activity, or is it regulated through cognitive processing, or do both occur? This chapter discusses these issues from a developmental perspective.

AFFECT THEORY

Tomkins (1962, 1963, 1991, 1992) expanded Darwin's observations on the expression of emotion in man and animals into an affect theory. Tomkins chose the term "affect" rather than "emotion" for the group of nine innate mechanisms he described because this term is used more commonly in the psychodynamic literature. He outlined nine innate affects believed to be triggered by alterations of physiologic parameters, such as the intensity and steadiness of central nervous system activation. According to Nathanson (1993), in affect theory, an innate affect is seen as an analogic amplifier of its stimulus condition. It calls attention to anything with which it becomes associated. In describing these innate mechanisms, two-word names are given. The first indicates the milder presentation of the affect, the second its most intense presentation. The affect *interest-excitement* is triggered by an increase in certain kinds of information, such as the experience of novelty. Mild interest is associated with a furrowed brow, which may be associated with paying specific attention to something. A description of the affect and the concurrent facial appearance is shown in the accompanying Table 14–1.

In the higher ranges of activity, with excitement, attention is intentionally focused on the stimulus. *Interest-excitement* would represent an analogic amplification related to an optimal rise in the stimulus density. If too much infor-

Table 14–1. The Innate Affects

Positive
  1. Interest-excitement
     Eyebrows down, track, look, listen
  2. Enjoyment-joy
     Smile, lips widened and out

Neutral
  3. Surprise-startle
     Eyebrows up, eyes blink

Negative
  4. Fear-terror
     Frozen stare, face pale, cold, sweaty, hair erect
  5. Distress-anguish
     Cry, rhythmic sobbing, arched eyebrows, mouth
     down
  6. Anger-rage
     Frown, clenched jaw, red face
  7. Shame-humiliation
     Eyes down, head down and averted, blush
  8. Dissmell
     Upper lip raised, head pulled back
  9. Disgust
     Lower lip lowered and protruded, head forward
     and down

From Tomkins, 1962; summarized by Nathanson, 1993.

mation is presented, the affect *fear-terror* is the programmed response and the facial appearance changes, with the eyes frozen in a stare and a pale face. On the other hand, information that comes to the infant more rapidly and then stops, such as a hand clap, may trigger *surprise-startle,* which is the analogic amplifier of a sudden or abrupt stimulus. This affect is brief, so it cannot be said to have any positive or negative quality of itself. Surprise indicates readiness to evaluate whatever has taken our attention, whether it is pleasant or unpleasant. The relief of a preexisting stimulus may produce a pleasant feeling. Tomkins refers to this affect as *enjoyment-joy,* which represents a common analogic amplification of the decrease in the stimulus. Milder arousal leads to a smile or pleasure, and a sudden decrease produces laughter. Affects are thought to match their stimulus in many ways so that sudden rise and fall of surprise-startle is recognized. Another stimulus with constant density, such as rhythmic crying or sobbing, is referred to as *distress-anguish.* Finally, if the stimulus is of constant density and even higher than necessary to produce the affect of distress, the innate affect of *anger-rage* results. During life, the amplified

analogs of high density constant stimulation include facial displays, such as a frown, clenched teeth, and reddening of the face in anger.

In Tomkin's view, there are two positive affects, namely, interest-excitement and enjoyment-joy; a neutral affect, surprise-startle; and six negative affects, fear-terror, distress-anguish, anger-rage, shame-humiliation, dissmell, and disgust. Each of these has a triggering stimulus and facial display. The affect *shame-humiliation* is thought to have evolved as an auxiliary to the affect system. Shame affect interrupts the interest or enjoyment, amplifying what had been going on by producing a change in muscle tone, gaze, and the blush. Finally, *dissmell* and *disgust* relate to environmental stimuli. They are initially triggered by food that smells or tastes bad and provide a primitive mechanism of rejection. Subsequently, they assume an interpersonal quality to maintain interpersonal distance.

DEVELOPMENT OF EMOTION EXPRESSION

The expression of emotion has been investigated in a variety of developmental studies. Izard et al. (1980) found that infants from 1 to 9 months of age showed facial expressions that could be discriminated when they were filmed while engaged in a variety of life experiences including playing with mother, receiving an injection, and other routine situations. The authors recorded emotional expressions of interest, surprise, sadness, happiness, fear, contempt, anger, and disgust. Independent raters agreed on the distinctness of emotions when shown slide pictures of these infants depicting various emotional states. Moreover, the infant's expression was linked to the context of the social situation. Expressions of emotion were both selective and discrete.

Such facial expressions as anger (eyebrows together making a vertical line, eyelids tensed, mouth compressed) and surprise (arched eyebrows, rounded eyes, and open mouth) were reliably identified. The authors suggest that these expressions begin from the first days of life and are not learned but are innate. The expressions are not imitated, but rather are released in specific eliciting situations that automatically produce them. Additionally, an infant can recognize that a facial expression goes with a particular tone of voice (Walker-Andrews, 1986). When presented with the sound of a happy or angry voice, infants tend to discriminate the face matching the voice. After ten weeks of age, an infant reacts differently depending on the mother's facial expression, whether it is happy or sad. This suggests that an infant not only responds to the mother's facial configuration but may attribute meaning to that expression. Buhler (1930) suggested that an infant responds to a pretend angry face as a game or joke and, once becoming accustomed to the pretend face, responds positively rather than negatively. Infants (Termine and Izard, 1988) also are more likely to turn away and play less with toys if the mother looks sad, or to freeze if she looks angry. This suggests a meaningful response to the mother's expression and not simple imitation. When the caretaker demonstrates an emotional expression toward a stranger, the infant is cued as to how to respond to that person.

Emotional expressions (facial and vocal) serve as cues to an infant faced with uncertainty. An infant who is uncertain will hesitate and look to his mother's face. The parent's expression encourages affective expression by the infant or inhibits it. The response to the facial expression is a specific rather than a general expression and may address a specific environmental object or event. This has been demonstrated through visual cliff experiments where the infant comes to a transparent plastic section of a table — the visual cliff. The infant will hesitate and then, on a signal from the mother, go over a visual cliff to her (Bradshaw, Campos, and Klinnert, 1986). The mother signals a happy face or a fearful one, and the infant shows a selective and appropriate response to these different facial expressions. The infant is also cued by the adult's expression toward events in the environment. By 9 months, the infant has begun to selectively point and by 12 months shakes the head "no," now showing nonverbal behavior more specifically. By a year, an infant can engage in a social dialogue and respond to an emotional expression. It is this moment-to-moment specific focusing and continuous self-referencing that maintains behavior. The sequence is from an initial adjustment of social behavior to emotional cues by the caretaker and selective focus on objects in the environment with an awareness of the adult's emotional response. Awareness of the intentionality of the emotion is conveyed to the infant. Approach and avoidance, encouragement and discouragement on the infant's part are responses to the emotional message provided by the adult.

The affective mechanisms involved in social referencing are unclear. The nativist explanation by Darwin (1872) suggests that there is an instinct for sympathy, an innate sense that tells the infant which feeling is being expressed by the adult and an instinctual arousal of the same feeling in the infant or child. Another view is that facial expressions have different behavioral consequences. For example, smiling faces are followed by good consequences and frightened faces by negative consequences. The adult's response, for example, smiling, elicits an appropriate positive emotion from the child. Laird (1974) has postulated that the development of affective expressions may be related to a feedback process, suggesting that when children imitate a facial expression of an adult, they receive feedback from their own facial muscles, which then leads to recognition of the emotional state. The infant might then come to associate his or her own facial expression with a particular emotional state. Laird's suggestions would indicate that facial expression is initially neutral without any affective meaning and subsequently acquires meaning for the child. However, his explanation is questionable because it is more likely that affective arousal precedes the facial muscle changes.

Harris (1989) suggests that an awareness of emotional expression (facial and vocal) is important for infants to begin to understand mental states of other people. Because there is a universal repertoire of discrete facial expressions, recognition of emotions may be the first step in becoming aware of the mental states in others. The infant's social behavior changes in an appropriate way, not simply in imitation of responses to the caretaker's facial expressions, after about 10 weeks of age. By the end of the first year, the infant may attach emotional meaning to objects in the immediate environment and can be cued by an adult in regard to the response to those objects. The beginning of social understanding seems to involve this initial awareness of emotional expression, which seems to help regulate the infant's social responsiveness to environmental experiences. As infants socially reference the adult, they begin to understand the intentionality and direction of the adult's emotional responses, although initially they do not bring about emotion but rather respond to it in others.

During the second year of life, there is an increase in social understanding. Children begin to comfort others and attempt to reduce others' distress. They may also provoke difficulties through teasing, physically hurting, and showing nuisance behavior. Children's awareness of their effects on others suggests that they are beginning to understand how their behavior can initiate, inhibit, or reduce the emotional state of another person. Efforts to change an emotional state among siblings have been studied by Dunn, Kendrick, and MacNamee (1981) and Dunn and Kendrick (1982). These authors studied child-sibling interactions and found that children may be helpful toward siblings, neutral toward them, seem to enjoy a sibling's distress, or become upset themselves when the sibling is upset.

Hoffer and Badzinski (1989) carried out developmental studies that may be pertinent when they studied children's integration of facial and situational cues to emotion. Children at four age levels (3 to 5, 6 to 7, 8 to 9, and 10 to 12) were shown pictures in which facial and situational cues were conflicting, congruent, or presented alone. The child was asked to rate whether the situation was happy or sad and the intensity of the emotion felt by characters in the pictures. There were developmental changes in the weights assigned to facial and situational cues, indicating that children's reliance on situational cues increased with age and reliance on facial expression decreased with age. There was a developmental increase in the tendency to integrate facial and situational cues. The child's ability to resolve the conflicting cues through stories increased with age. However, there were no age differences in the types of resolutions that were used. Children at all age levels were less likely to resolve pictures that involved inconsistent positive expression than pictures showing inconsistent negative expression. These investigations and others suggest that children's ability to interpret emotional

communications and their ability to decode nonverbal emotional cues may affect their ability to empathize with others and may be necessary for successful interpersonal relationships. As children age, they become better at detecting and interpreting nonverbal messages that are discrepant. They come to understand and infer how other people feel by considering how most people respond in a particular situation. Both situational and expressive cues are indicators of other's emotions, and their integration is a developmental advance in social understanding. In the study mentioned, 89% of the 3- to 5-year-olds focused almost entirely on facial expression and 67% of the next age group relied more on facial expression than using both facial and situational cues. By 8 to 9, the majority of subjects responded to both facial and situational cues. The developmental shift is from reliance on facial expression to simultaneous use of both situational and facial expression. Emotions are characterized by unique patterns of facial movements and the relationship between facial expression and common emotions, such as happy and sad, is present in infants, yet because the same emotion may be elicited in a variety of different situations and some situations may elicit more than one emotion, basing judgments on situations requires more complex processing. Children's stories also reflect how they interpreted emotions in that younger children's stories mentioned only facial expression, whereas older children suggested that the emotion was consistent with the particular situation.

EMOTION REGULATION

Although emotion regulation is closely related to social understanding, the emotional response to the environmental stimuli occurs at several levels. Lang (1968) proposed a tripartite model to account for them. The first level is neurophysiological or biochemical. Although many systems are involved, the most clearly understood responses take place in the autonomic nervous system and in psychoneuroendocrine activation. These include heart rate variability — i.e., vagal tone (parasympathetic activation) (Porges, 1991), endocrine response, and cortisol measurement in blood or saliva (Gunnar, 1986). Heart rate and vagal tone have been used as

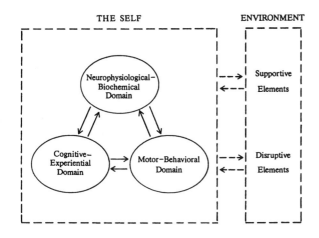

THE SELF   ENVIRONMENT

Figure 14–1. A scheme for conceptualizing the regulation of emotion. Emotion regulation is organized into three domains as shown (from Dodge and Garber, 1991).

indicators of the state of emotional response and as trait indicators of temperament. Changes in adrenaline and norepinephrine may have an important role in the regulation of social attachment. This has been demonstrated in rhesus monkeys where mother-deprived infants had lower levels of cerebrospinal fluid norepinephrine than mother-reared infants. Changes were also associated with social separation and social group formation, suggesting that the brain norepinephrine system appears to be sensitive to changes in the social environment (Kraemer et al., 1989; Kraemer, 1992).

The second level is the motor or behavioral expressive level. Emotional arousal or responsiveness is recognized through facial expression (frown, fear expression, happy face) (Ekman and Friesen, 1975; Izard, 1972), and through interactive expressive behavior, such as crying and nutritive sucking, play face, redirection in responding (social withdrawal) to peers, and by focusing or directing attention. These responses have also been used in describing the psychopathology of emotional expression.

A third means of emotional expression is subjective and experiential. It is found in verbal responses of feeling states provided in personal interviews (Dunn, Bretherton, and Munn, 1987). The language for emotion develops early, so words can be used to express feelings (Dunn and Brown, 1991). Children learn cognitive and behavioral strategies to alter their internal state and change their subjective experiences.

Darwin (1872) had observed that some forms of emotional expression are based on their functional and regulatory aspects (Dodge and Garber, 1991). Dodge (1989) defines emotion regulation as "the process by which activation in one response domain serves to alter, titrate, or modulate activation in another response domain."

The tripartite response model shown in Figure 14–1 suggests that emotional regulation may occur within domains, such as the regulation of the heart rate via respiratory activity, or between domains. Emotion regulation may also occur by way of interactions with the environment, which emphasizes the importance of interpersonal emotion regulation. The earliest forms of emotion regulation may involve soothing and environmental manipulation by the caregiver (Kopp, 1989). As the infant matures, he may actively involve the mother to help provide orienting information about the characteristics of an environmental event. The differentiation of affect is a developmental process that emerges from the tension between physiological and cognitive domains. Affective differentiation is also aided by the infant's involvement with the interpersonal environment.

Overall, the regulation of emotional response is a developmental accomplishment because it is not present at birth but is acquired in the early years of life. Initially (Kopp, 1989), regulation is provided by the caregiver, and one of the first developmental tasks is to transfer this control to the infant. In the first months of life, the infant discovers that certain motor activities, such as sucking, maternal contact, and hand-to-mouth activity, may modulate negative arousal states. These activities gradually are conditioned by association and become voluntary. Further development of sensory systems and motor skills enhances an infant's capacity to modulate negative states. With maturation, cognitive developments, such as selective attention, discrimination, and planning are used to regulate emotions. Each of these activities is facilitated and monitored by a caregiver. Early distress and separation cries are the first communicative signals for external regulation by the caregiver. Cries gradually evolve into nonverbal signals as the infant turns to the parent for guidance in novel or ambiguous situations.

Affective signals are the most direct forms of emotional expression as infants engage a caregiver, and infants are very sensitive to affective signals from others. Malatesta-Magai (1991) refers to these signals not simply as communicated information but as affective imperatives because affect has a "contagious" quality (Tomkins, 1962, 1963, 1991, 1992) for both partners. Behavioral expressions, such as compressing both lips or biting the lower lips, have been interpreted as efforts to regulate anger, a negative emotion. Moreover, social referencing, as described earlier, involves the infant's active movement to look at the mother during an arousing event and aids in guiding the infant's own affect and behavioral response to the event. Social referencing includes two aspects of social information processing: seeking information from another person and using it or not using it to regulate one's own behavior (Walden, 1991). Social referencing begins early in life as the infant, then preschool child, draws on observations of the behavior of others to regulate both affect and behavior. Most commonly, social referencing serves to reduce anxiety in a stressful situation, yet social referencing increasingly depends on the interpersonal context. Social context interacts with the environmental stimulus and the characteristics of the parental communicative behavior.

Infants become increasingly wary of acting without referencing their parents' responses. A mother's facial expressions of emotion influence children's behaviors differently at different stages of development and possibly utilize different mechanisms. By 6 months, social referencing is commonly used; however, older infants socially reference more frequently and more quickly. Walden (1991) suggests that infants less than 9 months of age reference primarily to check the adult's continuing presence. By the end of the first year, referencing also is to seek information. Infants of 17 or 18 months may manipulate a strange toy before referencing the mother's face, whereas children older than 18 months most commonly delay their behavior toward a strange toy until the mother's face has been referenced. With increasing age, both visual and verbal input is sought from the adult. Despite increased verbal ability, visual contact persists, perhaps because facial expression contains information not available by verbal means alone. The complexities of social references are only beginning to be understood.

Walden (1991) suggests that the time gap between the initial evaluation of an environmental stimulus or event and subsequent emotion-cognition-action sequence provides an opportunity for regulatory processes. These include obtaining information from a mother's emotional expression or for intentional, self-initiated action, such as modifying emotional expression (Izard and Kobak, 1991). Children then draw on biologically and socially based attachment relationships that foster searching for maternal guidance in situations of uncertainty as they learn intentional behaviors through experience.

As they grow older, children use language to understand and gain control over their own emotional responses and impulses. Developmentally, uninhibited anger/frustration decreases sharply in the second and declines in the third year (Goodenough, 1931). Children in the second and third year develop the ability to explain their own emotional state, to find comfort through requests to others, and to achieve their ends by persuading and deceiving others. Concurrently, there are changes in interpersonal relationships. This results in ability to control other emotional states. The role of talk about emotions and feeling states plays an important role in accomplishing this. Children use the ability to communicate feeling to regulate their affect. Stern emphasizes that with the acquisition of language children can be with others through "shared meanings."

With the growth of language ability, emotional relatedness may be enhanced and the ability to tolerate separation improved. Children increasingly influence their own emotional states and those of others and attempt to change their emotional state through others. Family discourse plays an important role in these developments.

Cognitive activity may serve to regulate emotion through the modification of emotional arousal, goals, experience, or expressive behavior. Cognitive understanding and behavioral expression of emotion interact to enhance emotion regulation. Reciprocally, cognitive activities may be altered through emotional states; in some instances, this may be regulatory, but in other instances, dysregulatory. The emergence of interpersonal dialogue is essential to reduce direct physical violence, to facilitate waiting before responding, and to control behavior in general. Cognitive controls assume additional importance in the behavioral expression of emotional responses as new cognitive capacities develop.

Finally, one would expect that an emotional system would have built-in regulatory mechanisms. Izard and Kobak (1991) suggest that emotions have the capacity to regulate one another such that anger attenuates fear and sadness, and in the process may decrease withdrawal and depressive tendencies. In addition, the individual personality with its multiple systems may have inherent regulatory mechanisms, such as the ability of the cognitive system to regulate the emotional system and, as a consequence, produce a coping strategy. In each of these instances, there is reciprocity among systems; for example, one emotion may influence perceptual and cognitive processes for information processing or appraisal, and these processes, in turn, may activate another emotion.

Intersystem Coordination: Play and Social Referencing

Play is one of the most important developmental processes involving the coordination of the various emotion regulatory systems (Izard and Kobak, 1991). The consistency with which infants and children begin to play suggests that play is partially a biological system with evolutionary roots. Playing is intentional and self-initiated, often social, and may facilitate the coordination of emotion, cognition, and action. In play, children have multiple opportunities to rehearse both verbal and motoric responses to their various emotion-feeling states. Through varieties of play, a child makes connections between feelings, thoughts, and activity. Because of the frequency in which children engage in play, it is thought to be a major setting to accomplish emotional integration.

Regulatory processes, such as active play and exercise, depend more on physical activity than do others. Play begins with simple, repetitive movements or circular reactions in infants, which help to maintain and enhance positive emotions of interest and enjoyment. Such positive emotional experiences then increase the infant's thresholds for negative emotions. Those positive emotional experiences, combined with play, create a strong emotion regulatory process or feed-forward/feed-back loop. The emotion of interest is engaged to motivate play and various aspects of play, including novelty, change, and complexity, and incongruities in themselves intensify this interest. Additional aspects of play, such as skill development and mastery of goals, produce the emotion of joy. A child's interest in the world of objects and in the social world is enhanced through the personal-environmental exchanges which take place during play.

Play involves several of the regulatory systems mentioned before, such as the play-face signal and social referencing, which occurs during exploratory play. Like other behaviors, play is influenced by ongoing social referencing. During social referencing, emotion regulation involves the coordination of several regulatory systems. The emotions that lead children to look toward the mother for additional emotional information are most likely rooted in attachment behavior. The importance of referencing is highlighted by the fact that when younger children are engaged intensively in play activities, they continue to periodically reference the parent who is nearby. The child's response to the mother's facial expression of emotion varies at different stages of development and possibly involves different mechanisms as the child grows older. The frequency and intensity of referencing may be linked to individual differences in temperament and personality, particularly related to fearfulness or shyness in children (Izard and Kobak, 1991). The child's response may also be linked to the quality of the previous relationship and intentional behaviors that are learned through life experience.

EMOTION DYSREGULATION

Emotion regulation is a developmentally acquired process, and experiences during development of children in high-risk populations may show failures in the development of emotion regulation. The effects of heightened arousal on cognitive processes have generally been found to be disruptive. Negative arousal-inducing stimuli may impair problem-solving accuracy, the ability to delay gratification, resistance to temptation, selectivity of attention, and hostile misinterpretation of others' gestures (Dodge, 1991). Tantruming, social withdrawal, and the response to severe pain may all be failures in regulation, or dysregulation. In these cases, the emotion response systems have not been able to effectively facilitate coping. Transient emotion dysregulation may occur in acute anxiety or pain states. Chronic emotion dysregulation may be evident in psychopathology; for example, in childhood depression. Such instances might be considered failures in behavioral and/or affective regulation of emotional response systems.

Aggressive conduct disorders have been considered as examples of chronic dysregulation of anger and impulsivity and also may demonstrate emotional vulnerability. "Emotional vulnerability" is a term that was coined (Masters, 1991; Masters, Felleman, and Barden, 1981) to designate children who were predisposed, because of prior socialization or temperament, to become debilitated with arousing stimuli. Aggressive children may be unable to regulate their emotional responses and utilize cognitive mechanisms to reduce their responses to provocation by peers. Moreover, aggressive children may become cognitively disorganized when provocative situations occur and show severe aggressive responses. Depressed children are demonstrating emotion dysregulation when they fail to ameliorate negative affective states. On the other hand, children who are the offspring of depressed mothers and children who have chronic depressive syndromes may not acquire effective emotion regulation strategies or may doubt their effectiveness if they attempt to implement them (Garber, Braafladt, and Zeman, 1991). Disorders of conduct and affect, when seen as failures in the development of emotion regulation, are examples of developmental psychopathology.

EMOTION REGULATION IN HIGH-RISK POPULATIONS

A developmental perspective for children with developmental neuropsychiatric disorders must consider emotion regulation and dysregulation as a central issue in their interpersonal and environmental adaptation. If development is considered as a series of qualitative reorganizations among and within behavioral and biological systems, dysregulation of these systems may lead to behavioral and emotional disorders. In normal development, through the processes of differentiation and hierarchical integration, an individual child moves from a diffuse, undifferentiated condition to a state of increasingly organized behavioral complexity (Berger, 1990; Cicchetti, Ganiban, and Barnett, 1991). Throughout this developmental process, both intrinsic and extrinsic factors interact to determine developmental outcome. Such an orientation is not linear, but rather reflects transactions between people and in the environment that both direct and reorient a course of development.

During development, there are qualitative changes in ability and in behavior that allow mastery of new developmental tasks as the growing child incorporates the previous developmental advances to meet new challenges. Failure to master and integrate earlier developmental tasks may result in incompetence or maladaptation.

Viewed from the perspective of emotion regulation, intrinsic organizational changes and central nervous system functioning — which may involve neuronal migration, establishment of neurotransmitter pathways, and cerebral hemisphere lateralization — are primary considerations. Psychologically and psychosocially, the development of cognitive, representational, and metarepresentational skills and the establishment of a coherent self system are critical to the developmental course of emotion regulation and may be dysfunctional in disabled individuals.

Social and environmental factors in emotion regulation include the parental or caregiver response to affective expression and the capacity of the caregiver to channel socialization of an affective display during social interactions (Hesse and Cicchetti, 1982; Stern, 1985). The capacity to self-monitor emotion emerges from experiences of socialization, which are linked to receptive, expressive, and pragmatic language development (Bretherton and Beeghly, 1982; Kagan, 1981). Overall, the intrinsic factors that relate to neurobiological reorganizations and the psychological factors interact with the environmental provision to establish effective emotion regulation. The major risks evolve from developmental disorders that affect brain maturation along with a continuum of caretaking casualty (Sameroff and Chandler, 1975) in which the interpersonal environment fails in helping the growing child to master emotional responsivity.

Children with Down syndrome, physically and sexually abused developmentally disabled children, and children whose parents have a major mood disorder are among the groups at risk for disorders of emotion regulation. Children with a wide variety of mental retardation syndromes are also at risk.

Due to the frequency of neurological abnormalities that influence cognitive development and the intensity of their affective expression, biological vulnerability to maladaptation is high in children and adolescents with mental retardation. Down syndrome has been extensively studied in this regard (Cicchetti and Sroufe, 1978; Ganiban, Wagner, and Cicchetti, 1990). Those children with developmental disorders who are physically and sexually abused are at even greater environmental risk for dysfunctional regulation of emotion. Their primary difficulties as they grow older relate to self-control of anger with associated aggressive impulses. This group is an important target population because self-control of aggression is a major developmental task in early childhood (Cicchetti and Schneider-Rosen, 1984).

Children with developmental disorders whose parents have a mood disorder, either unipolar mood disorder or secondary mood disorders related to difficulty adapting to the child's handicap, may show emotional adaptive responses that limit the child's mastery of emotion regulation. A depressed parent may become preoccupied with negative thoughts, have a sense of hopelessness, and feel unable to modu-late these depressed feelings and their associated thoughts. If a depressed parent is a primary caregiver, the caretaking environment may not provide the environmental support to master phases of development related to emotion regulation. Moreover, negative transactions between the child and caregiver may produce additional problems and perpetuate those already present (Cicchetti and Schneider-Rosen, 1984).

Cicchetti, Ganiban, and Barnett (1991) have emphasized several areas of potential risk in emotion regulation related to various developmental stages. The first of these is homeostatic regulation (0 to 3 months); the second is differentiation of affect and management of cognitive and physiologic tension (4 to 9 months); the third is the development of secure attachments (9 to 12 months); and the fourth is the development of the self system, which involves self-awareness and self-other differentiation (18 to 36 months). Subsequently in the preschool years, developmental tasks that involve the emergence of play behavior as an aspect of mastery, the establishment of peer relations in the school-age years, and the mastery of adolescent tasks are all important considerations in dealing with developmental disorders.

Throughout the life cycle, emotion regulation becomes increasingly complex. Affect moves from being reflexive and guided only by physiologic discomfort to a reflective phase guided by one's own internal working models of attachment figures, the self, and expectations from the environment. With age, affect regulation becomes less susceptible to environmental influences and is increasingly controlled by understanding related to personal experience. With age, emotional representation differentiates as the child becomes better able to identify affects and direct them toward particular goals. As the child grows older, developmental tasks that are age-appropriate assume increasing importance. For the developmentally disabled child, difficulties in emotion regulation are a particular concern because neurobiological, psychological, and environmental factors may interact in ways that lead to emotion dysregulation.

ACHIEVING EMOTIONAL COMPETENCE

Effective emotion regulation leads to emotional competence. Saarni (1988) defines *emotional competence* as the demonstration of self-efficacy in mastering emotion-eliciting social transactions. Emotional competence is an important element in the validation of self-esteem. With enhanced self-esteem, regulating emotional experience is easier because anxiety about self-evaluation is reduced. A variety of components and skills are necessary for the establishment of socioemotional competence. These have been outlined by Saarni (1988) to include the following: (1) awareness of one's own emotional state with the capacity to recognize the experience of multiple emotions (moreover, one recognizes that feelings out of awareness may influence behavior); (2) an ability to recognize others' emotions based on their expressive behavior and situational cues to establish their emotional meaning; (3) the capacity to use the vocabulary of emotion and emotional expressions that are common to one's subculture; (4) the capacity to establish empathetic involvement in others' emotional experiences; (5) the ability to realize that inner emotional states may occur without apparent outward physical expression both in oneself and in others; (6) awareness and recognition of cultural display rules of emotional expression; (7) an ability to understand that unique personal information about an individual must be considered when inferring their emotional state; (8) an understanding that one's own emotional expressive behavior may affect others and to consider this in presenting oneself; (9) the capacity to adaptively cope with aversive or disturbing emotions, using self-regulatory strategies that reduce the intensity or duration of these emotional states; (10) an awareness that the structure of relationships is partially defined by emotional immediacy and genuineness of emotional expression; the extent of reciprocity within the relationship and sharing genuine emotions is an important aspect; and (11) the capacity for emotional self-efficacy, which means an acceptance of one's emotional experience that is concordant with one's beliefs about a desirable emotional "balance."

The development of each of these components and skills takes place during childhood and adolescence and achieves its completion in adulthood.

COGNITION AND EMOTION

The interaction of cognition and emotion has been considered by cognitive psychologists,

ethologists, personality and social psychologists, and neuroscientists. Consideration must be given to both the neural mechanisms that lead to behavioral expression and cognitive processes that are influenced by learning by the individual and family, and behavioral control based on language (Buck, 1986). The neural mechanisms that lead to emotional expression interact with cognitive and language systems. Cognition has been emphasized by some investigators, and emotion is considered the driving force by others. Emotion is related to motivation and provides the context for motivational potential. Buck (1986) suggests three functions of emotion; bodily adaptation, social communication, and subjective experience. How the individual responds to bodily arousal, uses social communication, and verbalizes his or her subjective experiences is important in understanding affective development in the developmentally disabled.

The function of emotion in bodily adaptation involves the regulation of the internal environment of the body to maintain homeostasis and facilitate adaptation. Homeostasis addresses the internal environment, and adaptation refers to the body's response to changes in the external environment. For both, steady states must be maintained at a uniform level. This corresponds to neurophysiological arousal in the tripartite model.

Social communication refers to responses that are accessible to others, such as facial expression, postures, and vocalization, which are comparable to the behavioral expressive level. Behavioral expression may be spontaneous when emotional expression is based on instinctive communication, which represents the "automatic" expression of internal/emotional/motivated states that are not under conscious control and are biologically structured (i.e., species-specific) rather than culturally structured. Here, communication is innate. Moreover, Buck (1986) points out that spontaneous expressions are not symbols because the relationship between the expression and the emotional state leading to it are linked and expressed as a sign to the observer.

There are "spontaneous" gestures that serve an early communicative focus. These gestures are designated as instrumental and expressive in nature. Instrumental gestures have an instrumental function; they make someone do something immediately (Attwood, Frith, and Hermelin, 1988). Examples are gesturing to look up, to come, signaling to be quiet with finger to mouth, and gesturing to leave. Instrumental pointing is not the same as pointing to get another person's attention, that is, to share the reference with them. In one instance, pointing makes one look at something they did not look at before. In the other, it addresses sharing an interest. This is a form of essential communication that does not require that the intention of the communication be evaluated. The response to an instrumental gesture is either/or, and one either complies or does not. With communication that requires an interpretation of intention, there is more flexibility in responding as one attempts to understand the intention. Intentional gestures may be considered as expressive gestures in that an affect is expressed toward another person. These gestures accompany states of mind. Examples include embarrassment, a physiological response to shame or social discomfort, consolation to someone in distress, hugging as an expression of concern or friendship, reaching out to shake hands as an act of friendship, and threatening gestures that are intentionally assumed. According to these authors, each of these gestures was shown in children with Down syndrome, indicating that a person with mental retardation can show both instrumental and expressive gestures. However, expressive gestures were rarely shown by subjects with autistic disorder. Other spontaneous gestures are shaking the head no, nodding yes, the shyness response, and gestures of shared referencing, referential looking, showing with pride, and offering comfort to another person in distress.

These social gestures evolve with development and acquire meaning. They gradually become linked with communicative gestures and thereby become linked to motivated behavior. The expressive gestures may involve subjective awareness of affect.

Affect begins to link with cognition as one is increasingly aware of one's mental state and has the facility to shift emotional state with this knowledge. An essential readout of emotions is by the cognitive system, and its importance is to inform the cognitive system about the emotions, e.g., happiness, surprise, and sadness. This is the subjective experience of motivation or emotional states. The cognitive system is sensitive to both the internal bodily environment and the external environment. The awareness of potentially dangerous situations through emotional cues and of emotions before they must be expressed are referred to as "feed-forward mechanisms" and facilitate planned responses based on emotional states. The subjective readout of emotions fosters more effective cognitive responses.

Cognition and the Self-Conscious Emotions

Lewis et al. (1989) have provided a general developmental model outlining the interface between cognition and the development of self-conscious emotions. These authors propose several stages in development. In the first stage, the primary emotions appear. Although the timing of the primary emotions has not been clearly determined, interest, joy, physical distress, and disgust expressions have been demonstrated at or shortly after birth (Izard, 1977). Anger expressions have been noted as early as 4 months of age (Stenberg, Campos, and Emde, 1983) and surprise has been identified by 6 months (Charlesworth, 1960). Lewis suggests that if the eliciting circumstances are clearly defined, expressions of surprise, anger, fear, and sadness may be observed as early as 10 weeks of age.

The second stage emerges with increased cognitive capacity as the infant develops a referential self. Now, the earliest development of *self-conscious emotions* becomes apparent, and the first evidence of embarrassment, empathy, and envy may be noted. Self-referential behavior appears between 15 and 24 months of age (Bertenthal and Fischer, 1978).

The consolidation of cognitive skills provides the background for the emergence of the third stage. Lewis refers to these as secondary emotions. In stage three, the first class of secondary emotions become established that are characterized by self-referential behavior and include the full development of empathy, embarrassment, and possibly envy. Such emotions appear before or near the second birthday. Around the same time, young children are learning about their social world and developing emotional scripts and those rules of conduct that allow them to evaluate their own behavior. With an awareness of standards and rules, the second class of self-conscious emotions—the self-evaluative emotions, shame, pride, and guilt, emerge. Greater cognitive capacity is needed for the self-evaluative emotions than for the self-conscious emotions. *Self-evaluative emotions* involve a set of standards, rules or goals that are culturally defined and are transmitted to the child. Standards, rules, and goals must be incorporated into the child's behavior so that the child does not need the actual presence of another person to respond to them. The child is able to build a representation of what he or she alone possesses about these standards, rules, and goals and what will happen if they are violated or successfully fulfilled. The process of incorporation begins early in life, so children before the age of 2 anticipate adult reactions, seek positive reactions to their successes, and avoid negative reactions to their failures. Subsequently, they begin to evaluate their performance and show emotional responses to success and failure independent of expectations of adults' responses. Children become capable of responsibility for their behavior as they become aware that they are the producers of particular patterns of behavior. Therefore, self-evaluation includes not only the standards, rules and goals but also an awareness of one's own action. For example, pride is the consequence of comparing one's actions against a standard and then believing that one is responsible. The same is the case for shame. Lewis, Alessandri, and Sullivan (1992) studied differences in shame and pride as a function of children's gender and task difficulty. In this study, children attempted easy and difficult tasks, and their emotional responses were recorded. Children at about 3 years of age were given easy and difficult tasks. They were significantly more likely to show pride when they succeeded on the difficult task. Shame was more likely to be shown when they failed on an easy task than when they failed on a difficult one. Interaction with parents leads to some transfer of the parents' self-conscious emotions to their children through emotional expression, which is, in turn, mediated by the child's cognitive and evaluative processes.

Shame and Guilt

In psychoanalytic theory, shame is usually subsumed under guilt, in which case it is either ignored or considered a lower-order amoral state related to the fear of getting caught. Lewis (1971) suggests that what is lacking in this theory lies in Freud's failure to formulate his discoveries theoretically in terms of emotions (particularly attachment emotions). She suggests that undischarged states of guilt and shame are of considerable importance in symptom formation. She goes on to point out that human social life is our species-unique adaptation to life and that shame and guilt are particularly important modulators of social life; that shame-guilt and guilt-shame cycles are common issues in working with parents and children and essential to understanding self-esteem.

Lewis (1971) suggests that these two states develop in tandem and relate to field dependence and independence. Field-dependent people are more prone to shame and field-independent people to guilt. She notes that there are sex differences in field dependence that parallel sex differences in proneness to shame. Shame refers to social anxiety; guilt refers to moral anxiety. Shame touches the vegetative nervous system and is associated with blushing and profuse perspiration; it is generally associated with anxiety. In the older child, shame often evokes guilt reactions. The self-blaming quality of shame is easily confused with guilt, and the punitive psychoanalytic superego can be confused with masochistic self-debasing tendencies of shame-prone individuals.

Shame refers to a family of affective-cognitive states in which humiliation, mortification, embarrassment, and chagrin are among the variants. Shame is connected with being a social being. Shame is about the self; shame can be evoked by being looked at; it speaks to the imagery of the other in shame experience. Shame is the vicarious experience of the other's disapproval of the self. Absence of eye contact is often indicative of social anxiety. Shame is evoked either by a moral transgression or the self's failure to keep up the good opinion of a significant other. Because it is only about the self, shame is felt simultaneously as an inappropriate subjective reaction, which evokes more shame. Shame evokes a particular kind of fury i.e., humiliated fury or shame-rage, which is felt as inappropriate. It may be a first step of recovery of the self, but it may be experienced as unjust.

In shame, we lose each other or, more correctly, we lose (or believe we lose) another's esteem or love. At the same time, we court his or her approbation. As we try to flee, we install the other as the judge of our worth. In shame, the other is not injured, but certain ideal norms have been violated, and this is related to a deeper fear than retribution or punishment. It is the fear of being excluded from human society. Shame implies total abandonment — not a fear of physical death but psychic extinction.

Guilt is likened to the idea of the subject injuring the object. The subject has a feeling of having committed a transgression and expects punishment by the object. With punishment, the matter comes to a close and there is reconciliation. Socially, a guilty person is punished according to the laws of society, but the person who is put to shame endangers his very membership in society. He is placed beyond the norms of society when it is said "He knows no shame."

Guilt is a family of affective-cognitive states such as fault, blame, responsibility, and obligation. Guilt is about things that are undone in the real world. It has an objective quality; there is less disorganization of the self, more rational ideation, and the feeling that the self should do something. In guilt, the other is less important than in shame. States of shame and guilt are described as differentiated emotions. Both are universal affective cognitive states essential to human development. They attempt, but often fail, to restore the affectional ties on which development and well-being rest. Moreover, they are both depressive affects. When they fail to restore peace with others and are undischarged, they lead to symptoms of anxiety.

Approach to Emotion and Cognition in Developmental Disorders

A developmental approach to the interface of emotion and cognition addresses continuity and discontinuity of emotional and cognitive development and may provide a key to their interrelationship. Cicchetti and Sroufe (1978) have considered the relationship of cognitive and affective development in Down syndrome, a mental retardation syndrome that is ordinarily recognized shortly after birth. They studied the emergence of laughter in children with Down syndrome and contrasted it with a nonhandicapped population. They found that laughter at physical stimulation and at incongruity in the environment followed the same sequence in both groups; however, children with hypotonia showed laughter less often, although they did demonstrate smiling. Overall, the authors reported that laughter in response to social stimulation and incongruity was related to mental age and that one sees the coemergence of affect and cognition in children with Down syndrome. They suggest that affectively eliciting stimuli leading to affective expression may provide landmarks for evaluation in Down syndrome, further suggesting that the fear response can be followed in a similar way to study the relationship of fear and cognition. They note that muscle tension is needed for laughter, as evidenced in the children with hypotonia. This finding and Buck's (1986) notion about emotional expression speak to the somatic arousal or bodily adaptation "readout" aspect of emotion. One needs cognitive awareness to appreciate incongruity in emotionally responding, sufficient muscle tension to offer the response, and sufficient sensory input for interpretation of tension.

Kasari et al. (1990) have deepened the focus on affect development in their studies of affective sharing through their investigations of joint attention interactions of normal, autistic, and mentally retarded children. These authors studied the association of shared positive affect in two different communicative contexts, joint attention and requesting. Normal children showed frequent positive affect that was displayed toward the adult during joint attention situations. In comparison, children with autistic disorder failed to display high levels of positive affect during joint attention whereas mentally retarded children displayed high levels of positive affect during both requesting and joint attention situations. They concluded that children with autistic disorder show joint attention deficits that are associated with a disturbance in affective sharing.

These studies emphasize the importance of investigating developmental disorders to better understand emotion regulation and dysregulation, and the interface of emotion and cognition. Attention should continue to be directed toward specific developmental disorders rather than general categories, such as mental retardation.

REFERENCES

Attwood, A.H., Frith, U., and Hermelin, B. (1988). The understanding and use of interpersonal gestures by autistic and Down's syndrome children. *Journal of Autism and Developmental Disorders,* 18:241–257.

Berger, J. (1990). Interactions between parents and their infants with Down syndrome. In D. Cicchetti and M. Beeghly (eds), *Children with Down syndrome: A developmental perspective,* pp. 101–146. Cambridge University Press, Cambridge.

Bertenthal, F.I., and Fischer, K.W. (1978). The development of self-recognition in the infant. *Developmental Psychology,* 11:44–50.

Bradshaw, D.L., Campos, J.J., and Klinnert, M.D. (1986). Emotional expressions as determinants of infants' immediate and delayed responses to prohibitions. Paper presented at Fifth International Conference on Infant Studies, Los Angeles.

Bretherton, I., and Beeghly, M. (1982). Talking about internal states: The acquisition of an explicit theory of mind. *Developmental Psychology,* 18:906–921.

Buck, R. (1986). The psychology of emotion. In J.E. LeDoux and W. Hirst (eds), *Mind and brain,* pp. 275–300. Cambridge University Press, Cambridge, MA.

Buhler, C. (1930). *The first year of life.* John Day, New York.

Charlesworth, W.R. (1960). The role of surprise in cognitive development. In D. Elkind and J.H. Flavell (eds), *Studies in cognitive development: Essays in honor of Jean Piaget,* pp. 257–314. Oxford University Press, London.

Cicchetti, D., and Schneider-Rosen, K. (1984). Theoretical and empirical considerations in the investigation of the relationship between affect and cognition in atypical populations of infants: Contributions to the formulation of an integrative theory of development. In C.E. Izard, J. Kagan, and R.B. Zajonc (eds), *Emotions, cognition, and behavior,* pp. 366–408. Cambridge University Press, Cambridge, UK.

———, and Sroufe, L.A. (1978). An organizational view of affect: Illustrations from the study of Down's syndrome infants. In M. Lewis and L. Rosenblum (eds), *The development of affect,* pp. 309–350. Plenum Press, New York.

———, Ganiban, J., and Barnett, D. (1991). Contributions from the study of high- risk populations to understanding the development of emotion regulation. In J. Garber and K.A. Dodge (eds), *The development of emotion regulation and dysregulation,* pp. 15–48. Cambridge University Press, Cambridge, UK.

Darwin, C. (1872). *The expression of the emotions in man and animals.* John Murray, London. (University of Chicago Press, 1965)

Dodge, K.A. (1989). Coordinating responses to aversive stimuli. *Developmental Psychology,* 25:339–342.

———. (1991). Emotion and social information processing. In J. Garber and K.A. Dodge (eds), *The development of emotion regulation and dysregulation,* pp. 159–181. Cambridge University Press, Cambridge, UK.

———, and Garber, J. (1991). Domains of emotion regulation. In J. Garber and K.A. Dodge (eds), *The development of emotion regulation and dysregulation,* pp. 3–11. Cambridge University Press, Cambridge, UK.

Dunn, J., and Kendrick, C. (1982). *Siblings: Love, envy and understanding.* Harvard University Press, Cambridge, MA.

———, and Brown, J. (1991). Relationships, talk about feelings, and the development of affective regulation in early childhood. In J. Garber and K.A. Dodge (eds), *The development of emotion regulation and dysregulation,* pp. 89–108. Cambridge University Press, Cambridge, UK.

———, Bretherton, I., and Munn, P. (1987). Conversations about feeling states between mothers and their young children. *Developmental Psychology,* 23:132–139.

———, Kendrick, C., and MacNamee, R. (1981). The reaction of first-born children to the birth of a sibling: Mother's reports. *Journal of Child Psychology and Psychiatry,* 22:1–18.

Ekman, P., and Friesen, W.V. (1975). *Unmasking the face.* Prentice-Hall, Englewood, Cliffs, NJ.

Frith, U. (1989). *Autism: Explaining the enigma.* Basil Blackwell, Oxford, U.K.

Ganiban, J., Wagner, S., and Cicchetti, D. (1990). Temperament in Down syndrome. In D. Cicchetti and M. Beeghly (eds), *Children with Down syndrome: A developmental perspective,* pp. 63–100. Cambridge, University Press, Cambridge, UK.

Garber, J., Braafladt, N., and Zeman, J. (1991). The regulation of sad affect: An information-processing perspective. In J. Garber and K.A. Dodge (eds), *The development of emotion regulation and dysregulation,* pp. 208–240. Cambridge University Press, Cambridge, UK.

Goodenough, F.I. (1931). *Anger in young children.* University of Minnesota Press, Minneapolis.

Gunnar, M.R. (1986). Human developmental psychoneuroendocrinology: A review of research on neuroendocrine responses to challenge and threat in infancy and childhood. In M.E. Lamb, L.A. Brown, and B. Rogoff (eds), *Advances in developmental psychology,* Vol. 4, pp. 51–103. Lawrence Erlbaum, Hillsdale, NJ.

Harris, P.L. (1989). *Children and emotion: The development of psychological understanding.* Basil Blackwell, Oxford.

Hesse, P., and Cicchetti, D. (1982). Toward an integrative theory of emotional development. *New Directions for Child Development,* 16:3–48.

Hoffner, C., and Badzinski, D.M. (1989). Children's integration of facial and situational cues to emotion. *Child Development,* 60:411–422.

Izard, C.E. (1972). *Patterns of emotions.* Academic Press, New York.

———. (1977). *Human emotions.* Plenum Press, New York.

———, and Kobak, R.R. (1991). Emotions system functioning and emotion regulation. In J. Garber and K.A. Dodge (eds), *The development of emotion regulation and dysregulation,* pp. 303–321. Cambridge University Press, Cambridge, UK.

———, Huebner, R., Risser, D., McGinnes, G., and Dougherty, L. (1980). The young infant's ability to produce discrete emotion expressions. *Developmental Psychology,* 16:132–140.

Kagan, J. (1981). *The second year. The emergence of self-awareness.* Harvard University Press, Cambridge, MA.

Kasari, C., Sigman, M., Mundy, P., and Yirmiya, N. (1990). Affective sharing in the context of joint attention interactions of normal, autistic, and mentally retarded children. *Journal of Autism and Developmental Disorders,* 20:87–100.

Klinnert, M., Campos, J.J., Sorce, J., Emde, R.N., and Svejda, M. (1983). Emotions as behavior regulators: Social referencing in infancy. In R. Plutchik and H. Kellerman (eds), *Emotions in early development.* Vol. 2, *The emotions.* Academic Press, New York.

Kopp, C.B. (1989). Regulation of distress and negative emotions: A developmental view. *Developmental Psychology,* 25:343–354.

Kraemer, G.W. (1992). A psychobiological theory of attachment. *Behavioral and Brain Sciences,* 15:493–541.

———, Ebert, M.H., Schmidt, D.E., and McKinney, W.T. (1989). A longitudinal study of the effect of different social rearing conditions on cerebrospinal fluid norepinephrine and biogenic amine metabolites in rhesus monkeys. *Neuropsychopharmacology,* 2:175–189.

Laird, J. (1974). Self-attribution of emotion: The effects of expressive behavior on the quality of emotional experience. *Journal of Personality and Social Psychology,* 29:475–486.

Lang, P.J. (1968). Fear reduction and fear behavior: Problems in treating a construct. In J.M. Schlien (ed), *Research in psychology,* Vol. 3, pp. 90–103. American Psychological Association, Washington, DC.

Lewis, H.B. (1971). *Freud and modern psychology,* Vol. 1, *The emotional basis of mental illness.* Plenum Press, New York and London.

Lewis, M., Alessandri, S.M., and Sullivan, M.W. (1992). Differences in shame and pride as a function of children's gender and task difficulty. *Child Development,* 63:630–638.

———, Sullivan, M.W., Stanger, C., and Weiss, M. (1989). Self development and self-conscious emotions. *Child Development,* 60:146–156.

Malatesta-Magai, C. (1991). Development of emotional expression in infancy: General course and patterns of individual difference. In J. Garber and K.A. Dodge (eds), *The development of emotion regulation and dysregulation,* pp. 49–68. Cambridge University Press, Cambridge, UK.

Masters, J.C. (1991). Strategies and mechanisms for the personal and social control of emotion. In J. Garber and K.A. Dodge (eds), *The development of emotion regulation and dysregulation,* pp. 182–207. Cambridge University Press, Cambridge, UK.

———, Felleman, E.S., and Barden, R.C. (1981). Experimental studies of affective states in children. In B. Lahey and A.E. Kazdin (eds), *Advances in clinical child psychology,* Vol. 4, pp. 91–114. Plenum Press, New York.

Nathanson, D. L. (1993). About emotion. *Psychiatric Annals,* 23: 543–555.

Porges, S.W. (1991). Vagal tone: An autonomic mediator of affect. In J. Garber and K.A. Dodge (eds), *The development of emotion regulation and dysregulation,* pp. 111–128. Cambridge University Press, Cambridge, UK.

Rieder, C., and Cicchetti, D. (1989). Organizational perspective on cognitive control functioning and cognitive-affective balance in maltreated children. *Developmental Psychology,* 25:382–393.

Saarni, C. (1988). Emotional competence: How emotions and relationships become integrated. In R. Dienstbier (series ed) and R.A. Thompson (volume ed), *Socioemotional development,* pp. 115–182. Nebraska Symposium on Motivation, 1988. University of Nebraska Press, Lincoln, NE.

Sameroff, A., and Chandler, M. (1975). Reproductive risk and the continuum of caretaking casualty. In F.D. Horowitz (ed), *Review of child development research,* Vol. 4, pp. 187–244. University of Chicago Press, Chicago.

Stenberg, C., Campos, J., and Emde, R. (1983). The facial expression of anger in seven-month-old infants. *Child Development,* 54:178–184.

Stern, D. (1985). *The interpersonal world of the infant.* Basic Books, New York.

Termine, N.T. and Izard, C.E. (1988). Infants' responses to their mothers' expressions of joy and sadness. *Developmental Psychology,* 24:223–229.

Tomkins, S.S. (1962). *Affect, imagery, and consciousness,* Vol. 1, *The positive affects.* Springer-Verlag, New York.

_____. (1963). *Affect, imagery, and consciousness,* Vol. 2, *The negative affects.* Springer-Verlag, New York.

_____. (1991). *Affect, imagery, and consciousness,* Vol. 3, *The negative affects: Anger and fear.* Springer-Verlag, New York.

_____. (1992). *Affect, imagery, and consciousness,* Vol. 4, *Cognition: Duplication and transformation of information.* Springer-Verlag, New York.

Walden, T.A. (1991). Infant social referencing. In J. Garber and K.A. Dodge (eds), *The development of emotion regulation and dysregulation,* pp. 69–87. Cambridge University Press, Cambridge, UK.

Walker-Andrews, A.S. (1986). Intermodal perception of expressive behaviors: Relation of eye and voice? *Developmental Psychology,* 22:373–377.

CHAPTER 15
EMERGENCE OF THE SELF

The social self was first proposed by William James (1890) and later by others (Cooley, 1902; Baldwin, 1895, 1906, 1911; Mead, 1934) to introduce the study of the self to empirical psychology. In psychiatry, the focus on self development arose independently in the early psychodynamic object relations schools. Object relations theorists, like social psychologists, emphasized that the self emerges from relations with others, particularly from the early mother-infant relationship (Winnicott, 1958). Bowlby (1969, 1973, 1980) expanded the early object relations approaches by developing an ethological model and subsequently incorporated research on internal representation, information processing, and memory formation into his model. Moreover, Bowlby emphasized the need to study healthy as well as disturbed children. He proposed that children construct "internal working models" of self and parent that derive from the infant/parent interaction. An "internal working model" may allow the infant to predict the parent's behavior. Developmental psychologists and cognitive psychologists have extended Bowlby's thesis beyond the attachment context of models of parental behavior to consider internal working models of the self. These psychologists suggest that attachment theory can be extended to expand our understanding of the concept of the social self (Bretherton, 1991). They emphasize script formation as an important element in the emergence of the social self.

This chapter reviews classical studies of the social self; the social self in attachment theory; working models of the self; individual differences in working models; cognitive, structural and motivational aspects of the self system; the development of the self; the emergence of a theory of mind; and issues related to the self in developmental disabilities.

HISTORY

Social Psychology

In classical psychological studies of the self, the self is considered both as object and as subject. In considering the social nature of the self, the unity of the self as well as the ideal or potential self are considered. The empirical self (as object) includes the body self and its possessions, the social self and its self-recognition, and the ethical self. Because the social self is derived from social experience, there are many social selves. In these analyses, *self-worth* is derived from the difference between the actual self and the potential self toward which one strives. Mead (1934) thought that the integration of the social selves occurs with the construction of a model of the self that considers how it is viewed by others.

From a developmental perspective, Mead suggests that children learn to take the role of particular others in pretend play by acting out individual adult attitudes as well as societal attitudes. In this way, the child may incorporate social roles and integrate the multiple selves originating in dyadic relationships with their parents into a unified self. The result is an understanding of self and others in relationship to oneself; the child learns to construct models of both self and parent.

Baldwin (1906) initially proposed that self and other are mutually interdependent. He suggested that, developmentally, children know others by their behavior and by their effects on them. The next milestone in the establishment of the self is the realization that others have bodies and experience them just as one experiences one's own body. An awareness of having similar experiences to others may lead to the eventual consolidation of prosocial feelings (i.e., caring for others and fairness, the emergence of empathy, and the establishment of justice). Children begin to understand others by focusing on their self-hood and, through imitation, may form internal representations of others as well as of themselves. In this way, patterns of behavior come to be understood through interactions with others.

Individual differences in relationships develop out of readjusting old experiential schemata with new ones. As relationships with others are assimilated and new learning from parents is accommodated, an ethical self forms as limits on social freedom are acknowledged. The active intervention of caregivers and other adults are crucial to the development of the ethical self. The ethical self is projected onto others whom the child expects to demonstrate behavior in conformity with his or her new social understanding. For example, children object to an adult ignoring rules and expect others to conform to the same rules that they have learned. In essence, Baldwin suggested that children acquire a sense of self through construction, impute subjectivity to others, expand their experience through imitation of others, and assimilate new experiences to the objective self (me) or to internal representations (self schemata) (Bretherton, 1991). Baldwin emphasized social reciprocity and feedback in the development of individual differences as well as in the establishment of the group self. He addressed the representational processes that underlie the sense of self.

Object Relations Schools

In classical social psychology, the emphasis is on general processes of social development rather than on a specific individual. However, the object relations school of psychoanalysis has placed its emphasis on the healthy versus pathological social development of the individual. Harry S. Sullivan (interpersonal theory) and Donald Winnicott are representative of these views; both emphasize individual differences in the development of the social self.

Sullivan (1953), the primary exponent of the interpersonal school, focused on individual differences in development through his emphasis on anxious caregiving. He suggested that the infant identifies the anxious caregiver as the "bad mother" and the sensitive caregiver as the "good mother," thereby incorporating two separate personifications or schemata of self experience (Bretherton, 1991). These personifications are created in periods of integrated caregiving experience with the "real" mother—not as a living person, but as "an elaborate organization" of the infant's mothering experience. It is the process of being cared for that is integrated. Subsequently, separate generalized good and bad person functions come to be differentiated and may be elaborated into representations of specific persons as good or bad. Later, in the first year, personifications of the self are created as "good me" and "bad me" depending on whether the parenting experiences were anxious ones or not. In addition, Sullivan postulates "not me" experiences which are so intensely anxious that they are not personified in awareness as "me" at all. In development, personifications of "me" and "mother" become part of the self. Sullivan suggests that the self-system protects itself through security operations (defense mechanisms or coping strategies) that repress "bad me" and "not me" experiences, yet defense mechanisms interfere with the integration of ongoing new experiences. Sullivan states that security operations "interfere with observation and analysis" of new experiences. He emphasizes that different forms of interpersonal relatedness are present at different times in the life cycle—with parents, best friends (chums) and with marital or intimate partners. However, during these relationships "me-you" patterns emerge that may be maladaptive schemata of the self or other. Moreover, these early dysfunctional relationships may negatively influence later relationships.

Winnicott (1958, 1965), an important representative of the object relations school, emphasized the quality of mother/infant relationships for the establishment of the self. He describes an unintegrated infant who, through the psychological "holding environment" provided by the emotionally attuned parent, eventually develops the psychological organization of a person. The parent is critical for this task of "self integration." Winnicott proposed a biological state in the early weeks after delivery (referred to as "primary maternal preoccupation") when the mother is physiologically sensitive to the infant's cry and biologically prone to be synchronized to the infant's needs. Moreover, by being continually available, she allows a sense of infantile omnipotence (competence) to develop. By also being nonintrusive, yet psychologically attuned, when the infant does need her, she provides the continuity that establishes the basis for the subsequent "capacity for aloneness" in later life. Winnicott considered the capacity for aloneness to be central to the integration of a stable self. This continual attunement by the mother allows the infant the ease and security to become attuned to his or her own bodily rhythms, processes, and urges.

Once infantile omnipotence, or competence (Bretherton, 1991), is fully established, the infant must learn that this sense of omnipotence is not complete. Winnicott (1965) suggests this understanding is realized gradually as the mother's responses decrease and she reduces her attunement to infant signals, moods, and needs. Such graduated failures in availability may have adaptive significance and play an essential role in the infant's self-differentiation, but they may also induce experiences of anger toward a mother who is no longer perfectly responsive. Now the mother's task is to show that she will not retaliate despite the infant's negative feelings of anger. By her consistency, she shows that she is not harmed by the infant's anger and, by being resilient, can survive his destructive negative affect (anger). Although no longer perfectly attuned, a "good enough mother" remains sufficiently responsive to maintain support for a healthy self in the growing child.

ATTACHMENT THEORY: THE SOCIAL SELF

In attachment theory, as in the approaches of Sullivan and Winnicott, the infant is thought to be prepared to engage in social interactions from birth. Moreover, in attachment theory, maternal responsiveness is essential for the development of the self, and actual mother-child transactions are reflected in mental representations of the self and mother. Moreover, subsequent patterns of relating between them are built on earlier ones. Bowlby (1969), as attachment theorist, places substantial emphasis on the emergence of the healthy self. In doing so, he proposed that the individual constructs "internal working models" to interact with the physical and personal world. These working models aid in perceiving and interpreting events, predicting the future, and devising new plans. An internal working model suggests dynamic mental structures that an individual may use to devise strategies for action. The model or the models are essentially a small-scale construction of external reality that includes the potential for future actions. Although not fully accurate or perhaps not very detailed, the relational structure of working models is consistent with the reality that they represent, for example, spatial, temporal, and causal relations. A working model, in a sense, is a description of the internal world that is created to represent the external world from stores of memories and earlier perceptions. These are representations of the self and others as internalized complexes of experienced relationships. Such formulations are similar to earlier theories. Sullivan (1953) had spoken of "personifications of mother and me" and "me-you patterns." Psychoanalysts, such as Sandler and Sandler (1978), write of "interactions between self and object representations that make unconscious dialogs possible." Kernberg (1976) describes self-object affective units that are "positively or negatively toned interaction schemata that become a basis of self and object representations." Conceptually, the working model offers advantages over static terms, such as "internal object" and "object representation."

Bowlby (1969) postulated that internal working models of self and attachment figures grew out of actual patterns of infant-caregiver transactions and emerge around the end of the first year of life when the infant has reached the developmental phase of object permanence and has begun to acquire language. Because of their origins in transactional patterns, these working models are established in close complementarity and, taken together, may represent the relationship. Such models of the self must be understood in the context of the relationships within which they emerged and are developing. A nurturant relationship with parents may construct a working model of the self as competent and loved, but if the attachment figures are rejecting, a complementary internal working model of the self as untrustworthy may form. When emotional support is insufficient but not rejecting, the child may potentially form working models of the world as dangerous and perceive the self as weak and helpless. In order to adapt to change and guide the interpretation of interpersonal transactions with the caregiver, working models of the self must be continuously deconstructed and reconstructed to accommodate changes that take place over development. With increasing competence and more highly developed thought processes, the child and caregiver respond differently to one another. This leads to greater complexity in content of both the child and parent's internal working models. In this process, internal working models of the self as competent and accepted may be maintained as the parent continues to be encouraging and supportive of autonomy, thus retaining the child's affective stability over time.

Although they do change over time, internal working models do not remain in continuous flux (Bretherton, 1991). Ways of acting and thinking that are initially deliberately chosen tend to become less accessible to awareness as automatic processing occurs when they enter long-term memory (see Chapter 13). Consequently, young people may focus their attention on unfamiliar or new situations. However, stability is achieved in relation to the interpersonal world with the risk of excessive simplification and possible distortions as models are generalized. Adaptations in working models must follow when new experiences do not fit the corresponding internal working models and previous adaptations are not adequate. In such situations, an individual may cling to outdated working models and use processes Bowlby (1980)

referred to as "defensive exclusion." This may take place when two incompatible interpersonal choices come into consciousness and one is chosen while the other is monitored outside awareness. That such processing occurs has been demonstrated in dichotic listening experiments, when incompatible messages are presented to both ears, yet the subject normally hears "only one message."

Defensive exclusion is most likely to occur in response to conflicting messages that produce mental pain; for example, if the parent continually ridicules the child's security seeking but the child reinterprets this rejection as motivated by parental love or in other ways denies negative feelings toward the parent. In these circumstances, the child may defensively exclude from awareness the working model of the "bad" unloving parent but retain in consciousness access to the "good" loving parent. Idealized models of unconditionally loving and of completely rejecting parents generally do not correspond to reality and often become maladaptive. The confusion that may ensue may lead an individual to attempt to operate with two or more conflicting working models of the same attachment figure and two or more conflicting models of the self. Models acquired earlier in life that are out of awareness may conflict with more recent, but incompatible, contemporary working models. In later life, through identification with their parents, children may adopt the same patterns of behavior toward his own children that they experienced during their childhood. In this way, patterns of interaction may be transmitted from one generation to the next. Bowlby (1973, p. 323) suggests that social transmission through the medium of family microculture is no less important than inheritance through the medium of genes.

Bretherton (1990, 1991) reports that findings from observational studies of parent-infant or parent-toddler attachments, and from attachment-related interviews involving the use of story telling with preschoolers, kindergarten children, and adults, are consistent with Bowlby's (1973) formulations. In observational studies, when children's attachment or autonomy signals are ignored or misread, the development of open communication between parent and child is affected (Ainsworth, Bell, and Stayton, 1974; Blehar, Lieberman, and Ainsworth, 1977).

Children who are securely attached are able to discuss attachment relationships without insisting that they or their attachment figures are perfect. However, insecure-avoidant children and adults tend to defend themselves against interpersonal closeness by restrictiveness when they discuss attachment relationships. They tend to be aloof and may have a strong tendency to idealize parents or themselves when making global judgments and are unable to find adequate examples of adaptation in their autobiographical memory (Main, 1990). Such memories may be absent or contradictory.

Before the infant is born, parents have internal working models of themselves as caregivers and working models of the unborn infant (Zeanah et al., 1985). These anticipatory working models may be influenced by the parents' own experiences in childhood; however, later relationship experiences certainly play a role in establishing these models. When encountering the real infant, anticipatory working models are imposed on the new relationship. To be adaptive, these must fit the temperament and needs of the new infant or child. If the parents' anticipatory working models are coherent, well-organized, and accessible to awareness without much defensive exclusion, the adaptation may take place smoothly. However, if parental internal working models are poorly organized and subject to extensive defensive exclusion, the parent may read the infant's cues selectively and may not be able to take the infant's perspective or recognize the infant's goals and respond to them empathetically (Ainsworth, Bell and Stayton, 1974). When the infants' or children's signals are not appropriately recognized, their own developing working models may become distorted and inflexible. Moreover, if the infant is developmentally disabled or handicapped, a discrepancy between the parents' working model of a child and the child's presentation may require that parents grieve the loss of the expected normal child in order to accept the infant that they have.

Developments in Attachment Research

Current attachment research focuses on issues of multiple attachments, the outcome of secure and insecure attachment, and the developing complexity of working models with age (Bretherton, 1991). The infant and child have multiple attachments and multiple social selves. Different attachment relationships call for different responses, so that the quality of an infant's relationship to the mother or to the father may vary. Main and Weston (1981) evaluated infants with their father and with their mother at 12 and 18 months. Concordant secure and insecure patterns of attachment with both parents were not demonstrated. Main, Kaplan, and Cassidy (1985) investigated the child's representation of attachment at six years of age in response to a family picture and to a projective test about separation. These authors found that responses were highly predictable from the early pattern of attachment with the mother but not with the father, suggesting that the principal attachment figure may be more influential than another in the construction of a working model of the self. In the Main and Weston (1981) study, it is suggested that models of the self in some circumstances may be averaged so that when the relationship to both parents is insecure, later outcome may be less favorable. Models of the self might be intermediate if the relationship to one parent is insecure and the relationship to the other is secure.

Other areas of ongoing research deal with the later outcome of insecure and secure attachment. Developmental progression in the differentiation and integration of the self in secure individuals has been studied extensively in specific age groups (Bretherton, 1987) and cross-culturally (Grossmann and Grossmann, 1990). Children with the secure pattern tend to develop competence in their explorations of the world. Children with insecure attachment may lack confidence that support will be available and may not seek out a caregiver when stressed (insecure-avoidant) or may be uncertain of the caregiver's availability and show separation anxiety symptoms (insecure-ambivalent pattern). A fourth group has been described by Main and colleagues (Main and Hesse, 1990; Main and Solomon, 1986), and designated the "insecure-disorganized" attachment pattern. These are children who are fearful of their caregiver. They may be unable to use their caregiver as a secure base and may be inhibited in their exploration of the world.

To investigate long-term psychological functioning, Jacobsen, Edelstein, and Hofmann (1993) have extended attachment studies beyond infancy and early childhood, focusing their study on the relationship between children's attachment representations and their cognitive functioning in middle childhood and adolescence. At age 7, 85 children were classified as securely or insecurely attached based on their discussion of a story that involved parental separation. The authors found three of the attachment groups — secure, insecure-avoidant, and insecure-disorganized. After controlling for the child's IQ and for attentional problems, these three groups were compared at ages 7, 9, 12, 15, and 17, using Piagetian tasks that assessed concrete and formal reasoning. Children with an insecure-disorganized representation showed the lowest scores on the deductive reasoning tasks at each of the age periods. These findings indicate that children with an insecure-disorganized attachment may be specifically disadvantaged in their subsequent cognitive functioning. Their negative self-concept and fears of their caregivers along with possible doubts about their own abilities may interfere with their deductive reasoning. The children with a secure attachment representation scored significantly better on the cognitive functioning tasks. These findings support a possible link between internal representations of attachment and long-term psychologic functioning, suggesting that attachment security may facilitate children's cognitive functioning.

Another area that is being investigated relates to the construction of a potential or ideal self in adulthood. Main, Kaplan, and Cassidy (1985) studied secure-autonomous adults who had insecure childhoods. They found that the parents' attitude toward attachment, in general, most strongly predicted child security and not necessarily the security or insecurity of the parents' own early relationships. Others (Grossmann et al., 1988) suggest that children are more secure if parents consciously express the desire that their own parents had been more supportive of them.

Another issue that is subject to ongoing research is the growing complexity of working models of the self with age. Attachment studies of children, young adults, and parents have emphasized qualitative stability in the presence of developmental changes. However, assessment tools have been chosen based on intuitive insight, in some instances, rather than systematic investigation (Bretherton, 1991).

Finally, although clinically it is useful to discuss representations of the self and other as "inner persons" who may engage in imaginary interactions, Bretherton (1991) suggests that research in this area may benefit from recent studies of mental representation. Among these are theories of event representation and social cognitive studies which emphasize the capacity for intersubjectivity.

COGNITIVE, STRUCTURAL, AND MOTIVATIONAL APPROACHES TO THE SELF

Object relations and attachment theories provide approaches to the social self. In summary, object relations theorists locate the self in social interactions and specify internalization of self-relevant information as a central developmental process. This involves the incorporation of affective, behavioral, and cognitive information that is communicated by significant adults in the mechanisms of changes in the self over time. Attachment theorists link the emergence and the quality of working models of the self to early and current experiences with caretakers. In these formulations, the responsivity and sensitivity of caregivers are the primary social interactive processes, leading to the individual's sense of self in relationship to others.

A second group of theorists approach the self through cognitive understanding. Cognitive approaches to understanding the self emphasize knowledge, beliefs, theories, and schema to describe what is known about oneself. As the self develops, it acquires and organizes this knowledge. This leads to structural approaches to the self that emphasize the ways such self-knowledge is organized, as in Piaget's description of the developmental progression of children's moral understanding. Others (McGuire, 1981) study organizational changes in the content of children's and adolescents' responses to the question, "Who am I?" and evaluate shifts in the thematic content of their answers. Structural theorists emphasize age-related changes in thematic content and complexity of self-knowledge. Those who study information processing use computer metaphors to describe how information about the self is processed.

A third group of self theorists emphasize motivationally based conceptions of the self

(Connell and Wellborn, 1991). Motivational approaches emphasize how self-related cognition and affect develop. In some instances, self-worth or self-esteem is taken as an organizational construct (Sroufe and Waters, 1977). Self-worth is hypothesized to relate to perceived confidence and to attributions of success and failure. On the other hand, psychodynamic theorists emphasize fundamental biological drives and identification processes in establishing self-esteem. Here, a sense of self emerges from a dynamic relationship between the constraints of the external world and instinctual drives. Others, such as Erikson (1950), emphasize identity formation through the mastery of a series of psychosocial crises. McClelland (1985) emphasizes power, achievement, and affiliation as distinct entities that are relevant to the development of the self. For motivational theorists, emotional processes and psychological needs are central in shaping the self, so self-actualization (Maslow, 1970), self-determination (Deci, 1980), and competence (White, 1959) are essential.

Connell and Wellborn (1991) integrate the various models of the self by suggesting a model with the following characteristics: (1) there are fundamental psychological needs for competence, autonomy, and relatedness; (2) the self system processes emerge from the interaction of psychological needs in social contexts; (3) aspects of social context most relevant to meeting psychological needs are the provision of structure, autonomy, support, and involvement; and (4) the inter- and intraindividual variation in the self system processes lead to various patterns of action. In their model, the developing person is an active partner in the construction of the self system from early life, and the self system itself is viewed as a set of appraisal processes in which the individual evaluates his or her status in a particular context with respect to the psychological needs mentioned (i.e., competence, autonomy, and relatedness). Their model provides a motivational perspective of the developing person. The need for competence involves the production of desired outcomes; the need for autonomy leads to the experience of choice in initiating, maintaining, and regulating activity along with the experience of there being connectedness between one's actions and personal goals

and values; relatedness refers to the need to feel securely connected to the social environment and to experience oneself as worthy of respect and love. Competence requires having the capacity and utilizing strategies to act effectively. Autonomy involves self-regulation and acknowledgment of what is important to the self. Relatedness emphasizes a wish for closeness to others and a sense of emotional security in relationship to them.

THE EXECUTIVE "I" AND INTERNAL WORKING MODELS

When considering the self, a distinction is drawn between the self as agent, "knower," or the "I," from the self as the object of knowledge or the "me." William James (1890) first presented this analysis of the self, which has continued to be instrumental in defining the self since his original proposal. The self has been viewed by some as having a central role in personality development, but by others as a source of confusion and complication. The disagreement largely is the result of failing to distinguish between the self as object and the self as agent. There has been little disagreement about the value of studying the self as object because people have views about themselves that influence their feelings and behavior. In regard to the self as object, it is possible to conduct research to measure people's views about themselves using self-report procedures, which are treated as objective data. However, the self as agent cannot be measured; it is a theoretical construct. Epstein (1991) suggests that there are two conceptual systems that contain selves as objects, a rational system and an experiential one. In the rational system, the views people hold about themselves can be readily reported. This is the self as measured by direct self-report in personality inventories and interviews. The experiential self consists of cognitions that come from emotionally significant experiences which the person may or may not be currently aware of. An individual may, on verbal self-report, identify himself as self-accepting and confident yet show through his nonverbal behavior evidence of low self-esteem through avoidance of eye contact, defensive aggression, and excessive bravado. On the other hand, the self as agent may be defined as an individual's self theory, which contains descriptive beliefs and motivational beliefs or beliefs about the outcome of self-initiated action.

This chapter emphasizes the interdependence between the "I" as "knower" and the "me" as representation or working model of the self. The dual nature of the self is not emphasized by Sullivan, Winnicott, or Bowlby, yet Epstein's rational and experiential selves must both be considered in assessment of both the child and the adult.

The relationship between the "I," as the executive operating system, and the "me," as the internal working model of the self or self-representation, deserves consideration. Johnson-Laird (1983) suggests that consciousness is our experience of our individual executive system. Using a computer model, he suggests that the executive or operating system is capable of monitoring and processing input from a large number of lower-level processes in sequence. Rather than operating serially, the lower-level processes are thought to operate in parallel, and the operating system has access to the output of these parallel systems but not to their internal working. The operating system gives higher-level commands to the lower-level processing systems, which produce specific actions.

Bretherton (1991) suggests that the executive system is more than a "knower," because it is a metasystem that sets priorities among inputs from various lower-level processes which may send conflicting commands. In Johnson-Laird's model, the lower-level processes maintain some autonomy, so there is "relative will power" based on the degree to which the operating system or the "I" can carry out its decisions. Executive plans may be disrupted by motivational systems that regulate survival behavior, including escape, attachment, or aggression. These are emergency signals that generally represent emotional responses of the body and the mind. Such cognitive-affective links are essential to adaptive functions. Maladaptive behavior may occur when the executive system is overwhelmed by the lower-level systems or when it overcontrols them, such as when survival signals are received. In each of these instances, incoming information is not appropriately processed.

In this model, the executive system would consult internal working models of the world and particularly those of the self system. If the working models are not adequate for adaptation or dissociated from one another, the executive system, or "I," cannot properly forecast and make interpretations to guide effective action. This model suggests that the correlation and interrelationship between the "I" and the "me" requires investigation in both secure and insecure relationships. One might consider that if attachment relationships are secure, the "I" and "me" will function well in relation to one another, but if attachment is insecure, then the integration of "I" and "me" may be disturbed.

The "I-me" relationship must also be considered in terms of social transmission of working models from the parent to the infant. The infant's executive operating system, or "I," is not developed and not well-coordinated, so internal working models may exist only at a sensorimotor level. As a result, the infant must rely on the adult to regulate external events in order to develop. Those who function as auxiliary "I's" to whom an infant is attached require integrated "I-me" systems to facilitate the infant's internal organization of "I" and "me." This formulation suggests that better understanding of the relationship of "I" and "me" throughout development is essential for understanding the establishment of the social self.

THE DEVELOPMENT OF A SENSE OF SELF

The self and its counterpart, the sense of other, are universal phenomena that crucially influence all of our social experiences. During development, several senses of self emerge. Stern (1985) describes these as the sense of self that is a single, distinct integrated body, that is an agent of actions, an experiencer of feelings, an establisher of intentions, a developer of plans, a transposer of experience into language, and a communicator who shares personal knowledge with another. Stern emphasizes that some senses of the self exist prior to self-awareness and language. Among these are the senses of agency, of physical cohesion, of a sense of continuity in time, and possibly of having intentions in mind. Through self-reflection and with the development of language, these preverbal existential senses of the self begin to reveal their own ongoing existence and are transformed into new experiences. If the sense of self begins before verbalization, then rather than looking for a time the sense of self begins, it is more productive to describe developmental continuities and changes. In regard to a preverbal self, Stern refers to "nonself reflexive awareness" that arises on the occasion of an infant's actions or mental processes. It may begin as the organizing subjective experience that will later be verbally referenced as the self. With the emergence of self, there is a sense of continuity, a sense of affective contact, a sense of intersubjectivity, a sense of creative organization out of disorganization, and a sense of transmitting meaning from one individual to another.

According to Stern, infants experience a sense of the emerging self from birth as they become aware of biologically based self-organizing processes. Consequently, the infant is selectively responsive to social events in the external environment. From 2 to 6 months, infants are thought to consolidate a sense of a core self as a separate, cohesive physical unit with the beginnings of agency, affectivity, and continuity in time. During these early periods, there is no autistic-like phase of development nor is there a symbiotic-like phase. The infant is actively involved in organizing and making sense of the environment and contacts with others.

From about 7 to 15 months, the sense of a subjective self is formed. Now the infant is devoted to seeking and creating intersubjective union with another. This process involves an awareness that one's subjective life, consisting of the mind's contents and the qualities of one's feelings, may be shared. This subjective self is emerging concurrently with the time when attachment and separation are beginning to take place.

The subjective self is followed by the establishment of the verbal self, which forms after 18 months. The verbal self does not replace the emerging self, core self, or subjective self, but each of these senses of self remain fully functional throughout life and continue to grow.

Stern suggests that affective experiences enter the intersubjective domain through a phenomenon called "affective attunement." The sharing of affective states is the most essential aspect of intersubjective relatedness. In affective attunement, contact is established between parent and infant not by imitation but through a kind of cross-modal matching. The modality of expression used by the parent to match the infant's behavior differs from that used by the infant. For example, the duration and intensity of an infant's vocalization may be matched by the mother's body movements or the infant's movements may be mirrored by the mother's voice. For example, a boy bangs his hand on a soft toy and sets up a steady rhythm; his mother begins to vocalize with the rise and fall of his hand in attunement. In affective attunement, what is matched is not another's behavior specifically but an aspect of the behavior that reflects the other person's feeling state, so what is matched is the feeling state rather than external behavior. As a result, there are matching expressions of an inner state. Such expressions may differ in their form, but in some sense, they exist as manifestations of a single and recognizable internal state. Such contact uses metaphor as behaviors are jointly expressed by parent and infant. The quality of feeling of a shared affective state is thus demonstrated through affective attunement (Stern, 1985).

It is during the second year of life that the infant's language begins to emerge and the process of senses of self and others takes on new meaning. With language, there is different and distinct personal word knowledge because language allows the creation of shared meanings. As language continues to emerge, the child begins to construct a narrative of his own life. Around 15 to 18 months, children begin to represent things in their minds in such a way that symbolic representation occurs. Symbolic play and language allow a child to refer to themselves as an external or objective entity. Now communication may take place about things and persons who are not present.

The infant develops the capacity to perform delayed imitations in that the representation of an original act is remembered as performed by someone else and the infant executes his own imitation of what was observed. In a sense, two versions of the event are adjusted—that observed and that accomplished. A psychological relationship develops to motivate delayed imitation. Representation of the self as an objective entity occurs and may be observed from the outside as well as felt subjectively from the inside. After age 18 months, infants develop an objective sense of self, which is evidenced by their behavior before a mirror, their use of names and pronouns for self-designation, acts of empathy, and the development of a core gender identity (Stern, 1985). For example, after age 18 months an infant with a colored rouge marker on his nose will point to himself rather than to his reflection, as is the case for younger infants. The infant touches his own face when he looks in the mirror rather than pointing to the reflection he sees in the mirror. Stern refers to this as the "objective self," whereas Lewis and Brooks-Gunn (1979) use the term "categorical self." Around the same time, the pronouns "I," "me," and "mine" are used to refer to the self. Empathetic acts may also be evidence of the emergence of self. To act empathetically, it is necessary to imagine the self as an object that may be experienced by another in the objectified other's subjective state.

With the establishment of a verbal self, language finally brings about the ability to narrate one's own life story. Narrative involves a different mode of thought from problem solving. To narrate, one must consider persons who act as agents with intentions and goals that are presented in a sequence, giving the narrative a beginning, a middle, and an end. Narratives are constructed or coconstructed with parents and begin to form an autobiographical history. In the development of a verbal self, the categorical, or objective, self labels and identifies and the narrated self creates a story from elements that describe the self in action, such as agency, intentions, and goals.

THE DEVELOPMENT OF A THEORY OF MIND

Bretherton (1991) acknowledges that human infants are prepared from birth to engage in social interactions with a caregiver and emphasizes the understanding of the self and other in the development of a theory of mind as infants begin to anticipate others' intentions. She describes the following phases: (1) interfacing of minds (preverbal stage, 9 to 14 months); (2) interfacing minds through language (the early verbal phase); (3) interfacing minds through language (transition to early childhood); and

(4) understanding mind (the preschool years and beyond).

Studies of infant memory have documented that cued recall of motor activity is possible as early as 3 months of age (Rovee-Collier and Fagan, 1981). Based on a better understanding of infant memory, Stern (1985) hypothesized that infants may register their daily interactional sequences with a parent as generalized episodes that store "small, coherent chunks of lived experience, including not only actions, but also sensations, goals and affects of self and other in a temporal-physical-causal relationship." He referred to these generalized structures in memory as representations of interactions that have been generalized (RIGs). Stern suggests that RIGs are accessed in memory when a familiar self-other episode occurs. Developmentally, the idea of RIGs is supported through research studies that show older infants can anticipate another person's behavior in context. For example, Izard (1978) found that 8-month-old infants showed fear when their arm is being prepared for an injection and subsequently refused to interact with the nurse who has given the injection. Moreover, infants at this age show an anticipatory smile during peek-a-boo games before a parent or playmate reappears from behind a cloth.

Interfacing of Minds (9 to 14 Months)

With the establishment of object permanence, there is a transition from reliance on RIGs, or sensorimotor interactional schemata, to working models, or representational schemata. At about 9 months, infants come to understand that intentions and affective states may be shared. At 9 months, infants may reliably follow their mother's line of visual regard (Scaife and Bruner, 1975). Before 9 months, this "shared reference" is only intermittently seen. Between 6 and 9 months, infants responds to an adult's negative facial-vocal displays with crying or frowning, but after 9 months they seem to understand that the adult partner's emotional expression may provide information about external events. The ability to understand communication about a joint topic is then evident. At this age, infants' affective, vocal, and gestural communications attract and direct others' attention to topics of mutual interest. Concurrently, infants begin to understand others' communications to them as messages. This suggests that by the end of the first year of life, infants have acquired an early "theory of mind" or ability to impute mental states to the self and others (Bretherton and Bates, 1979). One mind now can be interfaced with another through conventional comprehensible signals. Maternal affect attunement may be the caregiver's response to these changes in the infant's psychological understanding. Stern suggests these cross-modal experiences of attunement emphasize and focus the infant's attention on psychological, rather than behavioral, sharing of experience. Individual differences in affect attunement may be important factors in the development of individual differences in a working model of the self. A mother may underattune or overattune to certain infant behaviors. This poorly coordinated responding may undermine an infant's ability to attend to his or her own inner states. Findings on parent-infant communication and secure and insecure attachment relationships corroborate Stern's suggestions that exaggerated attunement may be detrimental (Grossmann and Grossmann, 1984). Overstimulating mothers may be engaged in overattunement, and mothers of insecure-avoidant infants may be nonattuned to distress signals (Escher-Graeub and Grossmann, 1983).

Interfacing Minds through Language (Early Verbal)

Intentional attention seeking and other communicative symbols deriving from the preverbal stage help to establish initial infant-parent contact. However, the emergence of single words into gestural messages leads to a more precise interface between parent and child. Once the child has gained object names and relational words, the capacity for intentional intersubjectivity becomes more apparent. Greenfield and Smith (1976) found that 2-year-olds used two types of words differentially such that if parent and child had established a focus of joint attention, children commented on the action component with a relational word. If a joint topic of attention had not been established, the object was labeled first. By the middle of the second year, simple conversations about absent objects

and people are possible. Moreover, by 18 months, some toddlers are able to label internal states if given in an appropriate context. Their first references are to hunger, pain, disgust, and moral approval (Bretherton, McNew, and Beeghly-Smith, 1981). This labeling ability along with the use of perspective-shifting pronouns (you and I) develops rapidly during the third year of life (Bretherton and Beeghly, 1982). Empathy toward distressed others, the use of dolls as active partners in symbolic play, and self-recognition in the mirror also are occurring at this time. The shift that occurs may represent a gradual transition from an implicit to an explicit theory of mind. The establishment of language may also result in some contradiction for children because verbal explanations to them may be simplified too much and may be at variance with the child's own interpretation. At the beginning of language, verbal working models, which are available to conscious reflection, and nonverbal working models may be in conflict.

Interfacing Minds through Language (Transition to Early Childhood)

During the second year of life, children may begin to entertain a more explicit theory of mind. This suggestion was based originally on data recorded from mothers who listed their children's utterances about internal states in everyday context (Bretherton and Beeghly, 1982). Dunn, Bretherton, and Munn (1987) later corroborated these utterances through direct observation. By 28 months, a majority of 30 infants studied had a vocabulary that allowed the discussion of internal states and were able to talk about perceptions, sensations, and volition. Approximately two thirds of the sample labeled some emotions. The use of terms for moral judgment and utterances about cognitive processes were rare at this age but became more common after 30 months (Shatz, Wellman, and Silber, 1983). Children in the middle of the second year of life sometimes made causal statements about internal states; for example, "Grandma mad; I wrote on wall." Causal statements reported by Bretherton and Beeghly (1982) included utterances about events or actions that precede a particular state, utterances about negative states that act as motivators or causes for later behavior, and utterances that explain an emotion in terms of another related mental state. Moreover, 2- and 3-year-olds may be able to impute emotions and intentions to themselves, to dolls, and to play mates during make-believe play (Bretherton et al., 1986).

Wellman (1988) suggests that the term "theory of mind" is appropriate to describe 2½-year-old toddlers' talk about internal states. He suggests several criteria must be met to demonstrate an explicit theory of mind: (1) basic categories for defining reality exist; (2) these basic categories are organized into a coherent system of interrelationships; and (3) a causal attributional framework of human behavior has been acquired by the individual. Some children at 28 months were able to distinguish real from nonreal (e.g., "It's not real; it's only pretend"), to define one mental state in terms of another, appearing unhappy and being sad and talking about the consequences of emotional states, such as happiness and anger. Therefore, children at this age quite frequently do distinguish between reality and internal states, in keeping with the theory of mind model.

Understanding Mind: Preschool Years and Beyond

Children can be more formally interviewed in regard to mind by age 3. Wellman (1988) reported that 3-year-olds could distinguish between concrete objects and thought objects. When asked about absent objects in contrast to "pictures in your head" (Estes, Wellman, and Wooley, 1988), 3-, 4-, and 5-year- old children gave different reasons for not being able to touch a real, absent object (i.e., because "it's not there") or a thought-object (because "it's not real"). Therefore, young children have categories for distinguishing mental and nonmental phenomena. Three-year-olds do define mental states in terms of other mental states, for example, "People can't see my imagination." Moreover, they use a causal explanatory framework and give causes for several positive and negative emotions. Consequently, 3-year-olds do demonstrate a theory of mind. In addition, they seem to think of intentions as causes of behavior. As they grow older, children seem to have different conceptions of mind such that younger

children think of mind as a container that holds information. By age 4, reasoning about cognitions and feelings is more in keeping with an implicit theory of mind as a processor that interprets information (Perner, 1988). Differences between 3-year-olds' and 4- and 5-year-olds' conceptions of mind are evident in their responses to false belief tasks. For example, in the theory of mind tasks, 4-year-olds who have looked inside a matchbox filled with candy can correctly predict that another child who does not know the secret of the candy being there would wrongly guess that it contained matches. Three-year-olds, in contrast, are incapable of imputing false beliefs. The 3-year-old says the other child will guess correctly. Moreover, 4- and 5-year-olds can impute knowledge to others that they do not possess. Older preschool children are able to grasp that their truth is not necessarily another's truth. Four- and 5-year-olds also can understand that two children who receive the same gift may feel differently about it (Gove and Keating, 1979).

Perner (1988) suggested that young infants have mental models but cannot manipulate them out of context. He referred to this as the level of representation. When preschoolers can rearrange the components of mental models and create alternative realities in pretense or anticipate the future, they have reached the level of representation. By age 4, an additional capacity, metarepresentation, may emerge. Older preschool children do not just manipulate alternative models of events, they can construct mental models of belief states about events. This is metarepresentation because they manipulate mental models of mental models.

After approximately 7 years of age, the capacity for metarepresentation becomes further developed. Now children think not only about what others believe or think but about what others think about them (Miller, Kessel, and Flavell, 1970). To do this requires an ability to manipulate a mental model of two individuals' belief states as they relate to each other. The capacity for metarepresentation may be necessary for a child to understand another's deceptive intentions in games that involve hiding and guessing, their ability to understand second-order false beliefs (Perner and Wimmer, 1985) and their awareness that others as well as the self can be deliberately fooled about what is felt about the self. The metarepresentational ability becomes further enhanced in dealing with abstractions during adolescence.

THE SELF IN DEVELOPMENTAL DISORDERS

The establishment of the self is influenced by general cognitive limitations and disordered development in specific domains, such as the phonologic, visuospatial, and social cognitive ones. Both executive and nonexecutive functions may be disturbed in the developmental disorders. Attachment and stranger anxiety may be delayed in mental retardation; language disorders may adversely influence the development of working models; visuospatial disturbance may influence the establishment of the body self; and theory of mind disturbance may be apparent in autistic disorder. Parental discrepant working models of the expected normal child may reduce the parents' capacity to become attuned and limit the emergence of an adaptive self system.

Cicchetti et al. (1990) point out the dearth of experimental studies of the development of the self during the transition from infancy to early childhood in the developmental disorders and in children who have been abused. They have studied the development and coherence of the self system in children with Down syndrome and in maltreated children. In the first instance, biological factors assume primary importance; in the second, environmental factors (parent-child interactions) are primary. These authors found that, during play, children with Down syndrome showed similar, but delayed, sequences in their conceptions of self and other when compared to nonhandicapped children. Those children with Down syndrome who utilized play to represent self and other in hypothetical situations were the most cognitively mature. Nonlinguistic representations of the self were more advanced than linguistic representations. In contrast, maltreated children showed poor-quality internal working models with regard to themselves and in their relationship to attachment figures. Deviations in self system processes were found in visual self-recognition, in linguistic representations of the self and others, and in perceived self-competence. Studies such as these highlight the

importance of investigating children with developmental disorders to understand the emergence of the self system and to provide guidelines for treatment.

REFERENCES

Ainsworth, M.D.S., Bell, S.M., and Stayton, D. (1974). Infant-mother attachment and social development. In M.P. Richards (ed), *The introduction of the child into a social world*, pp. 99–135. Cambridge University Press, London.

Baldwin, J.M. (1895). *Mental development of the child and the race: Methods and processes*. Macmillan, New York.

_____. (1906). *Social and ethical interpretations in mental development*, 4th ed. Macmillan, London.

_____. (1911). *The individual and society*. Goreham, Boston.

Blehar, M.C., Lieberman, A.F., and Ainsworth, M.D.S. (1977). Early face-to-face interaction and its relation to later infant-mother attachment. *Child Development*, 48: 182–194.

Bowlby, J. (1969). *Attachment and loss*. Vol. 1, *Attachment*. Basic Books, New York (2nd rev. ed., 1982).

_____. (1973). *Attachment and loss*. Vol. 2, *Separation*. Basic Books, New York.

_____. (1980). *Attachment and loss*. Vol. 3, *Loss, sadness and depression*. Basic Books, New York.

Bretherton, I. (1987). New perspectives on attachment relations: Security, communication, and internal working models. In J. Osofsky (ed), *Handbook of infant development*, pp. 1061–1110. John Wiley & Sons, New York.

_____. (1990). Open communication and internal working models: Their role in the development of attachment relationships. In R.A. Thompson (ed), *The Nebraska Symposium on Motivation, 1988*, pp. 57–113. University of Nebraska Press, Lincoln, NE.

_____. (1991). Pouring new wine in old bottles: The social self as an internal working model. In M.R. Gunnar and L.A. Sroufe (eds), *Minnesota Symposia on Child Development*, 23:1–42. Lawrence Erlbaum, Hillsdale, NJ.

_____, and Bates, E. (1979). The emergence of intentional communication. In I. Uzg (issue ed), 4:81–100.

_____, and Beeghly, M. (1982). Talking about internal states: The acquisition of an explicit theory of mind. *Developmental Psychology*, 18: 906–921.

_____, Fritz, J., Zahn-Waxler, C., and Ridgeway, D. (1986). Learning to talk about emotions: A

functionalist perspective. *Child Development,*
57: 529–548.

_____, McNew, S., and Beeghly-Smith, M. (1981).
Early person knowledge as expressed in verbal
and gestural communication: When do infants
acquire a "theory of mind"? In M.E. Lamb and
L.R. Sherrod (eds), *Infant social cognition,* pp.
333–373. Lawrence Erlbaum, Hillsdale, NJ.

Cicchetti, D., Beeghly, M., Carlson, V., and Toth, S.
(1990). The emergence of the self in atypical
populations. In D. Cicchetti and M. Beeghly
(eds), *The self in transition.* pp. 309–344. University of Chicago Press, Chicago.

Connell, J.P. and Wellborn, J.G. (1991). Competence,
autonomy, and relatedness: A motivational
analysis of self-esteem processes. In M.R. Gunnar and L.A. Sroufe (eds), *The Minnesota Symposia on Child Development,* 23:43–77
Lawrence Erlbaum, Hillsdale, NJ.

Cooley, C.H. (1902). *Human nature and the social
order.* Scribner's, New York.

Deci, E.L. (1980). *The psychology of self-determination.* D.C. Heath, Lexington, MA.

Dunn, J., Bretherton, I., and Munn, P. (1987). Conversations about feeling states between mothers
and their young children. *Developmental Psychology,* 23:132–139.

Epstein, S. (1991). Cognitive-experiential self theory: Implications for developmental psychology. In M.R. Gunnar and L.A. Sroufe (eds),
Minnesota Symposia on Child Development,
23:79–124. Lawrence Erlbaum, Hillsdale, NJ.

Erikson, E. (1950). *Childhood and society.* W.W.
Norton, New York.

Escher-Graeub, D. and Grossmann, K.E. (1983).
*Bindungssicherheit im zweiten Lebensjahr-die
Regensburger Querschnittuntersuchung
[Attachment security in the second year of life:
The Regensburg cross-sectional study].*
Research Report, University of Regensburg
(quoted by Bretherton, 1991).

Estes, D., Wellman, H.M., and Wooley, J.D. (1988).
Children's understanding of mental phenomena.
In H. Reese (ed), *Advances in child develop-
ment and behavior.* Academic Press, New York.

Gove, F.L., and Keating, D. (1979). Empathic role-
taking precursors. *Developmental Psychology,*
15:594–600.

Greenfield, P.M., and Smith, J.H. (1976). *The structure of communication in early development.*
Academic Press, New York.

Grossmann, K.E., and Grossmann, K. (1984, September). *The development of conversational
styles in the first year of life and its relationship to maternal sensitivity and attachment
quality between mother and child.* Paper presented at the Congress of the German Society

for Psychology, Vienna (quoted by Bretherton,
1991).

_____, and _____ (1990). The wider concept of
attachment in cross-cultural research. *Human
Development,* 33:31–47.

_____, Fremmer-Bombik, E., Rudolph, J., and
Grossmann, K.E. (1988). Maternal attachment
representations as related to patterns of infant-
mother attachment and maternal care during the
first year. In R.A. Hinde and J. Stevenson-Hinde
(eds), *Relationships within families,* pp.
241–260. Oxford University Press, Oxford.

Izard, C.E. (1978). Emotions as motivations: An evo-
lutionary-developmental perspective. In R.A.
Dienstbier (ed), *Nebraska Symposium on Motivation,* pp. 163–200. University of Nebraska
Press, Lincoln.

Jacobsen, T., Edelstein, W., and Hofmann, V. (1993).
Children's representations of attachment as
related to later cognitive functioning. Poster
presented at the 40th Annual Meeting of the
American Academy of Child and Adolescent
Psychiatry, October, 1993, San Antonio, TX.

James, W. (1890). *The principles of psychology,* Vol.
1. Henry Holt, New York.

Johnson-Laird, P.N. (1983). *Mental models.* Harvard
University Press, Cambridge, MA.

Kernberg, O. (1976). *Object relations theory and
clinical psychoanalysis.* Aronson, New York.

Lewis, M. and Brooks-Gunn, J. (1979). *Social cognition and the acquisition of self.* Plenum Press,
New York.

Main, M. (1990). *A typology of human attachment
organization with discourse, drawings, and
interviews.* Cambridge University Press, New
York.

_____, and Hesse, E. (1990). Parents' unresolved
traumatic experiences are related to infant disorganized attachment status: Is frightening and/or
frightened parental behavior the linking mechanism? In M. Greenberg, D. Cicchetti, and M.
Cummings (eds), *Attachment in the preschool
years,* pp. 161–182. University of Chicago
Press, Chicago.

_____, and Solomon, J. (1986). Discovery of an
insecure-disorganized/disoriented attachment
pattern: Procedures, findings and implications
for the classification of behavior. In M. Yogman
and T.B. Brazelton (eds), *Affective development
in infancy,* pp. 95–124. Ablex, Norwood, NJ.

_____, and Weston, D. (1981). The quality of the
toddler's relationship to mother and father:
Related to conflict behavior and the readiness to
establish new relationships. *Child Development,*
52:834–840.

_____, Kaplan, K., and Cassidy, J. (1985). Security
in infancy, childhood and adulthood: A move to

the level of representation. In I. Bretherton and E. Waters (eds), Growing points of attachment theory and research, *Monographs of the Society for Research in Child Development*, 50, Serial No. 209 (1–2), 66–104.

Maslow, A.H. (1970). *Motivation and personality*, 2nd ed. Harper & Row, New York.

McClelland, D.C. (1985). *Human motivation.* Scott, Foresman, Dallas, TX.

McGuire, W. (1981). The spontaneous self-concept as affected by personal distinctiveness. In A.A. Norem-Hebersen and M. Lynch (eds), *Self-concept.* Ballinger, Cambridge, MA.

Mead, G.H. (1934). *Mind, self, and society.* University of Chicago Press, Chicago.

Miller, P.H., Kessel, F.S., and Flavell, J.H. (1970). Thinking about people thinking about people thinking about . . . : A study of social cognitive development. *Child Development*, 41:613–623.

Perner, J. (1988). Developing semantics for theories of mind: From propositional attitudes to mental representations. In J.W. Astington, P.L. Harris, and D.R. Olsen (eds), *Developing theories of mind*, pp. 141–172. Cambridge University Press, New York.

———, and Wimmer, H. (1985). "John thinks that Mary thinks that . . . : Attribution of second-order beliefs by 5- to 10-year-old children. *Journal of Experimental and Child Psychology*, 39:437–471.

Rovee-Collier, C.K., and Fagan, C.W. (1981). The retrieval of memory in early infancy. In L.P. Lipsitt (ed), *Advances in infancy research*, Vol. 1, pp. 225–254. Ablex, Norwood, NJ.

Sandler, J. and Sandler, A. (1978). The development of object relationships and affects. *Journal of Psycho-Analysis*, 59:285–296.

Scaife, M., and Bruner, J.S. (1975). The capacity for joint visual attention in the infant. *Nature*, 253:265–266.

Shatz, M., Wellman, H.M., and Silber, S. (1983). The acquisition of mental verbs: A systematic investigation of the first reference to mental state. *Cognition*, 14:301–321.

Sroufe, L.A., and Waters, E. (1977). Attachment as an organizational construct. *Child Development*, 48:1184–1199.

Stern, D.N. (1985). *The interpersonal world of the infant.* Basic Books, New York.

Sullivan, H.S. (1953). *The interpersonal theory of psychiatry.* W.W. Norton, New York.

Wellman, H.M. (1988). First steps in the child's theorizing about the mind. In J. Astington, P. Harris, and D. Olson (eds), *Developing theories of mind*, pp. 64–92. Cambridge University Press, New York.

White, R.W. (1959). Motivation reconsidered: The concept of competence. *Psychological Review*, 66:297–333.

Winnicott, D.W. (1958). *From paediatrics to psychoanalysis.* Hogarth Press, London.

———. (1965). *The maturational processes and the facilitating environment.* International Universities Press, New York.

Zeanah, C.H., Keener, M.A., Stewart, L., and Anders, T.F. (1985). Prenatal perception of infant personality: A preliminary investigation. *Journal of the American Academy of Child Psychiatry*, 24:204–210.

EVOLUTION OF LANGUAGE AND THE DEVELOPMENT OF REPRESENTATION

From the standpoint of evolution and ethology, the emergence of language is a crucial event in the establishment of the mind and distinguishes humans from other higher animals. Bickerton (1990), a linguist, points out that language is necessary to the development of consciousness and the emergence of mind. Although commonly thought of as a communicative device, language is more than that. Most basically, it is a system of representation—a means to sort and manipulate information. To understand social communication disorders in development, it is necessary to understand the evolutionary importance of representation. Representations, when established, can be used in a variety of ways. With the establishment of representation, pretense is possible as is play, but so also is deception. How the language system came about from our evolutionary past is a critical element in understanding the continuity between higher primates and humans and is the subject of this chapter.

DEVELOPMENT OF REPRESENTATION

Chrysippus, a philosopher who lived in the third century B.C., was one of the Greek stoics who was interested in how the world is represented by human beings to other human beings. The stoic philosophers may have been the first to invent the terminology for events and processes that occur when one thing is used to stand for another thing. Their word was *lekton*, which

was thought to signify a hidden process that must take place in an interpreter when one thing (*semaione*) is understood to take the place of or represent another thing (*tugchonon*). This process allows the interpreter to make the assumption that one thing is another thing. The stoics considered this a physical, concrete process, but hidden from direct view rather than an idea or concept. In his book *Embodiments of Mind,* McCulloch (1965) says, "What's in the brain is the stoic *lekton.*" This representational ability is basic to understanding the role of language in evolution and in developmental disorders. Representation is particularly important in regard to human relations and individual experience as it relates to beliefs, desires, and intentions. Primary representations are established through sensory experience, but secondary representations, or metarepresentation, require a process unique to humans—the capacity to reflect and reconstruct experiences. The ability for metarepresentation allows metaphorical and symbolic processes to be possible. The emergence of these ways of understanding is of particular importance in developmental disabilities, especially in severely retarded individuals and in those with autistic disorder.

THE EVOLUTION OF LANGUAGE

To understand the evolution of language and its uses, we must begin with the higher primates, who share 98% to 99% of human genes, with a particular focus on how the organization of their brains may differ from our own. MacLean (1990) has described an evolutionary or neuroethological perspective on brain development. He describes three characteristic formations: the protoreptilian formation, the paleomammalian formation (limbic system), and the neomammalian formation.

The evolutionary link between mammals and reptiles, the mammal-like reptiles (therapsids), are extinct. Yet reptiles and lizards are abundant, and observations of their behavior do provide evidence of an early link to social communication. Lizards give birth to many young, then destroy them immediately after birth unless they escape; here, parental behavior is absent. Parental attachment to the young is facilitated by sounds made by the newborn. Perhaps the earliest example of this kind of recognition is in the crocodile, which, possibly after hearing the sound of the egg cracking, moves forward with its snout to allow the newborn to break free. Although reptiles are nonverbal, they do have a substantial behavioral repertoire that includes at least 25 special forms of behavior, and at least 6 kinds of interoperative forms of behavior that are also characteristic of mammals.

A major physical change in the evolution from reptiles to mammals was a change in the articulation of the jaw that was followed by the establishment of the bones of the inner ear such that chewing and listening could occur simultaneously, enabling the parent to hear the infant's sounds. With the recognition of the infant cry, mother-infant behavior was transformed. The origin of suckling behavior and the delivery of milk from the mother led to prolonged contact and increased possibilities for individual recognition between mothers and infants and gave rise to the establishment of affiliative bonds. Moreover, audiovocal communication, particularly the infant cry, maintains maternal-offspring contact. This early vocalization, the separation or isolation call, is continuous throughout from mammalian species up to the human infant (MacLean, 1990, p. 401). With the development of these first vocalizations, vocal calls become extended such that a variety of calls are produced. In squirrel monkeys, the alarm call, the isolation call, and the twitter (an affiliative call) are examples. These differentiated calls may represent the first examples of a cognitive-affective link in evolution. Territorial and courtship displays may become linked not only through vision and smell but also through sound, as the defense of a newborn becomes a characteristic response.

The use of vocalization in defense of a newborn can be demonstrated in the vervet monkey in East Africa, whose alarm calls have been extensively studied (Cheney and Seyfarth, 1980). There are three alarm calls: one for predators on the ground (e.g., pythons), leading other monkeys to survey the ground when they hear this call; one for terrestrial predators (e.g., leopards); and a third for predators from the sky (e.g., martial eagles). Behavior occurs in other members of a troop corresponding to the type of alarm call. Those alerted to the snake look to the ground, to the leopard climb to the trees, and to the eagle descend to hide in bushes.

Newborns produce alarm calls but only later learn how to specify them. For example, a young monkey may make the eagle call for other large birds, such as owls and vultures, until it can become specified through experience (Cheney and Seyfarth, 1990, p. 129). Furthermore, it is the female monkey adults who primarily make the python and eagle calls, and the males who primarily make the leopard call. This may be the result of early socialization experiences, as the females remain with their mothers while the young males participate with the adult males in explorations that make it more likely that they would come in contact with leopards, who represent the greatest danger. Interestingly, there are anecdotal reports that these monkeys may use the alarm call to deceive other members of the troop or to distract them from aggression or to remove food competitors (Cheney and Seyfarth, 1990, p. 184; Leakey and Lewin, 1992, p. 242.). The alarm call may communicate an internal representation of a dangerous situation and produce the effect of others moving away (it is not known if this is a deliberate response or an associational response to clear the area of others). Experimental evidence is lacking that any animal species regularly manipulates the rate and context of false signals. Through more systematic experiments, it should become possible to determine whether these anecdotal reports do indeed reflect intentional signal falsification and to clarify the constraints under which deceptive communication arises. These alarm or panic calls have a survival function; vervet monkeys do not have specific sounds to identify nonpredators.

That these early vocalizations are representational is demonstrated by monkeys responding to audiotaped calls when there are no predators nearby. This early representational function of the call is basic and provides an evolutionary link, leading to continuity between higher primate and human behavior. How the vocal information is structured and how it is encoded is not yet known, but the benefit of the behavior can be demonstrated by its survival function. Simply describing and listing behaviors does not provide an adequate description. Instead, the more abstract social relationship that underlies the representation is more efficient. Relationships can be defined in terms of the content, quality, and patterning of interaction between two individuals over time. What matters in defining behavior is not only the behavior but the temporal relationship among behaviors and the context in which an activity is conducted.

Cheney and Seyfarth (1980, 1990) suggest that monkeys evolved the ability to represent social relationships because this offers the most accurate means of predicting the behavior of others. Rather than remembering discrete characteristics of each interaction based on patterns observed once or twice, a prediction can be made about the next interaction. Furthermore, vocal communication has meaning, so the representation or meaning of the vocalization can be understood by those who can interpret the sounds.

Moving up the phylogenetic tree to the chimpanzee, a higher level of representation is noted. Chimpanzees seem to recognize thoughts as agents of actions, and their behavior seems focused on altering or controlling others' states of mind. They seem to understand that other chimpanzees have beliefs, but they do not distinguish between different beliefs and no beliefs. The attribution of a mental state to another is not taught by vervet monkeys to their young. These younger monkeys rely on observational learning; perhaps the parent monkey fails to recognize that knowledge possessed by others differs from one's own. These monkeys' activities focus on

changing behavior of others, not on changing beliefs. The inability to attribute mental states is important in regard to empathy or compassion. Although grief has been noted in chimpanzees (Goddall's Flint avoided others, sat alone rocking, stopped eating, and eventually died following the death of his mother), other chimpanzees do not show sympathy or seem to recognize a mental state, so sorrow is not shared. This is a fundamental difference between human and nonhuman primates in social behavior.

Even though 98% to 99% of human genes are shared with the chimpanzee, there are remarkable differences in mental functioning between humans and the higher primates, particularly in language. The evolution of language must have occurred fairly recently because it is thought that our common ancestor emerged only about five million years ago. In fact, anthropological studies suggest that brain weight may have been greater in early man. However, it is not the weight of the brain but how it is organized that is critical in regard to language development. Children with macrocephaly and recent descriptions of the brains of children with autistic disorder suggest that brain weight or size are not the critical factors.

Three main sources point to the early establishment of spoken language in human evolution: anatomical evidence on the organization of the human brain and the vocal system; the products of the human mind that might require the use of language to communicate with others, for example, the use of tools; and last, the more abstract products of communication, such as image production and ritualistic behavior.

As noted in Chapter 11, consciousness cannot be specifically and precisely located in a particular brain region; it requires utilization of several brain areas. Other functions, such as language, that have been considered to be localized are not fully localized. An individual may lose large sections of the brain with no loss of language or cognitive function. During evolution, the brain has increased in size, yet the larger brain does not seem to be simply made up of a cumulation of functional units. When the human brain is compared with that of higher primates, differences in the size of the various lobes are the most apparent. In humans, the temporal and parietal lobes are prominent, whereas the occipital lobe is reduced in size when compared to other primates. Most pronounced is the frontal lobe, which is approximately double the size of that in apes. Consequently, brain lobes have a human organization (or in the primates, an apelike organization). The prominence of the various lobes allows us to study fossil brain casts to understand the evolutionary changes that have taken place. Particularly, these differences in brain regional development make it possible to look back to determine the earliest time that the humanlike brain organization became apparent.

In the human brain, two language centers are particularly prominent, namely, Wernicke's area and Broca's area. Wernicke identified damage to the upper posterior part of the left temporal lobe as leading to difficulties with language comprehension wherein the patient might speak fluently but not make sense. On the other hand, Broca demonstrated that damage to the lower posterior part of the left frontal lobe produced difficulties in speech production, with intact comprehension. As a result of the development of language, the left hemisphere is larger than the right. This left hemisphere dominance is associated with handedness. In humans, it is assumed that left hemisphere dominance is the consequence of language development and that handedness has accompanied it. In higher primates, one hemisphere may be larger than the other, but this effect is not as apparent as in humans. Although in nonhuman primates handedness preference has not been demonstrated at the population level, the use of hand preference has been reported in language-trained chimpanzees (*Pan troglodytes*) in both naturalistic and experimental paradigms (Hopkins and Morris, 1993; Morris, Hopkins and Bolser-Gilmore, 1993). Moreover, Hopkins et al. (1992) demonstrated hemispheric asymmetries for processing communicative symbols in language-trained chimpanzees.

In the human brain, there is a distinct prominence over Broca's area, the region involved in language production. The Broca's area prominence may be demonstrated in fossil brain casts and is sought by paleoanthropologists. In human evolution, the clear rise seen over Broca's area is taken as a physical signal of language ability, although it is an uncertain one. In viewing human evolution in paleoanthropology, the skull of *Homo habilis* was found to have evidence of Broca's area. Although this is not proof that language evolved with *Homo habilis*, it is important to recognize that this is the first known hominid species in which brain expansion has occurred. *Homo habilis* lived approximately 2 million years ago. The evidence for language before *Homo habilis* has not been demonstrated. For example, a distinct Broca's area has not been noted in australopithecus. Therefore, although some vocalization is expected, no paleoneurological evidence is available to suggest language areas developing in the brain before *Homo habilis*. Moreover, Leakey and Lewin (1992) suggest that human language, in its earliest stages, was an extension of vocal abilities, so a range of sounds were expressed along with some structure in their expression. Vocal noise, then, was associated with primate sociability.

Besides physical evidence, the creation of stone tools may provide cues to brain organization. It has been suggested that the use of stone tools may provide a guide to handedness. Toth (1987) found that the pattern of flakes recovered from the earliest archeological sites is similar to the pattern produced when a right-handed person makes tools. He speculates that *Homo habilis* were primarily right-handed, suggesting left hemispheric dominance had emerged by this time, which would perhaps be associated with the evolution of language because right-handedness is associated with left hemispheric dominance. Still, the presence of left hemispheric dominance provides only indirect evidence of language evolution. It is most likely that language abilities emerged gradually during the hunting and gathering way of life. In primate evolution, there is some evidence that communication occurs. For example, a troop of baboons will split in two at the beginning of the day and travel in groups together; the parties will forage for food in different parts of their range. Yellow baboons come and go, visit or stay. They may relate to one another and even recognize a natal relationship even though there is not a coalition of the various troops. This establishment of groups for hunting and gathering seems associated with social communication, but is primarily nonverbal. However, among modern human hunter-gatherers, temporary aggregations of individuals are quite common. These periods of aggregation are associated with intense socializing, renewing and evaluating alliances, and searching for marriage partners. This social aggregation becomes part of tribal structure, and individuals become united by common language and culture. On the other hand, it is unlikely that the earliest hominids showed such extensive social organization. Leakey and Lewin (1992) suggest that it is not the case, that once characteristics of humanness emerged, all characteristics were present. It may well be that it was only with the emergence of *Homo sapiens* that social aggregation evolved.

Another anatomical approach to the emergence of language has to do with the vocal apparatus itself. This includes the larynx, the pharynx, the tongue, and the lips. In the basic mammalian pattern, the larynx is high in the neck. As a consequence, the larynx locks into the nasopharynx, the air space at the back of the nasal cavity. This allows animals to breathe and drink at the same time. As a result of this anatomical pattern, the range of sounds that an animal can make is limited because the pharyngeal cavity, which is necessary for sound amplification, is small. Consequently, vocalization depends primarily on the shape of the oral cavity and the lips, which modify sounds which are produced in the larynx.

On the other hand, in humans the structure is unique and very different from the animal world. In humans, the larynx is located much lower in the neck, so humans cannot concurrently drink and breathe without choking. Therefore, humans are more vulnerable to choking on food while swallowing it. Still, this lower position of the larynx produces a larger pharyngeal space above the vocal chords, which makes possible a greater range of sound modification and becomes the key to the production of articulate speech.

Laitman and colleagues (Laitman, Heimbuch, and Crelin, 1978; Laitman and Heimbuch, 1982; Laitman and Reidenberg, 1988) have investigated the development of the human vocal tract from infancy onward. They have demonstrated that human infants are born with the larynx in the typical mammalian position, which is high in the neck, so they can simultaneously breathe and drink, as they do during nursing. At about 1½ years, the larynx begins to migrate down the neck, but does not

reach the adult position until about 14 years. As a consequence of the migration of the larynx, there is increasing ability in sound production. The descent of the larynx in evolution provides an alternative way to look at the fossil records. For example, the high larynx in the human ancestor would imply apelike language ability, but a lower larynx would suggest human ability. Although much of the cartilaginous vocal tract decays during fossilization, the shape of the bottom of the skull, or basicranium, that is seen in fossils is related to the position of the larynx. The basicranium is the roof of the upper respiratory tract. In the basic mammalian pattern, the basicranium is essentially flat, but in humans it is demonstrably arched. In the australopithecus, a typical apelike basicranium is noted. This suggests that it would have been impossible to produce universal vowel sounds, which are characteristic of human speech. The earliest time in the fossil record that a fully flexed basicranium is seen is 300 to 400 thousand years ago. This pattern is maintained subsequently and clearly demonstrated in fully modern humans, who evolved about 100 thousand years ago. Laitman and Heimbuch (1982) suggest that the earliest *Homo erectus* shows evidence of flexion in the basicranial area. Based on this evidence, spoken language may have begun to evolve about 1.6 million years ago. These authors propose that in *Homo erectus,* the larynx may have been in an intermediate position between the ape configuration and what we see in modern humans, perhaps similar to children of about age six. It is presumed that the dangers of choking were present, but some selective advantage accrued due to a partially developed language ability. It has not been possible to use the basicranial information to look further back than *Homo erectus* to *Homo habilis* because none of the basal crania of the latter species are sufficiently intact.

Although fossil evidence suggests that spoken language may have emerged in early *Homo* species, to learn more about the emergence of language and mind, another approach is necessary. One approach is to study written language. The actual oldest records of language are no older than the first invention of written systems, which was 5,000 to 6,000 years ago, yet the physiological basis for language in earlier fossils suggests that human language roots extend back before this time. To answer this question, Isaac (1984) has evaluated the stone tool record by assessing the complexity of stone tools over time. Between 2 million and 50,000 years ago, stone tools became more numerous, and about 1.6 million years ago, and again about 250,000 years ago, major improvements in tools were noted. These dates coincide with the emergence first of *Homo erectus,* and subsequently, of the early archaic *Homo sapiens.* The improvement in stone toolmaking has been taken to suggest that ancestors became more skilled in their tool manufacture and were able to do more with them. With time, the fabric of culture seems more apparent in the design of tools and suggests innovation used in their production. However, Isaac doubts this assumption and does not feel that the increase in complexity necessarily indicates an increase in tasks performed with the tools. Changes and refinement in stone tool structure, on the other hand, may reflect cultural changes. It may be that toolmaking began to involve more complex rules. To communicate more complex rules, a more elaborate syntax and detailed vocabulary might be needed.

The presence of order and similarity in stone artifacts in the archeological record, then, may echo other societal changes. The changes in tool production may indicate clear designation of roles in the community. When modern foraging people have been evaluated, they have been noted to demonstrate elaborate kinship systems that dictate marriage, food sharing, and location of housing. The establishment of order would have substantially benefited from the emergence of language. Furthermore, the crafting of sculptures and the development of painted images seem to have involved esthetics, as these images are visually pleasing forms. The establishment of order in culture and the emergence of esthetics would potentially have required spoken language (Leakey and Lewin, 1992).

Isaac (1984) goes on to suggest that the augmented cultural milieu was essential to the further establishment of language. However, direct evidence of spoken language is not available so other approaches need to be considered. Anthropologists have looked for evidence of abstraction as evidence of language emergence, because a mind without language is locked into its own mental world. Words and reflective thought allow the exploration of the world and may create experiences through imagination and conceptualization. Visual images could be a unique product of such conceptualization.

When higher primates have been studied, none have been shown to paint images that can be accepted as representational. However, it seems that the emergence of the representation ability was an essential event in human history — perhaps related to the mental world's going beyond the individual through the emergence of language. Representational images in the archeological record may potentially be part of some earlier mythologies. Such representational and abstract images begin to appear in Africa and in Europe about 30,000 years ago. It is striking that image making enters the archeological record at about the same time in both places. Before this time, there are some scattered remnants of symbolic behavior, including an engraved ox rib from a 300,000-year-old site in France and a piece of sharpened ocher found near the coast dated to about 250,000 years ago in France. Although it is possible that earlier evidences of representation or symbolic behavior were made on materials that did not survive, one would expect that if images that were 30,000 years old were found on rock surfaces, earlier ones might have been found if they existed. The current evidence continues to suggest that the earliest representational images were produced approximately 30,000 years ago.

In addition to images, other symbolic means may be investigated. A specific example is the use of ritual burial, which is associated with Neanderthal people. The body of a hunter was found in a grave in a cave in La Chapelle-Aux-Saints in France that dates back 40,000 years. Accompanying the body was a bison leg, other animal bones, and some flint tools. Another example is a burial 60,000 years ago in the Zagros Mountains in modern Iraq. In this instance, the burial is laid out on plant material surrounded by spring flowers, thistle, grape hyacinth, and other plants. It is suggested that concern for the dead may be associated with language development and the emergence of consciousness of bereavement. The evidence suggests beyond chance that the associations of bodies with stone tools and specific alignments are consistent with the early emergence of burial rituals. Yet even though a *Homo sapiens,* i.e., *Homo sapiens neanderthalensis,* Lieberman (1991) suggests that language deficiency was a characteristic feature because the basicranium of the old man at La Chapelle does not show any more flexion than that seen in a 1.5-million-year-old *Homo erectus.*

Based on such studies, Lieberman (1991) suggests that language deficiency may have played a role in the extinction of the Neanderthals. Lieberman, Crelin, and Klatt (1972) used computer modeling techniques to determine the phonetic output of a reconstructed Neanderthal airway. They found that the reconstructed airway output was similar to that of nonhuman primates and human newborns. They postulate that Neanderthal speech would have been nasalized and would have resulted in a high number of phonetic errors. Still, Neanderthals are thought to have had the anatomical prerequisites to produce nasalized versions of all human speech sounds except *i, u, a* and velar consonants. Moreover, Neanderthal hominids seem to have had a fairly advanced culture in which elderly ill individuals could survive. They used complex stone tools and fire, most likely wore clothing, may have made wood-framed skin shelters, and may have produced art. However, they probably did not have modern human speech because they lacked a human vocal tract.

The acquisition of fully articulate spoken language with syntax was a major event in the origin of modern humans. The earliest fossil remains of anatomically modern *Homo sapiens* that can be accurately dated suggest they lived about 100,000 years ago. These early humans had modern supralaryngeal vocal tracts and the brain mechanisms that are necessary to produce human species syntax. They most likely had a language, or languages, that made use of complex syntax and reasoning ability (Lieberman, 1991), yet it is possible that human language and thought could be still older, and modern human beings might have appeared as early as 250,000 years ago. The earlier figure is based on tracing human efforts to establish the meaning of death through burial rituals and the conduct of life through religious and moral practices.

Leakey and Lewin (1992) suggest that the development of language represented an incremental change and that the critical advance may have been in sound perception and mental decoding rather than in the capability to rapidly produce sounds. Therefore, they suggest that both language production and perception may have evolved together. Human speech uses fifty sounds in contrast to only a dozen in other higher primates. This fourfold increase in humans is a consequence of a modified vocal tract. However, the advance in the breadth of communication is more than additional sounds. Most likely, it is the result of the remodeling of mental machinery within the brain, but this cannot be established from fossil evidence. The growth of language with the emergence of these capacities is remarkable in that there are approximately 5,000 languages, each of which has its basis in complex evolutionary relationships to what may have been an original mother tongue. These languages belong to a dozen or more language families. Yet the languages tend to be associated with separate cultures. The establishment of language allowed individuals to establish their own culture and their own environment. The role of culture, as established with language, is particularly important because it provides meaning; however, this comprehensive language development is the end product of an evolutionary line that links us with the rest of the natural world (Leakey and Lewin, 1992). The evolutionary record, which shows *Homo erectus* and *Homo habilis* preceding *Homo sapiens,* provides a link to the evolutionary record and puts human specialness in historical perspective.

Empathy, Representation, and Brain Evolution

Differences in the brain between man and higher primates require the study of both behavior and anatomy. Chimpanzees may carry out certain tasks in language studies, yet the highest-functioning apes are not capable of empathizing with another to the extent that they can understand the effect that their own actions may have on another's thinking or feeling. A capacity for empathy seems to form the basis of moral reasoning. Deacon (1983, 1990) has studied the evolutionary basis of how the brain developed the capacity to symbolically represent others' thoughts and actions, what he called "representational empathy." He suggests that the brain reorganized itself over 2 million years ago by expanding its ability to process language and to establish symbolic representation. Rather than the development of entirely new structures and novel neuronal connections, he suggests that there is a "systematic reorganization" in which the human brain gradually recruited and modified brain regions and circuits, which were once important for other functions, to use in establishing symbolic learning.

The primary evolutionary changes do occur in the prefrontal cortex, which is twice as large in humans as in other primates if adjustments are made for total brain size. Broca's area, which is involved in speech, is included in this expanded frontal region. Deacon (1983) suggests that the prefrontal cortex is particularly important and that it inherited space and circuitry that extends throughout the brain to regions that were once used for vision, smell, and specialized vocalizations — areas that have shrunk in size over time. How did this reorganization take place? What demands drove the reorganization? Deacon (1983) finds that the ability to think symbolically arose about 2 million years ago with the establishment of *Homo habilis.* He indicates that the increase in brain size in *Homo habilis* seems to signal a new reorganization of the brain, which may have occurred in response to some new cognitive demands, speculating that such essential change evolved from the need to facilitate communication with other early human ancestors. Social structure may have become more complex as stone tools were used to hunt game and to prepare meat. New ways may have been needed to publicly negotiate longer-term agreements with one another and to enter complex relationships, which involved hunting and sexual exclusion.

The complexity of the needed social learning may have driven the evolution of a distinctly human brain, leading to the highly complex specialized brain that allows humans to "represent to ourselves what goes on in others' minds." According to Deacon, this capacity becomes the "basis of moral decisions. Human compassion as well as intentional cruelty may have evolved in parallel with language ability." His view is consistent with the idea that an important evolutionary change that occurred was in the development of the representational ability used for language and for anticipating others' intentions.

The level of representation of another individual is not specifically a mental state, according to Brothers and Ring (1992), but rather the representation of a person. That representation includes intentional stances or attitudes and action tendencies that have an affective valence for the observer. What one person experiences is not simply another being with a mental life, but rather a person. The personal representation relates to an evolutionary view of social cooperativeness in evolutionary development.

Theory of Mind in Primates

Premack and Woodruff (1978) described "theory of mind" in chimpanzees. They used this term to describe the attribution of beliefs, knowledge, and emotions to both oneself and others. It is considered a theory because mental states are not directly observable in behavior; however, they can be used to make predictions about behavior. These authors and others (Astington, Harris, and Olson, 1988) suggested that an animal or human mind has first-order intentionality and experiences beliefs and desires. However, there is also a second-order intentionality whose origins are less clear. Second-order intentions refer to having a mental state about the mental state of another. The emergence of second-order intentions has been studied by primatologists and by developmental psychologists (Astington, Harris, and Olson, 1988). Metarepresentation, as proposed by Leslie (1987), is an essential concept in understanding the formation of second-order intentionality. Metarepresentation decouples descriptive mental states, such as belief, from the external world. From a developmental perspective, the sense of personal agency and goal-directedness appear first and belief appears later. There is a selective advantage of judging others by their motives rather than by their prior behavior, which allows better generalization of past experiences from one circumstance to another. The ability to predict whether another who has acted deceptively before will be deceptive again provides selective advantage.

Still, fundamental differences do exist

between human and nonhuman primates based on the presence, or lack, of a theory of mind, that is, the ability to recognize one's own knowledge and to attribute mental states to another. The latter's awareness of motives of another is based on experience of action, but not of thought and feeling. Although sensitive to other animals' behavior, they know little about knowledge and the motives that cause them to act as they do. In short, these nonhuman primates do not know what they know and are not able to recognize knowledge or lack of it in others. Cheney and Seyfarth (1990) conclude that monkeys see the world as made up of things that act but not things that think and feel.

Despite the importance and presence of representations in monkeys and higher apes, there is no evidence of communicative intent to change another's mental state or draw attention to one's own mental states. Lacking attribution of mental states to others, these primates do not recognize that mental states exist. In summary, chimpanzees are acute observers of others' behaviors but not of others' minds.

IMPACT OF EARLY EXPERIENCE ON LANGUAGE

Studies in Chimpanzees

Chimpanzees have been raised in a typical human language environment, thus providing them with the same environmental advantages that a young child enjoys. Although they lack a true theory of mind, chimpanzees can learn to sign single words and join different word classes into a consistent pattern. This may be as characteristic of them as it is in children under age two. The first ape-language studies utilized sign language with the chimpanzee Washoe, who, after four years of training, is recorded to have learned 132 hand signs (Gardner, Gardner, and Van Cantfort, 1989). Gardner and Gardner (1974) showed the similarity of utterances between children at the two-word stage of language development and the chimpanzee Washoe, who used American Sign Language (ASL) (Table 16–1).

These sets of examples show that both the child who is under two and the chimpanzee attribute qualities to objects, show location of actions, and express the relations of agents to actions, yet although the two sets of items are

formally identical, there are differences in the child utterances from those in the chimpanzee. Apes use sign language to talk only about objects they want or actions they want performed on them. On the other hand, the child seems to be categorizing for the sake of categorization. So, although there are no formal substantive differences between the utterances, it may be concluded that the children under two years of age at this stage in development may show evidence of a line similar to that of early ancestral forms of language.

Despite these findings, questions were raised about the technique used with Washoe and whether the signs were truly used to communicate. That is, were Washoe's signs language or were they operantly conditioned hand movements? The major concern is whether the signing had meaning. These early investigations of the linguistic capabilities of apes focused on the ape's ability to produce signs or even words rather than focusing on comprehension. To answer these questions about meaning and comprehension, subsequent studies were carried out. These studies were based on the premise that because comprehension precedes word production and may, in fact, guide production in normal human language development, it should be possible to assess language comprehension in chimpanzees if they have the cognitive ability to understand syntactic structure and word-referent relations.

To answer this question, Savage-Rumbaugh et al. (1993) carried out systematic experiments where they compared language comprehension skills of a 2-year-old child and an 8-year-old pygmy chimpanzee or bonobo (Pan paniscus), who was raised in a special language environment that was similar to that in which children are raised but modified for an ape. The child (Alia) and the bonobo (Kanzi) were exposed to spoken English and to lexigrams beginning in infancy, although neither was trained to comprehend speech. In these settings, which used a common caretaker, language acquisition was through observational learning. The authors asked both Alia and Kanzi to respond to the same 660 novel sentences. The responses were videotaped and scored for accuracy of English language comprehension. Both Alia and Kanzi were able to comprehend novel requests and simple syntax. Both performed equally well on

Table 16–1. Comparison of Child and Chimpanzee Utterances

Child Utterances	Washoe's Signed Utterances (ASL)
1. Big train; red book	1. Drink red; comb black
2. Adam checker; Mommy lunch	2. Clothes Mrs. G.; you hat
3. Walk street; go store	3. Go in; look out
4. Adam put; Eve read	4. Roger tickle; you drink
5. Put book; hit ball	5. Tickle Washoe; open blanket

From Gardner and Gardner, 1974.

sentences that required the ability to reverse word order. Kanzi showed higher accuracy than Alia in decoding the syntactic device of word recursion (repeated application or nesting of entities; e.g., the man who ate the apple that was on the tree that was on the hill that was near the lake that was . . .), whereas Alia was superior on the conjunctive, a structure which requires the greater use of short- term memory.

This study demonstrated that the comprehension of spoken English could be tested in a child and a bonobo raised in similar environmental settings. By testing them in a similar manner, a systematic comparison of the language capacities of an ape and a child was possible. In the past, the language capacity of apes has sometimes been attributed to imitation of their caregivers, and it has been suggested that they are not able to produce syntactically based sentences (Terrace et al., 1979). The findings with Alia and Kanzi challenge these assumptions. First, Kanzi's comprehension cannot be attributed to imitation because the experimenter did not perform a set of actions for Kanzi to imitate and then follow. Moreover, information processing at a syntactic level was demonstrated both in correct responses and in errors. Finally, comprehension was demonstrated not only for word order but also for word recursion. Comprehension was of spoken English, entailing the parsing of phonemes, words, and sentence structures (Savage-Rumbaugh et al., 1993).

Wallman (1992) acknowledges that Kanzi is able to put together the object or objects and the action mentioned in an appropriate manner when considering the properties of the objects involved. However, he suggests that Kanzi's performance does not provide evidence that he was attending to simple syntactic features, such as word order. Yet Bates (1993) does conclude

that Kanzi is capable of language comprehension that approximates the level of the abilities of a human 2-year-old who is on the verge of full-blown sentence processing.

Early Language Deprivation in Humans

Human language develops in a social context. There are rare examples of children being raised without language exposure from adults. These are ordinarily abusive situations, and it has been difficult to separate out the effects of abuse and preexisting mental retardation when interpreting the findings. One such case is that of a girl, Genie, described by Susan Curtiss (1977). This was a young woman who had been imprisoned alone in a bedroom from approximately 18 months of age until her early teens, without exposure to language during those years. Intensive speech and language therapy was initiated, but she did not fully acquire language. Although she demonstrated the pre-2-year-old stages of language, she did not move beyond what is referred to as *protolanguage*. Her language basically consisted of two or three content words loosely linked by meaning but without grammatical items.

Her lack of response to language training is not consistent with language being a unitary system. If language acquisition requires exposure to some form of linguistic input within a critical period, then Genie, who was not speaking previously, would not have acquired any language. However, if there is not a critical period for acquisition, she should have acquired language fully. Her response raises questions about why she acquired language and why her language acquisition stopped at a particular point. Furthermore, why language stopped where it did rather than at an earlier or later stage must be considered.

One explanation is that protolanguage is an early stage of language development that, although part of our biological endowment, lacks most of the distinguishing formal properties of language (Bickerton, 1990). If this is assumed, then Genie acquired protolanguage because it is more robust than formal language. It does not have a critical period, although some lexical input is necessary for it to develop. The explanation for her language development ceasing would be because protolanguage and formal language are separate or disjoint, so the acquisition of one does not involve the acquisition of the other. Her language would have ceased when it did because she had moved as far as she could in the development of protolanguage alone. In addition to protolanguage, she developed some rote learned phrases but did not develop the formal language that one would have expected. She represents a case of an individual who, even though mature, still employed a variety of language that, despite its content, is formally no more developed than children under two. Similar findings are seen with adults who have formal language but are forced to utilize protolanguage by social circumstances in new language environments.

Still, the Genie case presents the problem of studying children with severe sensory and social deprivation. She had hyperbilirubinemia at birth, was thought by her father to be mentally retarded, and was subsequently severely neglected. The extent of early brain dysfunction before the beginning of her severe neglect is unclear. Recent studies of some of Harlow's early isolated monkeys (Martin et al., 1991) show the impact of early deprivation on the organization of brain development. Given the fact that Genie apparently had abnormal brain development, Bickerton's (1990) speculations on protolanguage are pertinent in regard to how far therapy might go in a severely deprived child with brain dysfunction, but it is probably mistaken to generalize from this case about language development. Genie experienced both sensory and language deprivation, and it remains unclear whether there may have been prenatal or perinatal events that affected brain development in her case.

MENTAL EVENT REPRESENTATION

In humans, an individual with the capacity to mentally represent and construct mental models has considerable advantages in both understanding and planning behavior. Mental modules that can simulate relevant causal relationships are essential for potential future planning and the capacity to respond. Internal working models require a representational system that utilizes dynamic events or agent-action-object structures rather than simple static images or logical operations alone. Representational processes underlie the development of reflective self-awareness, of the ability to take perspective, along with the capacity for intersubjectivity. Mental models most likely occur at two levels. First, the model consists of dissociable elements that are stored in long-term memory; second, temporary mental models are constructed from working, or short-term, memory when new adaptations are required. Thus, mental models are constructed and revised in working memory from representational elements of people and objects and various relationships — spatial, temporal, and causal — which are stored in longer-term memory. Consequently, component events must be organized as representations and stored in long-term memory, and these components must be locatable and available for retrieval in temporary working memory to be manipulated and recombined (Johnson-Laird, 1983). The elements that are constructed in working, or short-term, memory must be eventually fed back to a longer-term representational system.

The schematic structure of long-term memory has been emphasized by several authors (Nelson, 1986; Nelson and Ross, 1982; Schank, 1982; Schank and Abelson, 1977). These authors suggest that representational systems consist of mental structures that incorporate information about recurrent similar events. These events have been referred to as "event schemata," or scripts, and have been defined as sequentially organized structures, which may incorporate specific agent roles, action sequences that are motivated by specific goals and emotions, the recipients of actions, and the locality in which it takes place. Schank (1982) has proposed that scripts are called up when an individual re-experiences a relevant event and, in doing so, may be helpful in making predictions. He suggested that information which derives from episodic, or autobiographical, memory for personal events is reprocessed, localized, cross-indexed, and produced as a variety of different schema categories. Each of these preserves some aspect of the spatio-temporal-causal structure of experiences. Some of these schemata are important in ordering mini-event representations into more coordinated, longer event sequences (scripts) and others provide summary information from similar mini-events or generalize across different event sequences. In this proposal, elements of old information may be recombined to create new mental models.

The study of mental representation in developmental disorders is just beginning. The investigation of social cognition of metarepresentation in autistic disorder is well under way. The developmental disorders provide an opportunity to study the various aspects of event representation as it applies to language, memory, and the self.

REFERENCES

Astington, J., Harris, P., and Olson, D. (eds). (1988). *Developing theories of mind.* Cambridge University Press, Cambridge, UK.

Bates, E. (1993). Comprehension and production in early language development. Commentary on Savage-Rumbaugh, E.S., Murphy, J., Sevcik, R.A., Brakke, K.E., Williams, S.L., and Rumbaugh, D.M. (1993). *Language comprehension in ape and child.* Monographs of the Society for Research in Child Development, 58(3–4, Serial No. 233):222–242.

Bickerton, D. (1990). *Language and species.* University of Chicago Press, Chicago.

Brothers, L., and Ring, B. (1992). A neuroethological framework for the representation of minds. *Journal of Cognitive Neuroscience,* 4:107–118.

Cheney, D.L., and Seyfarth, R.M. (1980). Vocal recognition in free ranging vervet monkeys. *Animal Behavior,* 28:362–367.

_____, and _____ (1990). *How monkeys see the world.* University of Chicago Press, Chicago.

Curtiss, S. (1977). *Genie: A psycholinguistic study of a modern-day "wildchild."* Academic Press, New York.

Deacon, T.W. (1983). Human brain evolution. I. Evolution of language circuits. In H.J. Jerison and I. Jerison (eds), *Intelligence and evolutionary biology,* pp. 363–382. Springer-Verlag, Berlin.

_____. (1990). The neural circuitry underlying primate calls and human language. In B.A. Chiarelli, P. Lieberman, and J. Wind (eds), *The origin of language, Proceedings of a NATO/Advanced Study Institute,* Il Sedicesimo,

Florence, Italy. (Referenced by P. Lieberman, in *Uniquely human.*)

_____ (in press). *Symbolic origins.*

Gardner, B.T., and Gardner, R.A. (1974). Comparing the early utterances of child and chimpanzee. In A. Pick (ed), *Minnesota Symposium on Child Psychology,* vol. 8:3–23. University of Minnesota Press, Minneapolis.

_____, _____, and Van Cantfort, T.E. (1989). *Teaching sign language to chimpanzees.* State University of New York Press, Albany, NY.

Hopkins, W.D., and Morris, R.D. (1993). Handedness in great apes: A review of the findings. *International Journal of Primatogy,* 14:1–25.

_____, _____, Savage-Rumbaugh, S., and Rumbaugh, D. (1992). Hemispheric priming by meaningful and nonmeaningful symbols in language trained chimps. *Behavioral Neuroscience,* 106:575–582.

Isaac, G. (1984).The archeology of human origins: Studies of the lower pleistocene in East Africa. *Advances in World Archeology,* 3:1–79.

Johnson-Laird, P.N. (1983). *Mental models.* Harvard University Press, Cambridge, MA.

Laitman, J.T., and Heimbuch, R.C. (1982). The basicranium of Plio-Pleistocene hominids as an indicator of their upper respiratory systems. *American Journal of Physical Anthropology,* 59:323–344.

_____, and Reidenberg, J.S. (1988). Advances in understanding the relationship between the skull base and larynx, with comments on the origins of speech. *Human Evolution,* 3:101–111.

_____, Heimbuch, R.C., and Crelin, E.S. (1978). Developmental change in a basicranial line and its relationship to the upper respiratory system in living primates. *American Journal of Anatomy,* 152:467–482.

Leakey, R., and Lewin, R. (1992). *Origins reconsidered.* Little Brown, London, UK.

Leslie, A. (1987). Pretense and representation in infancy: The origins of theory of mind. *Psychological Review,* 94:412–426.

Lieberman, P. (1991). *Uniquely human: The evolution of speech, thought, and selfless behavior.* Harvard University Press, Cambridge, MA.

_____, Crelin, E.S., and Klatt, D.H. (1972). Phonetic ability and related anatomy of the newborn, adult human, Neanderthal man, and the chimpanzee. *American Anthropologist,* 74:287–307.

_____, Harris, K.S., Wolff, P., and Russell L.H. (1972). Newborn infant cry and nonhuman primate vocalizations. *Journal of Speech and Hearing Research,* 14:718–727.

_____, Klatt, D.H., and Wilson, W.H. (1969). Vocal tract limitations on the vowel repertoires of rhesus monkey and other nonhuman primates. *Science,* 164:1185–1187.

MacLean, P. (1990). *The triune brain in evolution: Role in paleocerebral functions.* Plenum Press, New York.

Martin, L.J., Spicer, D.M., Lewis, M.H., Gluck, J.P., and Cork, L.C. (1991). Social deprivation of infant rhesus monkeys alters the chemoarchitecture of the brain: I. Subcortical regions. *Journal of Neuroscience,* 11:3344–3358.

McCulloch, W.S. (1965). "What's in the brain that ink may character?" In W.S. McCulloch (ed), *Embodiments of mind.* MIT Press, Cambridge, MA.

Morris, R.D., Hopkins, W.D., and Bolser-Gilmore, L. (1993). Assessment of hand preference in two language-trained chimpanzees (*Pan troglodytes*): A multimethod analysis. *Journal of Clinical and Experimental Neuropsychology,* 15:487–502.

Nelson, K. (1986). *Event knowledge: Structure and function in development.* Lawrence Erlbaum, Hillsdale, NJ.

_____, and Ross, G. (1982). The general and specifics of long-term memory in infants and young children. In M. Perlmutter (ed), *Naturalistic approaches to memory,* pp. 87–101. Jossey-Bass, San Francisco.

Premack, D., and Woodruff, G. (1978). Does the chimpanzee have a theory of mind? *The Behavioral and Brain Sciences,* 1:515–526.

Savage-Rumbaugh, E.S., Murphy, J., Sevcik, R.A., Brakke, K.E., Williams, S.L., and Rumbaugh, D.M. (1993). Language comprehension in ape and child. *Monographs of the Society for Research in Child Development,* 58(3–4, Serial No. 233):1–220.

Schank, R.C. (1982). *Dynamic memory: A theory of reminding and learning in computers and people.* Cambridge University Press, Cambridge, UK.

_____, and Abelson, R.P. (1977). *Scripts, plans, goals, and understanding.* Lawrence Erlbaum, Hillsdale, NJ.

Terrace, H.S., Pettito, L.A., Sanders, R.J., and Bever, T.G. (1979). Can an ape create a sentence? *Science,* 206:891–900.

Toth, N. (1987). The first technology. *Scientific American,* 256:112–121.

Wallman, J. (1992). *Aping language.* Cambridge University Press, New York.

CHAPTER 17
TEMPERAMENT AND PERSONALITY

Although it is generally agreed that people differ in their characteristic styles of behavior and that temperament is of constitutional origin, controversies continue about the scientific concept and definition of temperament. Moreover, although temperament, personality, and personality trait disorder have been viewed in sequential fashion, suggesting that one leads to the next, this view is also controversial. If such a sequence occurs, a personality disorder would represent an extreme form of genetically based temperamental traits that along with environmental experience shape personality during the developmental years. An alternative approach (Rutter, 1987) suggests that these three terms — temperament, personality, and personality disorder — describe different phenomena and different processes.

Developmental considerations are of considerable importance in assessing temperament. How much of an infant's behavior can be designated as temperament? From a developmental point of view, the questions that must be addressed are, How does temperament develop? and, To what extent is temperament an interactive construct versus a personological one? These questions are important for both social and cognitive development. Whether temperament is a measure of a child's own contribution to his or her development depends on the individual developmental course of the temperamental dimensions themselves.

In this chapter temperament, personality,

and personality trait disorder are reviewed utilizing a developmental perspective. The chapter includes an historical introduction and a review of various definitions of temperament. It then addresses temperament and neurobiology, cognition, and gender. It concludes with a discussion of the assessment of temperament, relationship of temperament to personality, and temperament in developmental disorders.

HISTORY

Concepts of temperament are rooted in ancient attempts to link individual characteristics to physiologic processes. Over 2,000 years ago, following the then-current belief, the Greek physician Hippocrates (c. 470–370 B.C.) taught that health was maintained by the balance of four bodily fluids, called "humors," that is, blood, phlegm, yellow bile, and black bile. Subsequently, both Galen (c. A.D. 130–200) and Vindician (A.D. fourth century) (Diamond, 1974) have been credited with elaborating on this theory and proposing that there were four personality styles, each reflecting a characteristic humor: the sanguine, buoyant type; the phlegmatic, sluggish type; the choleric, quick-tempered type; and the melancholic, despairing type. Moreover, Galen discussed temperament in young children (Rothbart, 1989) and stated that "the starting point of my entire discourse is the knowledge of the differences which can be seen in little children, and which reveal the faculties of the soul. Some are very sluggish, others violent . . . shameless, or shy." He went on to suggest that if their souls were interchangeable, they would be expected to act in similar ways from their earliest days, but since there are behavioral differences "the nature of the soul is not the same for all" (Diamond, 1974, p. 604). Subsequently, an aberration or eccentricity of personality was attributed to a humor.

The fourfold approach to temperament continued throughout the Middle Ages and Renaissance, when in literature a "humor character" was one where one passion predominated. Richard Burton (1621) provided a comprehensive overview in *The Anatomy of Melancholy;* this orientation was still being discussed by Emmanuel Kant in 1798. In medicine, the theory of humors lost currency in the 19th century with Virchow's theory of cellular pathology. By 1903 William Wundt had changed the emphasis from typologies of temperament to dimensions of individual variability. He proposed temperamental dimensions of feelings and addressed the strength and speed of change of feeling. Ebbinghaus proposed the dimensions of optimism-pessimism and emotionality (Eysenck and Eysenck, 1985). In the 20th century the Russians, exemplified by Pavlov, focused on properties of the nervous system (i.e., strong or weak) in response to environmental stimuli and related this to temperament, and the British began to derive temperamental factors from self-report measures. Webb (1915) used factor analysis to assess emotionality, activity, and self-qualities.

DEFINITIONS OF TEMPERAMENT

The word "temperament" originates from the Latin *temperamentum,* meaning "a mixture of the bodily humors," from *temperare,* "to mingle in due proportion" (Rothbart, 1989).

Definitions of temperament have been proposed by a number of authors (Campos et al., 1983; Goldsmith et al., 1987). Those suggested by Thomas and Chess (1977), Plomin (1986), and Rothbart (1981) are representative and are emphasized here.

Thomas and Chess

The modern study of child temperament was initiated by Thomas, Chess, et al. (1963) in their New York Longitudinal Study. Their focus on temperament emphasizes individual differences in development; the child is an active agent who shapes his or her environment. Temperament has a neurobiological basis that includes genetic influences. Their focus is on socioemotional aspects of development rather than cognitive aspects (Rutter, 1987).

Thomas and Chess (1977) conceptualize temperament as the stylistic component of behavior. They describe it as the "how" of behavior (style), rather than the "why" of behavior (motivation), or the "what" of behavior (type of performance or ability). They suggest that a group of individuals, children or adults, could have the same motivation to perform a task and have similar levels of ability to carry it out, but may differ in their performance in regard to temperamental features, such as the amount of motor activity, their intensity of activity, their quality of mood expression, their ease of adaptability in carrying out the task, their persistence, and the extent to which they are distracted from completing the task. Each of these characteristics is considered to be a component of temperament. For these authors, temperament is an independent psychological attribute that is not secondary to other attributes, such as cognition, arousal, motivation, or emotionality, yet temperament does reciprocally interact with other attributes. Consequently, a child with temperamentally low persistence could stick to a particular task with greater persistence if highly motivated.

Thomas and Chess (1977) differentiate temperament from motivations, abilities, and personality. Temperament is expressed as a response to an external stimulus, opportunity, demand, or expectation. The social context may intensify or minimize the expression of temperamental features. The influence of temperament is bidirectional in that the response to a particular environmental influence will be influenced by the child's temperament. In addition, the child's temperament will affect the judgments, attitudes, and behavior of significant individuals toward the child.

Plomin

Plomin and Dunn (1986) define temperament as a set of inherited personality traits that appear early in life and are genetic in origin. These traits appear during the first years of life, which distinguishes them from groups of personality traits. Individual differences that are not personality traits, such as intelligence and other individual abilities, are excluded, as are other individual differences that disappear with age and do not have an enduring effect on later personality, for example, rhythmicity in regard to eating and sleeping. These authors suggest that temperament traits that appear in infancy provide the foundation for later personality. Because inheritance is basic to this definition, traits that emerge from an environmental event are not included in their definition. Although Plomin and Dunn suggest that temperamental features have high heritability, are stable over time, and emerge early in life, it must be noted that behavioral characteristics that are heritable are not temperamental features. Moreover, some traits require environments to become manifest, so individual behavior does change with development.

Rothbart

Rothbart (1981) defines temperament as relatively stable, primarily biologically based, individual differences in reactivity and self-regulation. Reactivity refers to the excitability or arousability of behavioral endocrine, autonomic, and central nervous system responses. These are assessed in regard to threshold, latency, intensity, recovery, and rise times. Self-regulation refers to attention, approach, avoidance, and inhibition, which serve to modulate, that is, to enhance or inhibit, reactivity. Temperament is observed behaviorally as individual differences in patterns of emotionality, activity, and attention. From a phenomenological point of view, it is experienced by the individual as feelings of energy, interest, and affect. Rothbart studies activity level, smiling and laughter, fear, distress at limitations (frustration), soothability, and duration of orienting as temperamental variables.

In addition to these three approaches, several other authors have contributed to research in temperament. Goldsmith and Campos (1986) define temperament as individual differences in the probability of experiencing and expressing the primary emotions and general arousal. Their definition is confined to the behavioral level because they feel temperament is most meaningful in social context. Kagan, Reznick, and Snidman (1987) add a further element to temperament, that of behavioral inhibition to the unfamiliar.

Overview of Temperament

Overall, temperament is viewed as a relatively small number of simple, nonmotivational, noncognitive, stylistic features (Rutter, 1987). Emotionality, activity, and sociability are generally agreed to be aspects of temperament. Each of these characteristics may have neurobiological correlates.

The key definitional requirement is to clarify how to separate temperament from other aspects of personality. For example, emotional reactivity is a temperamental characteristic that shows how a child will respond to a new situation, but a specific fear is predictive of behavior only in limited situations. Negative mood may be a temperamental feature, but helplessness and depression are not, consistent with the focus on temperament as the style of interaction. In this way, nonmotivational and noncognitive factors, and noncomplex behavioral tendencies, are taken into account. Using the same line of thinking, activity level is an aspect of temperament, but suspiciousness and obsessionality are not.

The general consensus is that temperament refers to a group of related traits and not only to a single trait. The designation "temperament" may be analogous to the term "cognition," in that temperament, like cognition, refers to several phenomena (e.g., activity, emotionality, and sociability), whereas cognition includes attention, memory, comprehension, and problem solving. Viewing temperament as a group of related traits results in definitions that describe a class of temperamental features that may be described in structural terms or in functional terms. Structural approaches come largely from adult personality research, whereas functional thinking is applied to the internal regulatory roles of temperament. The importance of temperament in regulating social behavior has important roots in clinical research, in developmental behavioral genetics, and in developmental psychology.

Among these general approaches to temperament, there is agreement that temperamental dimensions reflect behavioral tendencies, and that there are biological underpinnings of temperament. Temperament refers to individual differences rather than species-specific characteristics, so stranger and separation anxiety, shame, guilt, and sadness are not aspects of temperament because they are universal (Kagan, Reznick, and Snidman, 1989). Yet there is continuity relative to other aspects of behavior, so the interface of temperament and behavior becomes more complex with maturation. In older individuals, temperamental expression may be apparent only at times when novel environmental challenges occur that render coping skills ineffective.

Because of changes with maturation, the issue of temperament being modifiable must be considered. Still, it may be that the core constructs of temperament show complete continuity, but the expression of temperament is modifiable over time. If so, temperamental traits have a dynamic quality. This modifiability, the dynamic changes, might be expressed genetically. The expression of genes would be one substrate for dynamic regulation of temperament during the life span.

Temperamental qualities like sociability or shyness are generally considered to be dimensional. Kagan, Reznick, and Snidman (1987) asked whether some temperamental features could better be dealt with in terms of physiobehavioral patterns that are qualitatively distinct. These authors treat temperamental constructs as categories of children instead of assuming a continuous dimension such as sociability. They suggest that their work on inhibition or lack of inhibition to the unfamiliar illustrates the value of this approach (Kagan, Reznick, and Snidman, 1989).

Differences among investigators who study temperament reflect different boundaries for defining temperament. Thus, their criteria for the qualities that make up behavioral style, for the relationship of temperament to emotional behavior, for stability of temperament over time, and for the inheritance of temperament vary among them.

In summary, several issues regarding temperament can be said to be established. First, individual children differ from one another in important ways, which can be assessed. These include activity level, autonomic and emotional reactivity, behavioral inhibition in social situations, and sociability (Goldsmith et al., 1987). Second, these differences are important in regard to later development and for psychiatric risk. Interview measurements of temperament predict emotional and behavioral disorders later in development for both high-risk and normal populations (Graham, Rutter and George, 1973; Kagan, Reznick, and Snidman, 1987; Maziade et al., 1989a and 1989b; McCall, 1986; Rutter et al., 1964; Wolkind and De Salis, 1982). For example, questionnaire studies demonstrate an association of difficult temperament with an increased rate of sleep disturbance, accidents, and colic (Bates, 1980; Carey, 1985). In addition, Dunn and Kendrick (1982) demonstrated an increased rate of emotional disturbance in a follow-up study of the impact of the birth of a sibling on a child's behavior. Rutter (1978) demonstrated that temperamental features reported by parents subsequently predicted behavioral disturbances in school one year later. Therefore, temperament has been shown to predict behavior at a later date and in new and different social contexts.

Another area of outcome research is in sex differences in temperament that may arise in early development. How does temperament affect outcome in boys and girls? For example, girls may be at less risk for negative outcomes until entry into adolescence. The study of temperamental influences on outcome in children at risk is of importance. Temperament exerts its effects through transactions with others and in combination with other risk or protective factors. Regarding outcome, the majority of research has focused on maladjustment, but temperament also is important in successful adjustment. This was demonstrated in the Werner and Smith (1982) population study on the Island of Kauai, which discussed the influence of an outgoing positive and social temperament in disadvantaged children. The study of protective factors in children's development (Garmezy, 1985; Garmezy, Masten, and Tellegen, 1984) emphasizes temperament as an important feature. Successful outcome studies of this type emphasize competence rather than psychopathology. An understanding of the importance of social competence in preventing poor developmental outcome is needed to apply research findings.

EFFECTS OF TEMPERAMENT ON OTHERS

Children's temperament influences the way others respond to them. For example, Lee and Bates (1985) demonstrated that temperamentally difficult infants had more confrontations with their mothers. Rutter (1978) showed that children with aversive temperament were more likely to be targeted for criticism by their parents. Children with negative mood, a feature of temperament, had greater likelihood of having mothers who were irritable and teachers who seemed to react hostilely. Although the effects do tend to be reciprocal, Stevenson-Hinde and Hinde (1986) found that the effect is greater for that of the child on the adult rather than the reverse. Additional clinical studies have demonstrated the effect of a child's behavior on others. For example, for children with hyperactivity, drug treatment leads to changes in parental behavior toward the child (Barkley, 1981). Furthermore, differences in parental behavior to children who have organically based disabilities has been demonstrated (Cross, Nienhuys, and Kirkman, 1985).

TEMPERAMENT AND NEUROBIOLOGY

The relationship of temperament to neurobiological processes has been suggested by several authors. This approach to looking at the neurobiology has been studied more commonly by adult personality theorists. For example, Cloninger (1986) has suggested that, among the personality dimensions, certain characteristics, for example, harm avoidance, are related to high serotonin activity; novelty seeking, to low baseline dopaminergic activity; and reward dependence to low basal noradrenergic activity. However, Kagan, Resnick, and Snidman (1987) studies of behavioral inhibition to the unfamiliar relate this characteristic to a low threshold of responsiveness in the limbic and hypothalamic structures, changes in autonomic reactivity and in cortisol levels. Although the reasons for lower thresholds in the limbic sites are not clear, and probably complex, one factor that is likely to contribute is tonically higher levels of central norepinephrine or a higher density of norepinephrine receptors (Kagan, Resnick, and Snidman, 1989). They suggest that the actualization of inhibited behavior may require some form of chronic environmental stress that interacts with the temperamental disposition; a diathesis-stress hypothesis.

The three temperamental traits (i.e., emotionality, activity, and sociability) suggested by Buss and Plomin (1984), and a fourth, impulsivity, might also be investigated in regard to neurobiological factors. These temperamental characteristics may be comparable to Eysenck's (1982) extraversion, neuroticism, and psychoticism.

TEMPERAMENT AND COGNITION

Whether temperament, the style of responding, is fully independent of cognitive processes has been considered by Prior (1992). She suggests that one cannot assume there is a period when behavior is not influenced by cognition. For example, when considering self-regulation, behavioral inhibition requires cognitive mediation. Furthermore, cognition influences approach, withdrawal, and sociability. Martin (1989) has reviewed studies that investigate the relationship between temperament, particularly adaptability and persistence, and IQ. One longitudinal study (Maziade et al., 1987) found difficult temperament linked to IQ, yet these studies still support the independence of temperament and cognitive factors in very young children. Overall, the interaction between temperament and cognition is increasingly important as the child grows older.

Some temperamental factors may be mediated more by cognition than others. Emotionality is likely to influence cognition because affect may be primary in directing or guiding behavior. Similarly, the feedback between emotionality and cognition must be considered when studying behavioral outcomes. Sociability may have nontemperamental characteristics because it is learned through repeated experiences along with cognitive re-evaluation (Chess and Thomas, 1989). However, individuals do seek out environments that match their temperamental traits, and there is an active role in sustaining temperamental characteristics through environmental feedback. As Scarr and McCartney (1983) have noted, "the genotype determines responsiveness of the person" to the environment. Parental approval or disapproval of temperamental expressions influence these "innate" predispositions, so the child learns to modify his interpersonal behavior.

Children do indeed adapt their reactions to who and what is involved in their conflicts. Furthermore, when children fail to develop flexible cognitive scripts, their behavior may become stereotyped. Maladaptive behavior with extreme aggression is an example. Therefore, it is difficult to think of temperament as occurring without cognition or being independent of cognition. Temperament and cognition work in parallel and modify one another. Developmental ideas about schemas and internal working models and cognitive scripts discussed in Chapter 16 are important in thinking about temperament. Culturally based schemas also contribute to cultural differences in temperament. In the future, cognitive scripts may be found to play a role in modifying temperament and provide conceptual bridges between temperament and personality. These scripts are thought to emerge and become elaborated over time throughout development (Prior, 1992). The interface of temperament as innate, biologically influenced, and genetically determined, its shaping by environmental experience, and subsequent cognitive interpretation of experience and modification of behavior lead to a broader view of temperament.

It is particularly important in developmental disabilities to understand the relationship between temperament and cognition. The interface of temperament and personality is an important consideration in the developmental disorders.

ASSESSMENT OF TEMPERAMENT

The assessment of temperament is essential in personality research, using behavior ratings and evaluations (Carey, 1983; Dunn and Kendrick, 1980; McDevitt and Carey, 1978). Further refinement of methodology to study temperament in children with disabilities and those without disabilities is under way, using a lifespan developmental approach, yet temperament has been difficult to evaluate because its measurement is not the assessment of a specific observable and discrete behavior, but rather the measurement of a pattern of behaviors typically seen in interactions

with others. Temperament ratings require that others rate the child's behavior, so biases in individual adult perceptions of a child's behavior or their attributions about the child may influence their rating. Moreover, temperament measures may encompass both objective and subjective factors (Bates and Bayles, 1984).

For behavior rating, the situation used to observe the child's behavior must be clearly defined by the rater. The behavior observed not only indicates personal traits but also a situation-specific reaction to the setting. Because testing usually occurs in a social context, the elicitation of temperament features depends on the properties of that social context. The context includes temperament characteristics in the observer or the person interacting with the child and their past history of interactions together (Dodge, 1980).

For evolutionary purposes, temperament traits have been regarded as aspects of behavior that are pervasive over situations and consistent over time, once bias and behavioral attributions by others have been excluded. The assessor must keep in mind that some behavior traits are only present in specific situations. For example, although emotional reactivity shows heritability and stability over time, it may be adequately measured only in stressful situations. This is the case even though temperament is ordinarily considered to be pervasive across all situations.

Kagan, Resnick, and Snidman (1987) report that behavioral manifestations of the same trait may change over the course of development. For example, behavioral inhibition may be expressed in an infant who is seeking close proximity to the mother, but in the school-age child, that same trait of behavioral inhibition may be expressed as caution in approaching new tasks. In addition, the elicitation of inhibition requires that the task must be meaningful to the child. Behavioral variation occurring with progressive development, in itself, makes it unlikely that a predisposition would be expressed in the same way throughout childhood.

The assessment of constellations of behaviors may be more meaningfully considered than a single dimension. In some circumstances, the association of two behaviors may change their meaning; for example, Kagan, Resnick, and Snidman (1987) demonstrated that, in general, heart rate measures as a dimension added nothing further to understanding and accounting for the variance in measures of behavioral inhibition, yet children who had both behavioral inhibition and a high stable heart rate differed from the others in the group. Another example is the combination of restlessness and aggressiveness, which have interactional effects.

TEMPERAMENT AND PERSONALITY

Although in younger children temperament can effectively be viewed as a nonplanned style of responding, it is most likely a pure construct only in very young children, whose behavior is less specifically guided by cognitive processes. When cognitive processes become involved, then the more comprehensive term "personality" must be considered, although temperament does endure, for the most part, as stable behavioral dispositions. Similar language is used by personality theorists and temperament researchers in dealing with older children, particularly for factors such as emotionality and sociability. In school-age children, it becomes more difficult to differentiate these factors. Goldsmith (1983) has suggested that the estimate of heredity for temperament and for personality dimensions is similar.

In comparing the major personality dimensions and temperament (Digman, 1989), an overlap between the two concepts has been noted. For example, sociability (approach/withdrawal tendencies), or extraversion, is included in both constructs. Another temperament factor, friendly/compliant/agreeable, may be similar to the personality factor of cooperation/manageability/positive mood (Prior, 1992). Consciousness/self-control, a third factor, may be like self-regulation (Rothbart and Posner, 1985). This factor includes persistence, regularity, or rhythmicity in behavioral style and may be compared to personality descriptions of careless, dependable, and disorderly, which form part of a conscientiousness/self-control factor. Emotional stability is very much like emotionality, an agreed-upon temperament factor, which includes qualities of mood and the intensity of emotional reactions. Among personality dimensions mentioned by Digman, intellect/curiosity may not have a parallel in temperament structures, although its roots may be in adaptability, if adaptability relates to intelligence (Prior,

1992). Among temperament features, activity tends not to be described, although it may be considered that activity level is part of the behaviors that make up personality.

TEMPERAMENT AND PSYCHIATRIC DISORDER

In children, extremes of temperament have been considered to constitute dimensional forms of psychiatric disorder; however, this position has not been demonstrated. Extremes of temperament do not, in themselves, constitute a disorder; furthermore, the majority of symptoms in child psychiatric patients are not related to temperament. Temperament follows an indirect path in regard to the mechanism of disorder through its influences on other people's reactions. In addition, effects of temperament may vary by gender. The exaggeration of a trait does not necessarily indicate psychopathology, because the effects of that trait on others depend on the social meaning that the other person gives to the behavior. Temperament traits may carry both positive and negative implications according to the circumstances. For example, overly active infants and children with difficult temperament may do better in situations where there is limited care available because their behavior draws more attention from others to them. Still, activity and difficult temperament may be psychiatric risk factors in other situations.

TEMPERAMENT AND DEVELOPMENTAL DISABILITIES

Several areas in temperament research need resolution. For example, few studies of temperament in children with developmental disorders have been completed (Goldberg and Marcovitch, 1989). Studies of temperament are especially important in predicting adjustment in children with developmental disabilities, particularly in regard to transactional effects between the child's strengths and weaknesses and the environment. Specific studies have been conducted in Down syndrome (Gunn and Berry, 1985a and 1985b, Gunn, Berry, and Andrews, 1981, 1983), in children with mild disabilities (Van Tassel, 1984), children with mixed disabilities, and children who are neurologically impaired (Heffernan, Black, and Poche, 1982). Moreover, temperament has been investigated in normal infants (Maziade et al., 1984) and in handicapped infants during interactions with their mothers (Greenberg and Field, 1982); in developmentally delayed preschool children (Marcovitch et al., 1986) in older mentally retarded children (Chess and Korn, 1970), and in blind children (Fraiberg, 1974). Few specific abnormalities were noted when comparing the handicapped/developmentally delayed children to normal population samples. Still, associated brain damage may increase the risk of interpersonal difficulties. Studies of temperament and adjustment for hearing-impaired children (Prior et al., 1988) show that interpersonal relationships have a multivariate nature. From these studies, it has generally been reported that temperament by itself is not a risk factor. However, in combination with other biological, environmental, and interpersonal variables, there may be a significant effect. Knowledge of a handicapped child's temperament and how it matches with the family and social environment may be helpful in reducing conflict for families. Family factors that mediate outcome include psychological functioning, marital adjustment, child-rearing attitudes and practices, social support, and social stress (Prior, 1992).

Although there has been considerable interest in establishing temperament profiles in children with clinically identified disorders, instruments for temperament research have not been widely used; most research has focused primarily on children who are developing relatively normally. Studies in developmental disorders deal primarily with Down syndrome.

A focus on Down syndrome was initiated because children with this disorder represent the largest homogeneous group of developmentally disordered children who may be studied from birth through infancy and into the school-age years (Cicchetti and Sroufe, 1978), yet the majority of developmentally delayed children are a heterogeneous population and differ from the Down syndrome group. Therefore, findings should be focused on the specific developmental disorder. In children with Down syndrome, as previously demonstrated in normally developing children, there is a shift toward easier temperament with increasing age. Older children with Down syndrome have been rated as being temperamentally easier than normally developing peers, although during their infancy they were rated as more difficult (Baron, 1972; Bridges and Cicchetti, 1982; Rothbart and Hanson, 1983). Because older children with Down syndrome may be temperamentally "easy" and infants with Down syndrome may be temperamentally "difficult," generalization is of limited utility to understand individual children. There is sufficient temperament variation among developmentally delayed children, and among those with Down syndrome in particular, that generalizations cannot be substituted for individual assessments.

Using temperament measures in children with disabilities is important because understanding a child's temperament can aid both the parent and clinician in understanding a particular child. The goal is to guide interventions to encourage positive parent-child interaction. Carey and McDevitt (1980) have focused on the hyperactive child and proposed that problems in behavior and learning be understood in terms of a profile that includes the child's temperament. This approach may also be applied to children with other handicapping conditions. Although there is limited literature that addresses the clinical utility of temperament in establishing interventions with developmentally delayed children, there is data available on parental stress. Relative to populations of normally developing children, children with developmental handicaps are perceived by parents as a greater source of stress than children without handicaps.

PERSONALITY

Personality refers to a coherence of functioning that derives from how people react to their own constitutional attributes (i.e., temperament, their view of themselves, and the conceptual whole that this creates). There is no one specific measure of personality. Some aspects of personality are described in terms of dimensional traits, which would include items like obsessionality; others are best described in terms of processes, for example, the social, emotional, and cognitive aspects.

How does personality differ from temperament? A concept of personality is broader than a list or collection of temperament traits. Allport (1937), in describing personality, focused on personality as a dynamic organization that includes an active mental role as well as developmental changes. For Allport, personality describes the patterning that thinking people develop as their way of dealing with traits that are part of their genetic endowment, those life experiences encountered in social contexts, and the external events that happen to them.

A definition of personality (Sroufe, 1979) addresses the integration of organizational functions, including cognitive and motivational features along with temperamental or dispositional ones. Nonbehavioral features provide the clearest differentiation between temperament and personality. Still, in personality, a consistent style of behavior is characteristic. Personality includes coherent and orderly patterns of behavior that have their origins in attitudes, patterns of thought, and motivations, in addition to dispositions. Personality differs from temperament in that meaningful patterns of behavior may become apparent despite a lack of behavioral generalization from one situation to the next. There is more to personality development than the stabilization of those temperament traits that may generalize from one situation to the next. It is not simply environmental influence; nonbehavioral components are also important (Rutter, 1987).

Personality is a way of describing a dynamic integration of biological endowments, chosen encounters with others, and the individual style of responding to external events. Personality considers the development of the self-concept and the development of attitudes towards the self, the self's way of relating to others, the self's efforts to project itself into the future, and the establishment of a meaningful philosophy of life. In this comprehensive way, the person organizes and integrates to find coherence in his life experiences and to come to terms with basic biological needs. In this sense, a person becomes his own life history, or as Adolph Meyer (1933) termed it, a "history making" individual.

Chess and Thomas (1989) do not advocate a temperament theory of personality; they define personality to be the structured composite of enduring attributes that constitute the individuality of the person. In their view, personality includes motivations and abilities, standards and values, and psychological defense mechanisms, as well as temperament. Different personalities may have similar temperaments, and similar personalities may have differences in temperament.

ASSESSMENT OF PERSONALITY

There is no one agreed-upon way of measuring personality. Some aspects of personality, such as obsessionality, may be dealt with as dimensional traits, but others are thought of in terms of processes that involve emotional, social, and cognitive mechanisms. Personality disorder includes several categories that may be considered variants of psychiatric conditions such as an affective disorder, schizophrenia, or autistic disorder. On the other hand, there is a group of personality disorders that are characterized by persistent and pervasive abnormality in social relationships and in general social functioning. Personality disorders are clinically important in regard to both their chronicity and their prevalence. The study of personality and its relationship to temperament and personality style require continuing investigation from the developmental perspective.

DEVIANT PERSONALITY TRAITS, BEHAVIOR, AND TEMPERAMENT

Temperament focuses on style, which is simple, nonmotivational, and noncognitive. Deviant personality traits — such as social isolation, and schizoid, paranoid, histrionic, and obsessional features — are not included as temperament because of their motivational qualities. Moreover, recent evidence suggests that these traits may have a genetic basis as part of a broad definition of a major mental disorder, such as schizophrenia.

However, some behaviors that relate to personality style must be considered in relation to temperament. For example, aggressivity has been considered a temperament feature because of its stability over time (Olweus, 1980). Still, Buss and Plomin (1984) consider that aggressivity can be accounted for in their scheme's three features: activity, emotionality, and impulsivity.

PERSONALITY AND LIFE HISTORY

Personality has been studied in a variety of ways, including depth psychology, which addresses the meaning that the person attaches to experiences and the role of intrapsychic processes. Depth psychology does not provide a classification of personality. Instead, it focuses on finding meanings and the various ways that individuals use coping strategies as they adapt to intrapsychic and interpersonal experiences. These approaches emphasize the meaningful, personal narrative in the life history and the mastery of developmental challenges. Still, how an individual copes with life events may lead to a classification of coping styles, which will be useful in understanding how a particular person attributes meaning to experiences.

Social relationships are crucial to personality development. Attachment in relationships, cognitive processing of life experiences, and personality traits must be studied in social context. Close, confiding relationships are essential for individual development, beginning with parent-child relationships and moving on toward peer relationships. If the origin of personality is in social relationships, then these early relationships will become crucial in understanding personality development. Interpersonal relationships in themselves are not personality traits, but rather through reciprocity in relationships and psychological factors, such as complementarity, relationships may be integrated and used as "internalized models" which influence later relationships. Sroufe and Fleeson (1986) suggest several pathways to development.

DEVELOPMENT OF PERSONALITY

The developmental process begins with the internal organization of beliefs, coping styles, and attitudes that lead to coherent personality functioning. This results in establishing expectations about relationships and understanding relationships as they occur in social encounters. Initial early attachment patterns related to security and insecurity are associated with patterns of peer relationships in subsequent years. Although continuities of this kind are not fully understood in terms of their mechanisms, Bowlby (1988) emphasizes the establishment of internal working models. These models derive from expectations about relationships with others and how others will respond to social initiations and social interactions. Expectations generally are based on previous parent-child bonding. In this way, children may shape their later relationships as a result of social understanding which originates in earlier experiences. On the other hand, subsequent relationships do modify these working models.

In personality development, cognitive processing of personal experience (Rutter, 1987) must be considered. Harter (1986) describes this processing as constituting the self system. Personality development includes cognitions or awarenesses about one's self, one's relationships to others, and one's environmental interactions. As a result of these awarenesses, a coherent self-concept emerges. Our concept of self extends to others based on our perceptions of what sort of people they may be. Therefore, we may respond to our perception of another person, not only their specific behavior. We allocate social roles to others, and that allocation influences our own behavior.

Self-esteem and self-efficacy are linked to social problem solving skills but may also be studied in their negative aspects. Self-concepts are not static but rather develop over time as they become integrated, yet cognitive processes involving the self system may be important in developmental psychopathology in maintaining psychiatric symptoms, such as depression. Seligman emphasized learned helplessness (Peterson and Seligman, 1984), and others have addressed cognitive styles of helplessness and hopelessness in describing how individuals become vulnerable to loss and subsequently depressed. Low self-esteem is an important issue in developmental disabilities and may mediate how early adverse experiences result in later vulnerabilities to symptoms, such as depression. Cognitive approaches can be utilized as an aspect of treatment to deal with low self-esteem.

The link between temperament and cognition (or the self system) may be useful in understanding whether a sense of helplessness is an important mechanism through which temperament may predispose to an emotional disorder. On the other hand, these cognitive features may be a cognitive representation or the epiphenomena of a personality trait, and it is that constitutional trait itself that leads directly to a disorder. Consequently, personality traits must be considered. Certain interpersonal traits, such as altruism, empathy, and nurturing others (Rushton et al., 1986), are positive traits, whereas others, such as suspiciousness and rebelliousness (Ahern et al., 1982), are considered to be negative traits.

Personality traits have been derived from several theoretical approaches, for example, sensation seeking and internal locus of control, yet traits such as these are qualities that may be static and do not result in a new understanding of developmental change. Despite this, personality traits do require developmental consideration in regard to continuity. The term "heterotypic continuity" is used to describe behavioral change that occurs over time even though individual traits seem stable. For example, Kagan and Moss (1962) noted that children who were passive in early life were noncompetitive as adults. A second developmental factor addresses the stability of personality functioning over time. For example, in one study (Block, 1971), individuals who changed over time differed from those who did not change by being less relaxed and in greater conflict with societal values. Developmental studies are needed to further investigate stability of traits over time.

Genetic contributions to personality traits need to be viewed developmentally as fluid rather than fixed. Not only may there be different kinds of gene environmental interactions, but the genetic effects may be amplified during development in that people may create their own environments. Here, nature shapes nurture (Scarr and McCartney, 1983), so the strongest environmental factors may be those that differentially affect different children in the same family.

Finally, some personality traits derive from psychiatric terms, such as hysterical features, obsessionality, and paranoid qualities. These traits are central to the study of personality disorder from the psychiatric perspective.

PERSONALITY DISORDER

Personality trait disturbances have their onset in childhood or adolescence and show persistence over time. These abnormalities seem to constitute a basic aspect of an individual's usual functioning. Rutter (1987) notes four trends in the approach to personality disorder.

First, personality types are linked with forms of mental illness; second, personality disorders may be defined in terms of a postulated psychological deficit; third, a disorder may be seen entirely in terms of social defiance or incompetence, as in a sociopathic personality; and fourth, there are psychodynamic approaches that focus on psychodynamic mechanisms as etiological. The first approach leads to designations, such as schizoid or obsessional personality; the second, to descriptions of the inability to form close affectional ties or an inability to experience remorse; the third, to the failure to conform to societal norms; and the fourth introduces terms, such as "oral character" or "borderline personality."

Personality disorders include categories that may in some instances be considered variants of psychiatric disorders, such as mood disorder, schizophrenia, and autistic disorder. In addition, a large group of disorders are characterized by pervasive abnormality in social relationships and social function in general. This latter group of personality disorders are also clinically important in terms of their incidence and their chronicity.

In the ICD-10 classification system (WHO, 1992), the focus is on extremes of particular traits, such as paranoid or obsessional personality. DSM-IV (APA, 1994) addresses three clusters of personality disorder (A, B, C). The first cluster (A) is based on odd and eccentric behavior (paranoid, schizoid, and schizotypal); the second cluster (B) addresses dramatic or emotional behavior and antisocial behavior (histrionic, narcissistic, antisocial, and borderline); and the third cluster (C) emphasizes anxious or fearful behavior and obsessive/compulsive behavior (avoidant, dependent, and obsessive/compulsive patterns).

There are ongoing efforts to find physiological bases for the personality disorder classifications as they are better defined. One dilemma in the classification system is that individual patients may meet the criteria for several subtypes. When this occurs, multiple diagnoses are made.

FUTURE RESEARCH

Future research with developmentally disabled persons includes the development of a normative data base of temperament and personality traits for specific disabled populations, improved documentation of developmental changes over time, clarification of the relationship of temperament factors to social interactions, and the use of parental stress indices to provide clinicians with temperament data (Goldberg and Marcovitch, 1989). With better understanding of temperament, the establishment of formal reports on the utility of temperament data in assessment and treatment might be incorporated into a standard assessment profile. The standardization of assessment of temperament will benefit additional study of personality and personality traits in the developmental disorders.

REFERENCES

Ahern, F.M., Johnson, R.C., Wilson, J.R., McClearn, G.E., and Vandenberg, S.G. (1982). Family resemblances and personality. *Behavioural Genetics,* 12:261–280.

Allport, G.W. (1937). *Personality: A psychological interpretation.* Holt, New York.

American Psychiatric Association, Committee on Nomenclature and Statistics. (1994). *Diagnostic and Statistical Manual of Mental Disorders,* 4th ed. Author, Washington, DC.

Barkley, R.A. (1981). The use of psychopharmacology to study reciprocal influences in parent-child interaction. *Journal of Abnormal Child Psychology,* 9:303–310.

Baron, J. (1972). Temperament profile of children with Down's syndrome. *Developmental Medicine and Child Neurology,* 14:640–643.

Bates, J.E. (1980). The concept of difficult temperament. *Merrill-Palmer Quarterly,* 26:299–319.

_____, and Bayles, K. (1984). Objective and subjective components in mothers' perceptions of their children from age 6 months to 3 years. *Merrill-Palmer Quarterly,* 30:111–130.

Block. J. (1971). *Lives through time.* Bancroft Books, Berkeley, CA.

Bowlby, J. (1988). Developmental psychiatry comes of age. *American Journal of Psychiatry,* 145:1–10.

Bridges, F.A., and Cicchetti, D. (1982). Mother's ratings of the temperament characteristics of Down's syndrome infants. *Developmental Psychology,* 18:238–244.

Burton, R. (1621). *The anatomy of melancholy.* Oxford University Press, Oxford.

Buss, A.H., and Plomin, R. (1984). *Temperament: Early developing personality traits.* Lawrence Erlbaum, Hillsdale, NJ.

Campos, J.J., Barrett, K.C., Lamb, M.E., Goldsmith,

H.H., and Stenberg, C. (1983). Socioemotional development. In M.M. Haith, and J.J. Campos (eds), P.H. Mussen (series ed), *Handbook of child psychology,* Vol. 2, *Infancy and developmental psychobiology,* pp. 783–915. John Wiley & Sons, New York.

Carey, W.B. (1983). Clinical assessment of behavioral style or temperament. In M.D. Levine, W.B. Carey, A.C. Crocker, and R.T. Gross (eds), *Developmental-behavioral pediatrics,* pp. 922–926. W.B. Saunders, Philadelphia.

_____. (1985). Clinical use of temperament data in pediatrics. *Journal of Developmental and Behavioral Pediatrics,* 6:137–142.

_____, and McDevitt, S.C. (1980). Minimal brain damage and hyperkinesis: A clinical viewpoint. *American Journal of Diseases of Childhood,* 134:926–929.

Chess, S., and Korn, S. (1970). Temperament and behavior disorders in mentally retarded children. *Archives of General Psychiatry,* 23:122.

_____, and Thomas, A. (1984). *Origins and evolution of behavior disorders.* Brunner/Mazel, New York.

_____, and Thomas, A. (1989). Issues in the clinical application of temperament. In G.A. Kohnstamm, J.E. Bates, and M.K. Rothbart (eds), *Temperament in childhood,* pp. 337–386. John Wiley & Sons, Chichester, UK.

Cicchetti, D., and Sroufe, L.A. (1978). An organizational view of affect: Illustration from the study of Down's syndrome infants. In M. Lewis and L. Rosenblum (eds), *The development of affect.* Plenum Press, New York.

Cloninger, C.R. (1986). A unified biosocial theory of personality and its role in the development of anxiety states. *Psychiatric Developments,* 4:167–226.

Cross, T.G., Nienhuys, T.G., and Kirkman, M. (1985). Parent-child interaction with receptively disabled children: Some determinants of maternal speech style. In K.E. Nelson (ed), *Children's language.* Lawrence Erlbaum, Hillsdale, NJ.

Diamond, S. (1974). *The roots of psychology.* Basic Books, New York.

Digman, J. (1989). Five robust trait dimensions: Development, stability and utility. *Journal of Personality,* 57:195–214.

Dodge, K.A. (1980). Social cognition and children's aggressive behavior. *Child Development,* 51:162–172.

Dunn, J., and Kendrick, C. (1980). Studying temperament and parent-child interaction: Comparison, interview and direct observation. *Developmental Medicine and Child Neurology,* 22:494–496.

_____, and _____. (1982). Temperamental differences, family relationships, and young children's response to change within the family. In R. Porter and G.M. Collins (eds), *Temperamental differences in infants and young children.* Pitman/Ciba Foundation, London.

Eysenck, H.J. (1982). *Personality, genetics and behavior: Selected papers.* Praeger, New York.

Eysenck, H.J., and Eysenck, M.W. (1985). *Personality and individual differences.* Plenum Press, New York/London.

Fraiberg, S. (1974). Blind infants and their mothers: An examination of the sign system. In M. Lewis and L. Rosenblum (eds), *The effect of the infant on its caregiver.* John Wiley & Sons, New York.

Garmezy, N. (1985). Stress-resilient children: The search for protective factors. In J.E. Stevenson (ed), *Recent research in developmental psychopathology,* pp. 213–233. Pergamon Press, New York.

———, Masten, A.S., and Tellegen, A. (1984). The study of stress and competence in children: A building block for developmental psychopathology. *Child Development,* 55:87–111.

Goldberg, S., and Marcovitch, S. (1989). Temperament in developmentally disabled children. In G.A. Kohnstamm, J.E. Bates, and M.K. Rothbart (eds), *Temperament in childhood,* pp. 398–404. John Wiley & Sons, Chichester, UK.

Goldsmith, H.H. (1983). Genetic influences on personality from infancy to adulthood. *Child Development,* 54:331–335.

———, and Campos, J.J. (1986). Fundamental issues in the study of early temperament: The Denver twin temperament study. In M. E. Lamb and A. Brown (eds), *Advances in developmental psychology,* pp. 231–283. Lawrence Erlbaum, Hillsdale, NJ.

———, Buss, A.H., Plomin, R., Rothbart, M.K., Thomas, A., Chess, S., Hinde, R.A., and McCall, R.B. (1987). Roundtable: What is temperament? Four approaches. *Child Development,* 58:505–529.

Graham, P., Rutter, M., and George, S. (1973). Temperamental characteristics as predictors of behavior disorders in children. *American Journal of Orthopsychiatry,* 43:328–339.

Greenberg, R., and Field, T. (1982). Temperament ratings of handicapped infants during classroom, mother, and teacher interactions. *Journal of Pediatric Psychology,* 7:387–405.

Gunn, P., and Berry, P. (1985a). The temperament of Down's syndrome toddlers and their siblings. *Journal of Child Psychology and Psychiatry,* 26:973–979.

———, and Berry, P. (1985b). Down's syndrome temperament and maternal response to descriptions of child behavior. *Developmental Psychology,* 21:842–847.

Gunn, P., Berry, P., and Andrews, R.J. (1981). The temperament of Down's syndrome infants: A research note. *Journal of Child Psychology and Psychiatry,* 22:189–194.

———, ———, and ——— (1983). The temperament of Down's syndrome toddlers: A research note. *Journal of Child Psychology and Psychiatry,* 24:601–605.

Harter, S. (1986). Processes underlying the construction, maintenance and enhancement of the self concept in children. In J. Suls and A. Greenwald (eds), *Psychological perspectives on the self,* Vol. 3. Lawrence Erlbaum, Hillsdale, NJ.

Heffernan, L., Black, F.W., and Poche, P. (1982). Temperament patterns in young neurologically impaired children. *Journal of Pediatric Psychology,* 22:189–198.

Kagan, J., and Moss, H.A. (1962). *Birth to maturity.* John Wiley & Sons, New York.

———, Reznick, J.S., and Snidman, N. (1987). The physiology and psychology of behavioral inhibition in children. *Child Development,* 58:1459–1474.

———, ———, and ——— (1989). Issues in the study of temperament. In G.A. Kohnstamm, J.E. Bates, and M.K. Rothbart (eds), *Temperament in Childhood,* pp. 133–144. John Wiley & Sons, Chichester, UK.

———, ———, Clarke, C., Snidman, N., and Garcia-Coll, C. (1984). Behavioral inhibition to the unfamiliar. *Child Development,* 55:2212–2225.

Lee, C.L., and Bates, J.E. (1985). Mother-child interaction at age two years and perceived difficult temperament. *Child Development,* 56:1314–1325.

Marcovitch, S., Goldberg, S., Lojasek, M., and MacGregor, D. (1987). The concept of difficult temperament in the developmentally disabled preschool child. *Journal of Applied Developmental Psychology,* 8:151–164.

———, ———, MacGregor, D., and Lojasek, M. (1986). Patterns of temperament variation in three groups of developmentally delayed preschool children: Mother and father ratings. *Developmental and Behavioral Pediatrics,* 7:247–252.

Martin, R. (1989). Activity level, distractibility and persistence: Critical characteristics in early schooling. In G.A. Kohnstamm, J.E. Bates, and M.K. Rothbart (eds), *Temperament in childhood,* pp. 451–462. John Wiley & Sons, Chichester, UK.

Maziade, M., Boudreault, M., Thivierge, J., Capera, P., and Cote, R. (1984). Infant temperament: SES and gender differences and reliability of measurement in a large Quebec sample. *Merrill-Palmer Quarterly,* 30:213–226.

———, Cote, R., Boutin, P., Bernier, H., and Thivierge, J. (1987). Temperament and intellectual development: A longitudinal study from infancy to four years. *American Journal of Psychiatry,* 144:144–150.

_____, _____, Thivierge, J, Boutin, P., and Bernier, H.B. (1989a). Significance of extreme temperament in infancy for clinical status in preschool years. I. Value of extreme temperament at 4–8 months for predicting diagnosis at 4–7 years. *British Journal of Psychiatry,* 154:535–543.

_____, _____, _____, _____, and _____. (1989b). Significance of extreme temperament in infancy for clinical status in preschool years. II. Patterns of temperament change and implications for the appearance of disorders. *British Journal of Psychiatry,* 154:544–551.

McCall, R.B. (1986). Issues of stability and continuity in temperament research. In R. Plomin and J. Dunn (eds), *The study of temperament: Changes, continuities, and challenges,* pp. 13–26. Lawrence Erlbaum, Hillsdale, NJ.

McDevitt, S.C., and Carey, W.B. (1978). The measurement of temperament in 3- to-7-year-old children. *Journal of Child Psychology and Psychiatry,* 19:245–253.

Meyer, A. (1933). British influences in psychiatry and mental hygiene. The Fourteenth Maudsley lecture. *Journal of Mental Science,* 79:435–464.

Olweus, D. (1980). Familial and temperamental determinants of aggressive behavior in adolescent boys: A causal analysis. *Developmental Psychology,* 16:644–660.

Peterson, C., and Seligman, M.E.P. (1984). Causal explanation as a risk factor for depression: Theory and evidence. *Psychological Review,* 91:347–374.

Plomin, R., and Dunn, J. (1986) (eds). *The study of early temperament: Changes, continuities, and challenges.* Lawrence Erlbaum, Hillsdale, NJ.

Prior, M. (1992). Childhood temperament. *Journal of Child Psychology and Psychiatry,* 33:249–279.

_____, Glazner, J., Sanson, A., and Debelle, G. (1988). Temperament and behavioural adjustment in hearing impaired children. *Journal of Child Psychology and Psychiatry,* 29:209–216.

Rothbart, M.K. (1981). Measurement of temperament in infancy. *Child Development,* 52:569–578.

_____. (1989). Biological processes in temperament. In G.A. Kohnstamm, J.E. Bates, and M.J. Rothbart (eds), *Temperament in childhood.* John Wiley & Sons, Chichester, UK.

_____, and Hanson, M.J. (1983). A caregiver report comparison of temperament characteristics of Down's syndrome and normal infants. *Developmental Psychology,* 19:766–769.

_____, and Posner, M.I. (1985). Temperament and the development of self-regulation. In L.C. Harlage and C.F. Telzrow (eds), *The neuropsychology of individual differences: A developmental perspective,* pp. 93–123. Plenum Press, New York.

Rushton, J.P., Fulker, D.W., Neale, M.C., Nias, D.K.B., and Eysenck, H.J. (1986). Altruism and aggression: The heritability of individual differences. *Journal of Personality and Social Psychology,* 50:1192–1198.

Rutter, M. (1978). Surveys to answer questions. In P. Graham (ed), *The epidemiological approaches in child psychiatry.* Academic Press, London and New York.

_____. (1987). Temperament, personality and personality disorder. *British Journal of Psychiatry,* 150:443–458.

_____, Birch, H., Thomas, A., and Chess, S. (1964). Temperament characteristics in infancy and the later development of behavior disorders. *British Journal of Psychiatry,* 110:651–661.

Scarr, S., and McCartney, K. (1983). How people make their own environments: A theory of genotype environment effects. *Child Development,* 54:424–435.

Sroufe, L.A. (1979). The coherence of individual development. *American Psychologist,* 34:834–841.

_____, and Fleeson, J. (1986). Attachment and the construction of relationships. In W.W. Hartup and Z. Rubin (eds), *Relationships and development.* Lawrence Erlbaum, Hillsdale, NJ.

Stevenson-Hinde, J., and Hinde, R.A. (1986). Changes in associations between characteristics. In R. Plomin and J. Dunn (eds), *The study of temperament: Changes, continuities and challenges.* Lawrence Erlbaum, Hillsdale, NJ.

Thomas, A., and Chess, S. (1977). *Temperament and development.* Brunner/Mazel, New York.

_____, _____, Birch, H., Hertzig, M., and Korn, S. (1963). *Behavioral individuality in early childhood.* New York University Press, New York.

Van Tassel, E. (1984). Temperament characteristics of mildly developmentally delayed infants. *Developmental and Behavioral Pediatrics,* 5:11–14.

Webb, E. (1915). Character and intelligence. *British Journal of Psychology Monographs,* Nos. 1, 3.

Werner, E.E., and Smith, R.S. (1982). *Vulnerable but invincible: A study of resilient children.* McGraw-Hill, New York.

Wolkind, S.N., and De Salis, W. (1982). Infant temperament, maternal mental stage and child behavioural problems. In R. Porter and G.M. Collins (eds), *Temperamental differences in infants and young children,* CIBA Foundation Symposium 69, Pitman, London.

World Health Organization. (1992). *The ICD-10 Classification of Mental and Behavioural Disorders: Clinical descriptions and diagnostic guidelines.* Author, Geneva.

Wundt, W. (1903). *Grundzuge der physiologischen Psychologie,* Vol. 3, 5th ed. W. Engelmann, Leipzig. Cited by H.J. Eysenck and M.W. Eysenck (1985).

CREDITS

The author is indebted to the following for permission to reproduce copyrighted material.

Figure 1–1 reprinted by permission of the author from *Technologies for detecting heritable mutations in human beings.* Washington, DC: Office of Technology Assessment. Copyright © 1986.

Figures 1–2 and 1–3 reprinted by permission of the publisher from SA Whatley et al., The new genetics and neuropsychiatric disorders, *The Bridge Between Neurology and Psychiatry.* (EH Reynolds and MR Trimble, eds). Edinburgh: Robert Stevenson House. Copyright © 1989.

Figure 1–4 reprinted by permission of the author from *Technologies for detecting heritable mutations in human beings.* Washington, DC: Office of Technology Assessment. Copyright © 1986.

Figure 1–5 reprinted by permission of the publisher from SA Whatley et al., The new genetics and neuropsychiatric disorders. *The Bridge Between Neurology and Psychiatry.* (EH Reynolds and MR Trimble, eds). Edinburgh: Robert Stevenson House. Copyright © 1989.

Chapter 1 Glossary modified from MW Thompson et al., Patterns of single gene inheritance. *Genetics in Medicine.* © 1991 W.B. Saunders Company. Reprinted by permission.

Table 2–1 reprinted by permission of the author and publisher from JLR Rubenstein et al., The neurobiology of developmental disorders. *Advances in Clinical Child Psychology,* Vol. 13. (BB Lahey and AE Kazdin, eds). New York: Plenum Publishing Corporation. Copyright © 1990.

Table 2–2 reprinted by permission of the authors and publisher from JH Martin and TM Jessell, Development as a guide to the regional anatomy of the brain. *Principles of Neural Science,* 3rd edition. (ER Kandel, JH Schwartz, and TM Jes-sell, eds). Norwalk, CT: Appleton & Lange. Copyright © 1991.

Table 2–3 reprinted by permission of the author and publisher from HT Chugani, Functional brain imaging in pediatrics. *Pediatric Clinics of North America* 39:4. Copyright © 1992 by W.B. Saunders Company.

Figure 2–1 (left half) reprinted by permission of the authors and publisher from ER Kandel, Nerve cells and behavior. *Principles of Neural Science,* 3rd edition. (ER Kandel, JH Schwartz, and TM Jessell, eds). Norwalk, CT: Appleton & Lange. Copyright © 1991. Figure 2–1 (right half) author's adaptation reprinted by permission of the authors from ER Kandel, Nerve cells and behavior. *Principles of Neural Science,* 3rd edition. (ER Kandel, JH Schwartz, and TM Jessell, eds) .Norwalk, CT: Appleton & Lange. Copyright © 1991.

Figure 2–2 reprinted by permission of the author and publisher from PD MacLean, *The Triune Brain in Evolution: Role in Paleocerebral Functions.* New York: Plenum Publishing Corporation. Copyright © 1990.

Figure 2–3 reprinted by permission of the authors and publisher from I Kupfermann, Hypothalamus and limbic system: Peptidergic neurons, hemeostasis, and emotional behavior. *Principles of Neural Science,* 3rd edition. (ER Kandel, JH Schwartz, and TM Jessell, eds). Norwalk, CT: Appleton & Lange. Copyright © 1991.

Figure 2–4 reprinted by permission of the author and publisher from PD MacLean, *The Triune Brain in Evolution: Role in Paleocerebral Functions.* New York: Plenum Publishing Corporation. Copyright © 1990.

Figure 2–5 reprinted by permission of the authors and publisher from L Cote and MD Crutcher, The basal ganglia. *Principles of Neural Science,* 3rd edition. (ER Kandel, JH Schwartz, and TM Jessell, eds). Norwalk, CT: Appleton & Lange. Copyright © 1991.

Figure 2–6 reproduced, with permission, from the Annual Review of Neuroscience, Vol. 15. © 1992 by Annual Reviews Inc.

Figure 2–7 reprinted by permission of the author and publisher from HT Chugani, Functional brain imaging in pediatrics. *Pediatric Clinics of North America* 39:4. Copyright © 1992 by W.B. Saunders Company.

Table 3–1 (data on dopamine, norepinephrine, and serotonin) modified by permission of the authors and publisher from GA Rogeness et al., Neurochemistry and child and adolescent psychiatry. *Journal of the American Academy of Child and Adolescent Psychiatry* 31:5. Copyright © 1992 by Williams & Wilkins Publishing Company.

Table 3–2 reprinted by permission of the publisher from JR Cooper et al., Neuroactive peptides. *The Biochemical Basis of Neuropharmacology,* 6th edition. New York: Oxford University Press. Copyright © 1991.

Figure 3–1 reprinted by permission of the author from JT Coyle and JC Harris, The development of neurotransmitters and neuropeptides. *Basic Handbook of Child Psychiatry,* Volume 5, *Advances and New Directions.* (JD Noshpitz, editor-in-chief). New York: Basic Books, Inc. Copyright © 1987.

Figures 3–2, 3–3, 3–4 (right) reprinted by permission of the author from JT Coyle and JC Harris, The development of neurotransmitters and neuropeptides. *Basic Handbook of Child Psychiatry,* Volume 5, *Advances and New Directions.* (JD Noshpitz, editor-in-chief). New York: Basic Books, Inc. Copyright © 1987.

Figures 3–2, 3–3, 3–4 (left) reprinted by permission of the publisher from GA Rogeness et al., Neurochemistry and child and adolescent psychiatry. *Journal of the American Academy of Child and Adolescent Psychiatry* 31:5. Copyright © 1992 by Williams & Wilkins Publishing Company.

Figure 3–5 reprinted by permission of the author from JT Coyle and JC Harris: The development of neurotransmitters and neuropeptides. *Basic Handbook of Child Psychiatry,* Volume 5, *Advances and New Directions.* (JD Noshpitz,

editor-in-chief). New York: Basic Books, Inc. Copyright © 1987.

Figure 3–6 reprinted by permission of the author and publisher from AB Young and GE Fagg, Excitatory amino acid receptors in the brain: Membrane binding and receptor autoradiographic approaches. *Trends in Pharmacological Sciences,* A Special Report, pp. 18–24. Copyright © 1990 by Elsevier Trends Journal.

Figure 3–7 reprinted by permission of the authors and publisher from JD Barchas et al., Localization of the enkephalins and of β-endorphin in rat brain. *Science* 200:964–973. Copyright © 1991 by the AAAS.

Figures 3–8, 3–9, 3–10 reprinted by permission of the authors and publisher from ER Kandel et al., Synaptic transmission. *Principles of Neural Science,* 3rd edition. (ER Kandel, JH Schwartz, and TM Jessell, eds). Norwalk, CT: Appleton & Lange. Copyright © 1991. Figure 3–9 also reprinted by permission of the publisher from S Chien: The β-adrenergic receptor and other receptors coupled to guanine nucleotide regulatory proteins. *Molecular Biology in Physiology.* (S. Chien, ed). New York: Raven Press. Copyright © 1991.

Figure 4–1 reprinted by permission of the authors and publisher from DD Kelly, Sleeping and dreaming. *Principles of Neural Science,* 3rd edition. (ER Kandel, JH Schwartz, and TM Jessell, eds). Norwalk, CT: Appleton & Lange. Copyright © 1991.

Chapter 4 Glossary reprinted by permission of the author from *International Classification of Sleep Disorders: Diagnostic and Coding Manual.* Rochester, MN: American Sleep Disorders Association. Copyright © 1990.

Figure 5–1 reprinted by permission of the author and publisher from MW Thompson et al., Patterns of single-gene inheritance. *Genetics in Medicine,* 5th edition. Philadelphia: W.B. Saunders Company. Copyright © 1991.

Figures 6–1 and 6–2 reproduced, with permission, from the Annual Review of Neuroscience, Vol. 13. © 1990 by Annual Reviews Inc.

Figure 7–1 reproduced, with permission, from the Annual Review of Neuroscience, Vol. 15. © 1992 by Annual Reviews Inc.

Table 9–1 reprinted by permission of the author and publisher from RG Maurer, Disorders of memory and learning. *Handbook of Neuropsychology: Child Neuropsychology,* Vol. 6. (I Rapin and SJ Segalowitz, eds). Amsterdam: Elsevier Science Publishers BV. Copyright © 1992.

Table 9–2 reprinted by permission of the publisher from E Tulving, Concepts of human memory. *Memory: Organization and Locus of Change.* (LR Squire et al., eds). New York: Oxford University Press. Copyright © 1991.

Figure 9–1 reprinted by permission of the author and publisher from LR Squire and S Zola-Morgan, The medial temporal lobe memory system. *Science* 253:1380–1381. Copyright © 1991 by the AAAS.

Figure 9–2 adapted from ER Kandel and RD Hawkins, The biological basis of learning and individuality. Copyright © 1992 by Scientific American, Inc. All rights reserved.

Figure 10–1 reprinted by permission of the publisher from GE Hinton, How neural networks learn from experience. Copyright © 1992 by Scientific American, Inc. All rights reserved.

Figures 10–2 and 10–3 reprinted by permission of the publisher from D Van Kamp, Neurons for computers. Copyright © 1992 by Scientific American, Inc. All rights reserved.

Figure 13–1 reprinted by permission of the publisher from JB Sincoff and RJ Sternberg, The development of cognitive skills: An examination of recent theories. *Acquisition and Performance of Cognitive Skills.* (AM Colley and JR Beech, eds). Sussex, England: John Wiley & Sons, Ltd. Copyright © 1991.

Table 14–1 used by permission of the publisher from SS Tomkins, *Affect, Imagery and Consciousness,* Vol. 1. Springer Publishing Company, Inc., New York 10012. Copyright © 1962.

Figure 14–1 from J Garber and KA Dodge: Domains of emotion regulation. *The Development of Emotion Regulation and Dysregulation.* Copyright © Cambridge University Press 1991. Reprinted with the permission of Cambridge University Press.

Table 16–1 reprinted by permission of the publisher from BT Gardner and RA Gardner, Comparing the early utterances of child and chimpanzee. *Minnesota Symposium on Child Psychology,* Vol. 8. (A Pick, ed). Copyright 1974 by the University of Minnesota. Published by the University of Minnesota Press.

INDEX